1998
YEAR BOOK OF
SPORTS MEDICINE®

Statement of Purpose

The YEAR BOOK Service

The YEAR BOOK series was devised in 1901 by practicing health professionals who observed that the literature of medicine and related disciplines had become so voluminous that no one individual could read and place in perspective every potential advance in a major specialty. In the final decade of the 20th century, this recognition is more acutely true than it was in 1901.

More than merely a series of books, YEAR BOOK volumes are the tangible results of a unique service designed to accomplish the following:

- to *survey* a wide range of journals of proven value
- to *select* from those journals papers representing significant advances and statements of important clinical principles
- to provide *abstracts* of those articles that are readable, convenient summaries of their key points
- to provide *commentary* about those articles to place them in perspective

These publications grow out of a unique process that calls on the talents of outstanding authorities in clinical and fundamental disciplines, trained literature specialists, and professional writers, all supported by the resources of Mosby, the world's preeminent publisher for the health professions.

The Literature Base

Mosby and its editors survey approximately 500 journals published worldwide, covering the full range of the health professions. On an annual basis, the publisher examines usage patterns and polls its expert authorities to add new journals to the literature base and to delete journals that are no longer useful as potential YEAR BOOK sources.

The Literature Survey

The publisher's team of literature specialists, all of whom are trained and experienced health professionals, examines every original, peer-reviewed article in each journal issue. More than 250,000 articles per year are scanned systematically, including titles, text, illustrations, tables, and references. Each scan is compared, article by article, with the search strategies that the publisher has developed in consultation with the 270 outside experts who form the pool of YEAR BOOK editors. A given article may be reviewed by any number of editors, from one to a dozen or more, regardless of the discipline for which the paper was originally published. In turn, each editor who receives the article reviews it to determine whether or not the article should be included in the YEAR BOOK. This decision is based on the article's inherent quality, its probable usefulness to readers of that YEAR BOOK, and the editor's goal to represent a balanced picture of a given field in each volume of the YEAR BOOK. In addition, the editor indicates when to include figures and tables from the article to help the YEAR BOOK reader better understand the information.

Of the quarter million articles scanned each year, only 5% are selected for detailed analysis within the YEAR BOOK series, thereby assuring readers of the high value of every selection.

The Abstract

The publisher's abstracting staff is headed by a seasoned medical professional and includes individuals with training in the life sciences, medicine, and other areas, plus extensive experience in writing for the health professions and related industries. Each selected article is assigned to a specific writer on this abstracting staff. The abstracter, guided in many cases by notations supplied by the expert editor, writes a structured, condensed summary designed so that the reader can rapidly acquire the essential information contained in the article.

The Commentary

The YEAR BOOK editorial boards, sometimes assisted by guest commentators, write comments that place each article in perspective for the reader. This provides the reader with the equivalent of a personal consultation with a leading international authority—an opportunity to better understand the value of the article and to benefit from the authority's thought processes in assessing the article.

Additional Editorial Features

The editorial boards of each YEAR BOOK organize the abstracts and comments to provide a logical and satisfying sequence of information. To enhance the organization, editors also provide introductions to sections or individual chapters, comments linking a number of abstracts, citations to additional literature, and other features.

The published YEAR BOOK contains enhanced bibliographic citations for each selected article, including extended listings of multiple authors and identification of author affiliations. Each YEAR BOOK contains a Table of Contents specific to that year's volume. From year to year, the Table of Contents for a given YEAR BOOK will vary depending on developments within the field.

Every YEAR BOOK contains a list of the journals from which papers have been selected. This list represents a subset of the approximately 500 journals surveyed by the publisher and occasionally reflects a particularly pertinent article from a journal that is not surveyed on a routine basis.

Finally, each volume contains a comprehensive subject index and an index to authors of each selected paper.

The 1998 Year Book Series

Year Book of Allergy, Asthma, and Clinical Immunology: Drs. Rosenwasser, Borish, Boguniewicz, Nelson, Routes, and Spahn

Year Book of Anesthesiology and Pain Management®: Drs. Tinker, Abram, Chestnut, Roizen, Rothenberg, and Wood

Year Book of Cardiology®: Drs. Schlant, Collins, Gersh, Graham, Kaplan, and Waldo

Year Book of Chiropractic®: Dr. Lawrence

Year Book of Critical Care Medicine®: Drs. Parrillo, Balk, Calvin, Franklin, and Shapiro

Year Book of Dentistry®: Drs. Meskin, Berry, Jeffcoat, Leinfelder, Roser, Summitt, and Zakariasen

Year Book of Dermatologic Surgery®: Drs. Greenway, Barrett, Papadopoulos, and Whitaker

Year Book of Dermatology and Dermatologic Surgery: Drs. Thiers and Lang

Year Book of Diagnostic Radiology®: Drs. Osborn, Groskin, Dalinka, Maynard, Pentecost, Rebner, Ros, Smirniotopoulos, and Young

Year Book of Drug Therapy®: Drs. Lasagna and Weintraub

Year Book of Emergency Medicine®: Drs. Wagner, Dronen, Davidson, King, Niemann, and Roberts

Year Book of Endocrinology®: Drs. Bagdade, Braverman, Horton, Kannan, Landsberg, Molitch, Morley, Nathan, Odell, Poehlman, Rogol, and Ryan

Year Book of Family Practice®: Drs. Berg, Bowman, Davidson, Dexter, and Scherger

Year Book of Gastroenterology®: Drs. Aliperti and Fleshman

Year Book of Geriatrics and Gerontology®: Drs. Burton, Beck, Ostwald, Rabins, Reuben, Roth, Shapiro, and Whitehouse

Year Book of Hand Surgery®: Drs. Amadio and Hentz

Year Book of Hematology®: Drs. Spivak, Bell, Ness, Quesenberry, Wiernik, and Horowitz

Year Book of Infectious Diseases: Drs. Keusch, Barza, Bennish, Poutsiaka, Skolnik, and Snydman

Year Book of Medicine®: Drs. Cline, Frishman, Jett, Klahr, Malawista, Mandell, McCallum, and Utiger

Year Book of Neonatal and Perinatal Medicine®: Drs. Fanaroff, Maisels, and Stevenson

Year Book of Nephrology, Hypertension, and Mineral Metabolism: Drs. Schwab, Bennett, Emmett, Hostetter, Kumar, and Toto

Year Book of Neurology and Neurosurgery®: Drs. Bradley and Gibbs

Year Book of Nuclear Medicine®: Drs. Gottschalk, Blaufox, Neumann, Strauss, and Zubal

Year Book of Obstetrics, Gynecology, and Women's Health: Drs. Mishell, Herbst, and Kirschbaum

Year Book of Occupational and Environmental Medicine®: Drs. Emmett, Frank, Gochfeld, and Hessl

Year Book of Oncology®: Drs. Ozols, Eisenberg, Glatstein, Loehrer, and Tallman

Year Book of Ophthalmology®: Drs. Wilson, Augsburger, Cohen, Eagle, Grossman, Laibson, Maguire, Nelson, Penne, Rapuano, Sergott, Spaeth, Tipperman, Ms. Gosfield, and Ms. Salmon

Year Book of Orthopedics®: Drs. Morrey, Beauchamp, Currier, Tolo, Trigg, and Swiontkowski

Year Book of Otolaryngology–Head and Neck Surgery®: Drs. Paparella and Holt

Year Book of Pathology and Laboratory Medicine®: Drs. Raab, Cohen, Olson, Sirgi, and Stanley

Year Book of Pediatrics®: Dr. Stockman

Year Book of Plastic, Reconstructive, and Aesthetic Surgery®: Drs. Miller, Bartlett, Garner, McKinney, Ruberg, Salisbury, and Smith

Year Book of Psychiatry and Applied Mental Health®: Drs. Talbott, Ballenger, Frances, Lydiard, Meltzer, Schowalter, and Tasman

Year Book of Pulmonary Disease®: Drs. Jett, Maurer, Ryu, Strollo, and Wenzel

Year Book of Rheumatology®: Drs. Panush, Hadler, LeRoy, Liang, Reichlin, Simon, and Weinblatt

Year Book of Sports Medicine®: Drs. Shephard, Drinkwater, Eichner, Torg, Alexander, and Mr. George

Year Book of Surgery®: Drs. Copeland, Bland, Deitch, Eberlein, Howard, Luce, Seeger, Souba, and Sugarbaker

Year Book of Thoracic and Cardiovascular Surgery®: Drs. Ginsberg, Wechsler, and Williams

Year Book of Urology®: Drs. Andriole and Coplen

Year Book of Vascular Surgery®: Dr. Porter

1998

The Year Book of SPORTS MEDICINE®

Editor-in-Chief

Roy J. Shephard, M.D., Ph.D., D.P.E.

Professor Emeritus of Applied Physiology; Faculty of Physical Education and Health, University of Toronto

Editors

Marion J.L. Alexander, Ph.D.

Professor, Faculty of Physical Education and Recreation Studies; Research Associate, Health, Leisure and Human Performance Research Institute, University of Manitoba, Winnipeg, Manitoba

Barbara L. Drinkwater, Ph.D.

Research Physiologist, Department of Medicine, Pacific Medical Center, Seattle, Washington

Edward R. Eichner, M.D.

Professor of Medicine, University of Oklahoma Health Sciences Center; Team Internist, University of Oklahoma Varsity Athletes, Oklahoma City, Oklahoma

Francis J. George, A.T.C., P.T.

Head Athletic Trainer, Brown University, Providence, Rhode Island

Joseph S. Torg, M.D.

Professor of Orthopedic Surgery, and Director of the Joe Torg Center for Sports Medicine and Athletic Trauma, Allegheny University-Hahnemann, Philadelphia, Pennsylvania

American College of Sports Medicine Liaison Representative

Kent B. Pandolf, Ph.D.

Director, Environmental Physiology and Medicine Directorate, U.S. Army Research Institute of Environmental Medicine, Natick, Massachusetts

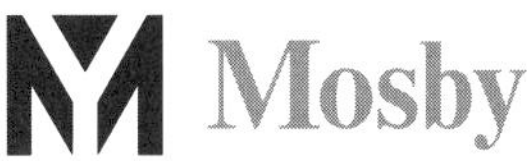

St. Louis Baltimore Boston Carlsbad Naples New York Philadelphia Portland London
Madrid Mexico City Singapore Sydney Tokyo Toronto Wiesbaden

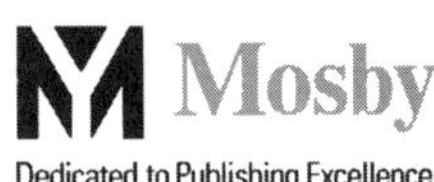

Dedicated to Publishing Excellence

Publisher: Theresa Van Schaik
Developmental Editor: Jaime Pendill
Manager, Periodical Editing: Kirk Swearingen
Production Editor: Amanda Maguire
Project Supervisor, Production: Joy Moore
Project Assistant, Production: Laura Bayless
Manager, Literature Services: Idelle L. Winer
Illustrations and Permissions Specialist: Steve Ramay

1998 EDITION
Copyright © 1998 by Mosby, Inc.

Printed in the United States of America
Composition by Reed Technology and Information Services, Inc.
Printing/binding by Maple-Vail

Mosby, Inc.
11830 Westline Industrial Drive
St. Louis, MO 63146

International Standard Serial Number: 0162-0908
International Standard Book Number: 0-8151-9740-3

Table of Contents

Journals Represented

Mosby and its editors survey approximately 500 journals for its abstract and commentary publications. From these journals, the editors select the articles to be abstracted. Journals represented in this YEAR BOOK are listed below.

Acta Neurologica Scandinavica
Acta Paediatrica
American Journal of Cardiology
American Journal of Clinical Nutrition
American Journal of Epidemiology
American Journal of Physical Medicine & Rehabilitation
American Journal of Physiology
American Journal of Respiratory and Critical Care Medicine
American Journal of Roentgenology
American Journal of Sports Medicine
Annals of Allergy, Asthma, & Immunology
Annals of Epidemiology
Archives of Pediatrics and Adolescent Medicine
Archives of Physical Medicine and Rehabilitation
Arthroscopy
Athletic Therapy Today
British Journal of Radiology
British Journal of Sports Medicine
British Medical Journal
Chest
Circulation
Clinical Biomechanics
Clinical Chemistry
Clinical Science
Contraception
Diabetes Care
European Heart Journal
Fertility and Sterility
Foot & Ankle International
Heart
International Journal of Obesity
International Journal of Sports Medicine
Journal of Applied Physiology: Respiratory, Environmental and Exercise
   Physiology
Journal of Athletic Training
Journal of Bone and Joint Surgery (American Volume)
Journal of Bone and Mineral Research
Journal of Cardiopulmonary Rehabilitation
Journal of Clinical Endocrinology and Metabolism
Journal of Clinical Investigation
Journal of Family Practice
Journal of Gerontology
Journal of Neurology, Neurosurgery and Psychiatry
Journal of Neurosurgery
Journal of Oral and Maxillofacial Surgery
Journal of Orthopaedic Research
Journal of Orthopaedic Trauma

Journal of Orthopaedic and Sports Physical Therapy
Journal of Pediatrics
Journal of Spinal Disorders
Journal of Sports Medicine and Physical Fitness
Journal of the American Geriatrics Society
Journal of the American Medical Association
Journal of the National Cancer Institute
Lancet
Medical Journal of Australia
Medicine and Science in Sports and Exercise
Metabolism: Clinical and Experimental
Neurosurgery
New England Journal of Medicine
Orthopedics
Physical Therapy
Physician and Sportsmedicine
Radiology
Science
Skeletal Radiology
Spine
Sports Medicine
Sports Medicine and Arthroscopy Review
Thorax
Transplantation Proceedings
Western Journal of Medicine

STANDARD ABBREVIATIONS

The following terms are abbreviated in this edition: acquired immunodeficiency syndrome (AIDS), cardiopulmonary resuscitation (CPR), central nervous system (CNS), cerebrospinal fluid (CSF), computed tomography (CT), deoxyribonucleic acid (DNA), electrocardiography (ECG), health maintenance organization (HMO), human immunodeficiency virus (HIV), intensive care unit (ICU), intramuscular (IM), intravenous (IV), magnetic resonance (MR) imaging (MRI), and ribonucleic acid (RNA).

NOTE

The YEAR BOOK OF SPORTS MEDICINE is a literature survey service providing abstracts of articles published in the professional literature. Every effort is made to assure the accuracy of the information presented in these pages. Neither the editors nor the publisher of the YEAR BOOK OF SPORTS MEDICINE can be responsible for errors in the original materials. The editors' comments are their own opinions. Mention of specific products within this publication does not constitute endorsement.

To facilitate the use of the YEAR BOOK OF SPORTS MEDICINE as a reference tool, all illustrations and tables included in this publication are now identified as they appear in the original article. This change is meant to help the reader recognize that any illustration or table appearing in the YEAR BOOK OF SPORTS MEDICINE may be only one of many in the original article. For this reason, figure and table numbers will often appear to be out of sequence within the YEAR BOOK OF SPORTS MEDICINE.

Introduction

Each year, our editors face the challenge of choosing among many (approximately 500) excellent articles. There are a multitude of exciting new developments in sports medicine—we barely have room to cover the highlights of this new research. The selections for 1998 include not only the usual topics of injury prevention and treatment, but also offers a better basic understanding of our discipline, new insights into the determinants of fitness and training response, new approaches to tackling the scourge of doping, and new programs that promise effective prevention and treatment of various chronic diseases.

Epidemiological reports continue to explore new sources of injury: this year, studies examine problems experienced by performers in Broadway shows, as well as injuries suffered by off-road cyclists, snowboarders, luge enthusiasts, rowers, in-line skaters, childhood and adolescent skiers, and cardiovascular outpatients. Three articles report on experience of sports physicians at the Olympic Games in Atlanta. Other selections discuss primary sports medicine in the context of managed health care. Near-infrared spectroscopy is attracting attention as a method of monitoring tissue oxygenation in chronic compartment syndrome; however, the diagnostic value of magnetic resonance imaging continues to attract much discussion. New therapeutic options include a collagen-calcium phosphate graft material for acute fractures, and a new biological glue for cartilage/cartilage interfaces. Attention is drawn to lighting standards in injury prevention. The deceptive advertising of footwear is discussed as a possible cause of injuries.

One study describes a case of pneumomediastinum in a surf lifeguard. The natural progression of lumbar spondylosis is reviewed. The handlebars of mountain bikes are identified as a cause of hepatic hematomas. Shoulder problems continue to be a source of pain in competitive swimmers, and two reports discuss failed repairs of shoulder instability. Subacromial impingement syndrome also continues to be a topic of interest. Adverse neural tension as a possible factor in repetitive hamstring strain is discussed. There is the usual batch of articles on the knee, covering both patello-femoral pain syndrome and ligament lesions, with new concepts on meniscal regeneration. Further reports discuss the problem of chronic pain following ankle sprains.

The impact of restricted knee flexion on vertical ground reaction force is studied. Gait in an athlete with shortened gastronemius muscles is described. The influence of flexibility on susceptibility to joint injury is examined. Myofibrillar disruption after repeated eccentric exercise, as well as the place of aquatic-based rehabilitation are considered.

Salivary lactate determinations are shown to allow multiple measurements without finger pricks or a need for rapid analysis of specimens, a boon to those regulating high-performance training by the monitoring of anaerobic effort. Urinary norepinephrine may provide a useful marker of overtraining. Saliva also offers a good method of determining testosterone/

cortisol ratios in the assessment of overtraining. Hydroxyurea has been found to enhance anaerobic and aerobic performance in individuals with sickle-cell anemia. Glucose supplements reduce the epinephrine and cortisol response to endurance running, and thus cause lesser changes in neutrophil and monocyte counts.

A longitudinal study of distance runners shows the ability of prolonged bouts of exercise to control body fat for many years. The amount of exercise needed for good health may be less than previously thought, as the estimated energy cost of stair climbing has proved to be less than assumed in one popular activity questionnaire. The human genome project is finally beginning to uncover genetic markers that identify an appreciable portion of the variance in aerobic power. Gene therapy is also beginning to be disussed in the context of sports medicine. Perhaps because of decreasing secretion of testosterone and growth hormone, even men who are running 80 km per week accumulate abdominal fat as they get older. Exercise alone is suggested to be as effective as a combination of exercise and dieting in a 12-week study of reductions in blood pressure. Further support is found for the concept that fat is lost more readily in men than in women. A massive prospective study from China shows that in patients with impaired glucose tolerance, the risk of developing diabetes is attenuated by exercising, and exercise alone is better than diet or diet plus exercise in the control of this disorder.

A follow-up of track athletes who maintained high-intensity conditioning indicates that they lost aerobic power as fast as sedentary individuals over the 20 years of observation. Spinal mobility does not appear to be adversely affected by either soccer playing or weight lifting through late middle-age, although participants in these two types of activity do experience their first episodes of back pain at a somewhat earlier age than those who are involved in shooting competitions.

Basic fibroblast growth factor appears in the urine within a few hours of myocardial ischemia, and, in future, it may offer a useful early warning of myocardial damage. Women respond less well to postcoronary rehabilitation than do men, although the reason for this seems to be that family responsibilities keep them from attending exercise classes on a regular basis. Those who do attend faithfully can achieve large gains in aerobic power, with resulting enhancement of the quality of life. A peak oxygen intake of less than 15 ml/[kg.min] and a ventilatory equivalent for CO_2 in excess of 50 are warning signs that cardiac transplantation is needed urgently. Descriptions of dyspnea are shown to differ between healthy exercisers and those with chronic airway disease. In supposedly asthmatic athletes, the secretion of catecholamines during all-out effort is sufficient to reverse any bronchospasm, without recourse to the inhalation of drugs such as salbutamol. Spasm is more likely with running than with involvement in power sports. Patients with exercise-induced anaphylactic reactions can exercise safely, provided allergy-generating foods are avoided. Contrary to some earlier views, progressive aerobic exercise appears helpful in the treatment of those patients (50%) who have chronic fatigue syndrome without any obvious psychiatric disorder. However, also contrary to popular wisdom, involvement in sport does not seem to be a panacea for juvenile delinquency.

Adequate fluid replenishment is reported as important to avoidance of heat stress under warm conditions, but no advantage is gained from hyperhydration. A relationship is shown between hyperthermia and sleepiness. Slow hill-walkers are shown in laboratory experiments to generate insufficient heat for safety under cool, wet, and windy conditions. The normal rise of core temperature during exercise can be prevented by immersing a person in a bath of cold water; this is a useful technique for determining which of the responses to exercise are thermally mediated. Competitive cycling is shown to decrease sperm motility, possibly through local microtrauma or a rise of intrascrotal temperature, rather than through hormonal changes associated with a negative energy balance.

In future, filter paper samples of capillary blood may offer a viable field method of testing for steriod abuse. A recent survey shows that many physicians still lack the basic knowledge of doping rules that is essential to avoid disqualification of the athletes for whom they are responsible. Attempts to detect administration of exogenous testosterone by the ratio of testosterone to luteinizing hormone seem to yield even more false positive tests than when using the ratio of testosterone to episterone. A study of mice found a substantial shortening of lifespan in animals that were given steroids for 6 months, with death attributable to tumors of the liver and kidneys, lymphosarcomas and cardiac abnormalities.

A 2.5 hour run leads to a dramatic decrease in the ratio of reduced to oxidized glutathione in the runner, implying that the activity led to a substantial increase in the formation of reactive species. Such changes may contribute to structural changes in the red cells of distance runners. Despite a high immunoglobulin content, bovine colostrum does not appear to increase salivary immunoglobulin A levels. Exercise appears to change the immunoglobulin composition of milk in lactating women, and they are advised to nurse before an exercise bout. Prolonged, intense exercise may also cause a temporary impairment of the response to vaccination. Reports that exercise may reduce the incidence of cancer of the breast and of the endometrium continue to be plagued by effects that are clinically interesting but statistically insignificant. Although exercise stimulates coagulation, this is well-balanced by activation of the fibrinolytic system; nitric oxide may be implicated in these changes.

Factors contributing to gender differences in injury experience are reviewed. Two articles examining the response of young girls to training help to address the deficit of research on preadolescent girls. One article describes the effects of oral contraceptives on delayed muscle soreness. An energy deficit rather than the stress of exercise is shown to be responsible for changes of LH pulsatility in exercising women. Osteoporosis continues a concern in older women, and a number of articles discuss the value of exercise with and without hormone replacement therapy. After adjusting for differences of lean body mass, old people are shown to have a substantially lower maximal oxygen intake than younger individuals, suggesting that either the pumping ability of the heart or local muscle blood flow decreases with age. Information from restrospective questionnaires challenges the traditional view that a vigorous exercise program is always helpful in preventing falls among the elderly. However, there is new evidence that exercise may enhance cognitive function.

Rehydration following heat exposure is delayed by the consumption of alcohol in concentrations of over 2%. Type II muscle fiber dominance appears to increase susceptibility to thermal stress. Testing of the living high/training low regimen shows that it confers a significant advantage in track performance to college level runners, relative to the older living high/training high regimen. Magnetic resonance imaging shows a surprisingly high incidence of osteonecrotic lesions in scuba divers.

Such is just a foretaste of the exciting developments that readers can explore in this year's edition of the Year Book. I hope that you will find the material just as fascinating as have the editors and abstracters.

Roy J. Shephard, M.D., Ph.D., D.P.E.

Exercise, Aging, and Immune Resistance to Infections and Neoplasms

Roy J. Shephard, M.D., Ph.D., D.P.E.
School of Physical & Health Education and Department of Preventive Medicine & Biostatistics, Faculty of Medicine, University of Toronto; Defence and Civil Institute of Environmental Medicine, North York, Ontario; Health Studies Programme, Brock University, St. Catharines, Ontario.

Aging is associated with a deterioration in elements of the immune system that offer resistance to infection and neoplasms.[22, 23, 25, 34, 35] So, it is not surprising that suceptibility to both infections and cancer increase with age, and that morbidity and mortality should be related to the loss of immune function. However, recent data suggest that regular exercise may help to delay the deterioration in immune function,[34, 38] raising the question as to how far this response may protect older individuals against both infection and cancer.

Infections

Susceptibility of the elderly to infections.—Elderly people are more prone to infections than young adults.[43] However, epidemiological data suggest that the vulnerability is not generalized. Much of the increase in susceptibility is attributable to certain types of infection, as listed in Table 1.

TABLE 1.—Important Infections in the Elderly

Site	Organism	Disease
Urinary Tract	Gram negative bacteria (mainly E. coli)	Cystitis, renal infections, bacteremia, sepsis
Bronchi and Lungs	Strep. pneumoniae H. influenzae Staph. aureus Gram negative bacteria	Pneumonia
	Tubercle bacillus	Tuberculosis
Intra-abdominal	Gram negative bacteria	Appendicitis Cholecystitis Diverticulitis Hepatic abcess
Skin and soft tissues	Staphylococcus Pseudomonas	Cellulitis Pressure sores
Sepsis	Gram negative bacteria	Sepsis
Endocardium	Strep. pneumoniae Staph. aureus	Infective endocarditis
Meninges	Meningococcus Mycobacteria	Meningitis
Joints	Staph. aureus Streptococcus	Septic arthritis
Peripheral nerves	Herpes virus	Herpes zoster
Central nervous system	Tetanus bacillus	Tetanus

Two points regarding the immune defenses stand out. First, much of the increase in susceptibility is due to bacterial, rather than viral, disease. Second, there are often specific, nonimmunological concomitants of aging that predispose to the infections we observe.

Urinary infections.—A high proportion of elderly individuals show a bacteriuria. Urinary tract infections account for between 30% and 50% of all cases of bacteremia or sepsis in the elderly.[6, 19] In many patients an obvious mechanical explanation of disease can be found without invoking immune malfunction. Urinary stasis may be caused by prostatic hypertrophy or calculi. The bladder may suffer from malfunction because of diabetic neuritis or other forms of neuronal degeneration. Exposure to microorganisms may be increased by frequent catheterization of the bladder. Nevertheless, Kasviki-Charvatin et al.[19] argue that in a number of cases there is no obvious mechanical or circulatory explanation of susceptibility to disease. They suggest that in such individuals a deterioration of immune function is the likely explanation.

Pulmonary disease.—A history of chronic lung disease, immobility, feeble coughing, and aspiration of food are all nonimmunological factors that contribute to the prevalence of pneumonia in the elderly. Nevertheless, a poorly functioning immune system leaves the old person more vulnerable to secondary bacterial infection following an upper respiratory tract viral infection.[21]

Skin diseases.—The skin is another site that becomes increasingly vulnerable to infection in the elderly. Immobility, peripheral vascular disease, diabetes mellitus, peripheral oedema, and trauma are all nonimmunological mechanisms contributing to a high incidence of skin lesions.[42] Again, the impact of these various mechanical and systemic problems can be exacerbated by a deterioration in immune response.

Primacy of immune aging.—Assuming that there is an age-related increase in susceptibility to disease, the next question has to do with the primacy of the immune dysfunction. Has disease led to a suppression of immune function, or is the decrease in immune function the primary event that has increased susceptibility to disease?[22]

Chronic disease is commonly associated with, and is sometimes preceded by, factors that have adverse effects upon the immune system. For example, nutrition is often impaired in advanced disease,[27] which leaves the body deficient in the amino acids necessary for leukocyte proliferation. Likewise, both chronic lung disease and the skin infections secondary to a poor circulation are usually preceded by many years of cigarette smoking, which itself impairs immune function.[7, 8, 38]

Nevertheless, several pieces of evidence indicate that the primary event is a deterioration in immune function, rather than the onset of disease.

1. The waning of immune function begins in adolescence, long before most people have any substantial burden of chronic disease.[1]
2. In patients who have undergone organ transplantation, the immune system is aged prematurely by immunosuppressant drugs, and such individuals develop a high susceptibility to infection.[9]

3. Patients with a primary constitutional immune deficiency are vulnerable to infections from an early age.[1]
4. The progressive depression of immune function by HIV predisposes a person to a host of opportunistic infections.[24]

Mechanisms of Immune Resistance

Viruses.—What are the mechanisms of immune resistance to viruses? Early resistance depends mainly upon the lytic action of natural killer (NK) cells. NK cell numbers are generally unchanged or even slightly increased by aging.[12] However, some authors have found a diminished affinity for the target cells,[26] and a decrease in cytolytic activity per cell.[31] Such changes could be due to an aging of NK cells, but they could also be secondary to an impairment of the T cell cascade that Shinkai et al.[38] have described, particularly a reduced production of interleukin-2.[12]

The main long-term defence against viruses comes from a proliferation of specific cytotoxic lymphocytes. This process peaks some seven days after infection. Lymphocyte proliferation depends upon a lengthy sequence of events, including macrocytic phagocytosis of the virus, presentation of viral proteins to the T cells, and the secretion of key cytokines that together form the T cell cascade.[2] In addition to a decreased production of IL-2, the number of IL-2 receptors on the target cells is decreased in the elderly.[25] Alterations in calcium availability or kinetics also slow the cytokine activation of T and B cells.[23]

Bacteria.—Immune defenses against bacteria include the phagocytic action of macrophages and neutrophils and the production of specific antibodies. The antibodies opsonize the bacteria, marking them as targets for phagocytosis. They also activate the complement cascade, and sometimes neutralize specific toxins.[1]

Macrophages from older animals show a decreased ascorbic acid content, and an increased content of reactive oxygen.[10] Functional changes include a slower rate of chemotaxis, but a greater tendency to adhere to target cells.[14]

However, the main adverse effect upon bacterial defenses arises from a suppression of the T cell cascade. In consequence, there is a reduced proliferation of B-cells, and a reduced production of immunoglobulins.

Protection from regular physical activity.—Does regular physical activity protect against infection? In young adults, the relationship between regular physical activity and infection is said to follow a J-shaped curve.[5] Moderate exercise and/or a period of moderate training has a positive influence, increasing resistance to infection. In contrast, a single very strenuous bout of exercise or a sustained period of very heavy training increases vulnerability to microorganisms.[28, 34]

There is little empirical information on how physical activity and training affect the susceptibility of older adults. Shephard et al.[37] questioned Master's athletes, and found that 76% considered themselves less vulnerable to infections than their sedentary peers. However, some 16% of endurance competitors were also conscious of a critical running mileage above which they became more susceptible to infections. The modal distance in the elderly was 50 km/week, substantially less than the figure of 97 km noted by Nieman et al.[28] for those aged 34–39 years. Karper and Boschen[18] carried out a prospective trial of moderate training in 10 women and 6 men aged 65 years. They saw a reduction in the number and severity of upper respiratory infections relative to pretraining data. However, seasonal variations in the prevalence of upper respiratory infections make it difficult to evaluate an uncontrolled study such as this.

Plainly, we need much more empirical information on reactions in the elderly, particularly with respect to the changes introduced by exercise and training. Nevertheless, available data suggest the response is similar to that observed in younger adults—an enhancement of protection with moderate physical activity, but a worsening of prognosis if exercise is too prolonged or intense. In particular, Master's athletes have a much better resting immune function than the sedentary elderly, and, indeed, many parameters in the Master's competitors match those observed in sedentary young adults.[38]

Neoplasms

Susceptibility of the elderly to cancer.—Cancer is largely a disease of the elderly. This reflects in part a cumulative exposure to carcinogens, but an age-related waning of immune function could also be a contributing factor. In support of the immune hypothesis, vulnerability to cancers is increased in patients who have received prolonged courses of immunosuppressant drugs following organ transplants. Patients with advanced HIV infection also become vulnerable to tumours. The main argument against immune involvement is the site of the lesion. The lungs, skin, colon, stomach, breast (in women) and prostate (in men) are the main tumor sites in those over the age of 50, whereas HIV infection leads to lymphoid tumours and Kaposi's sarcoma.

Mechanisms of immune resistance.—Likely immune mechanisms modulating defenses against cancer include an exercise- or training-induced increase in the number and/or activity of macrophages, natural killer and or lymphokine-activated killer cells and their regulating cytokines. Suceptibility to neoplasms might also be influenced by factors that modify the adherence, penetration, or multiplication of tumour cells.

C-reactive protein.—Endurance running increases concentrations of C-reactive protein, sometimes for several days. The C-reactive protein has a chemotactic effect, drawing monocytes to active muscle. It also makes tumour cells more vulnerable to phagocytosis, perhaps by binding with their surface proteins.[34]

Macrophages.—The activated macrophage plays a dominant role in protection against tumour cells. It is the initial phagocytic agent, it serves as an antigen-presenting cell, and it is the initial source of interleukin-1 and tumour necrosis factor. The anti-tumour activities of the macrophages are in turn regulated by IL-1, IFN-gamma, TNF-alpha, and macrophage activating factor.[1]

Some authors have suggested that not only moderate exercise, but even an exhausting 15 km run enhances the antitumour activity of human macrophages.[11] However, animal studies by Wood and Davis (1994) and observations on humans after a brief but exhausting bout of maximal running[3] each tend to support a J-shaped response. According to this latter view, macrophage function is stimulated by moderate physical activity, but is inhibited by exhausting exercise, probably because of a down-regulation by PGE-2.[34]

Aging in itself has a variety of effects upon the macrophages. To the extent that a given intensity of physical activity is more stressful for an older person, and more likely to induce tissue microtraumata, we might expect a greater production of PGE-2, and thus a greater suppression of macrophage function.

Natural killer cells.—NK cells destroy certain types of tumour cell. Moderate training increases both the number of NK cells and their cytotoxic activity, at least between exercise bouts.[30] However, NK numbers are decreased immediately following a bout of heavy physical activity.[34] Typically, normal values are restored within 24 hours, but in at least one study immunosuppression persisted for as long as 7 days. The depression of function postexercise is probably due to release of PGE-2, with suppression of the T cell cascade. To the extent that a given absolute intensity of exercise causes more prostaglandin release, the elderly are again likely to show a larger and more prolonged depression of NK function than younger individuals following a bout of very strenuous exercise.

LAK cells.—Moderate training has a favourable effect upon the cytotoxicity of lymphokine-activated killer (LAK) cells in mice,[16] but LAK activity is suppressed for at least 48 hours following a period of very strenuous training.[4] Again, the main blame probably lies with a suppression of the T cell cascade, so there is a potential for effects to be greater in an older person.

Neutrophils.—Neutrophils destroy tumour cells by producing peroxides and free radicals. Acute exercise induces a prolonged increase in neutrophil count,[34] but this change is often offset by a decrease in cytotoxic activity per cell.[20] Cytotoxic activity per cell also seems to be lower in athletes than in nonathletes.[39]

Protection from physical activity and training.—Many of the immune mechanisms that protect a person against invading microorganisms can also ingest and destroy tumour cells. Thus, we might anticipate similar effects of physical activity and training upon susceptibility to infections and to tumours: a reduced susceptibility with moderate exercise, but a worsening of prognosis once a cristical dose of physical activity has been surpassed.

Animal studies provide some support for a J-shaped relationship.[34, 36] Moderate exercise protects against carcinogens and implanted tumors, but heavy exercise has an adverse effect. Human epidemiological studies have focused on moderate occupational or leisure activity rather than intense exercise. Moderate physical activity is associated with a decrease in all-cause cancer rates, and specific protection against tumours of the descending colon. There are also suggestions of benefit at other sites, including the lungs, and, in women, the cervix and the breast.[40]

However, it is difficult to be certain whether benefit has been gained from changes in immune function or from some other variable associated with an active lifestyle.[33, 34] Colon tumors may be avoided because of a speeding of gastrointestinal transit, or the choice of a high-fiber diet. Tumors of the reproductive tract are influenced by a reduction of obesity, or a decrease in circulating estrogen levels. Finally, many athletes are nonsmokers, and many have a high intake of antioxidants.

In most instances, cancer develops at a relatively advanced age. However, we know little about interactions between aging and exercise. Some studies have found differences of risk between premenopausal and postmenopausal women. For example, Kampert et al.[17] noted that an excess body mass protected against breast cancer before the menopause, but it had an adverse effect in older individuals. Wu et al.[42] limited their observations to a retirement community, but they found that the association of colon cancer with a sedentary lifestyle was very similar to that described in younger individuals. Likewise, Albanes et al.[2] found no change in risk ratios after adjusting their data for age.

A number of studies of exercise and cancer have covaried for age.[15] Unfortunately, few have tested whether there is an age-exercise interaction term. Thus, it remains unclear how far a decrease in immune function is responsible for the increased risk of cancer in the elderly. More study is also needed to determine whether aging influences the protection that is derived from moderate exercise. However, available information suggests the benefit at any given relative intensity of activity is just as great in the elderly as in younger individuals.

Conclusions

An age-related deterioration in immune function may contribute to the increased susceptibility of older individuals to both acute infections and neoplasms. Moreover, the tissue damage associated with disease or neoplasia can suppress immune function. As in younger individuals, regular moderate physical activity induces changes of immune function that are likely to have a beneficial influence upon susceptibility to both types of conditions. Clinical data support this viewpoint. At any given relative intensity of effort, the effects of exercise and training seem comparable to those observed in a younger person. However, a single bout of prolonged, exhausting exercise, or a period of over-heavy training can have an adverse effect on the immune system; decreases in T cell function and an increased vulnerability to micro-trauma can make an older person more susceptible to acute infections, and possibly also to neoplasms.

Acknowledgment.—Dr. Shephard's studies are supported in part by funding from the Defence and Civil Institute of Environmental Medicine, and Canadian Tire Acceptance Limited.

References

1. Abbas AK, Lichtman AH, and Pober JS *Cellular and Molecular Immunology*, 2nd ed. Philadelphia: Saunders, 1995.
2. Albanes D, Blair A, Taylor PR: Physical activity and risk of cancer in the NHANESI Population. *Am J Publ Hlth* 79:744–750, 1989.
3. Bieger WP, Weiss M, Michel, G, et al: Exercise-induced monocytosis and modulation of monocyte function. *Int J Sports Med* 1:30–36, 1980.
4. Blank SE, Johansson J-O, Origines MM, et al: Modulation of NK activity by moderate intensity endurance training and chronic ethanol consumption. *J Appl Physiol* 72:8–14, 1992.
5. Brenner IKM, Shek PN, Shephard RJ: Infection in athletes. *Sports Med* 17:86–107, 1994.
6. Bryan CS, Reynolds KL: Hospital-acquired bacteremic urinary tract infections; epidemiology and outcome. *J Urol* 132:494–498, 1984.
7. Burton RC, Ferguson P, Gray M, et al: Effects of age, gender and cigarette smoking on human immuno-regulatory T cell subsets: Establishment of normal ranges and comparison with patients with colorectal cancer and multiple sclerosis. *Diagn Immunol* 1:216–233, 1983.
8. Carel RS, Eviatar J: Factors affecting leukocyte count in healthy adults. *Prev Med* 14:607–619, 1985.
9. Cooper, DKC, and Lanza, RP *Heart Transplantation*. Lancaster: MTP Press, 1984.
10. DeLaFuente M, Hernanz A, Collazos, ME et al: Effects of physical exercise and aging on ascorbic acid and superoxide anion levels in peritoneal macrophages from mice and guinea pigs. *J Comp Physiol B*, In press.
11. Fehr HG, Lötzerich H, Michna H: Human macrophage function and physical exercise: Phagocytic and histochemical studies. *Eur J Appl Physiol* 58:613–617, 1989.
12. Fiatarone MA, Morley JE, Bloom ET, et al: The effect of exercise on natural killer cell activity in young and old subjects. *J Gerontol* 44:M37–M45, 1989.
13. Fong TC, Makinodan T: In situ hybridization analysis of the age associated decline of IL-2 mRNA expressing murine cells. *Cell Immunol* 118:199–207, 1989.
14. Forner MA, Collazos ME, Barriga C, et al: (1994). Effect of age on adherence and chemotaxis capacities of peritoneal macrophages. Influence of physical activity stress. *Mech Ageing Dev* 75:179–189, 1994.
15. Gerhardsson M, Norell SE, Kiviranta H, et al: Sedentary jobs and colon cancer. *Am J Epidemiol* 123:775–780, 1986.
16. Hoffman-Goetz L: Exercise, natural immunity and tumor metastasis. *Med Sci Sports Exerc* 26:157–163, 1994.
17. Kampert JB, Whittemore AS, Paffenbarger RS (1988). Combined effects of childbearing, menstrual events, and body size on age-specific breast cancer risk. *Am J Epidemiol* 128:962–979, 1988.
18. Karper WB, Boschen MB: Effects of exercise on acute respiratory tract infections and related symptoms. *Geriatric Nursing* 14:15–18, 1993.
19. Kasviki-Charvati P, Droletti-Kafakis B, Papanayiotou PC, et al: Turnover of bacteriuria in old age. *Age Ageing* 11:169–174, 1982.
20. Koliada TI, Abzaeva LN, Baboshko IA: Effect of exposure to physical loading, hypoxia, and hyperthermia on the cellular and anti-infection resistance factors of the body. *Zh Microbiol Epidemiol Immunobiol* 2:76–79, 1988.
21. MacFarlane JT, Finch RG, Ward MJ, et al: Mourae A.D. Hospital study of community acquired pneumonia. *Lancet* ii:255–257, 1982.
22. Makinodan T, Bloom ET, James J et al: Immunity and ageing. In: M.S.J. Pathy. *Principles and Practice of Geriatric Medicine*, 2nd Ed. Chichester; John Wiley, pp 3–12, 1991.
23. Miller, RA: Accumulation of hyporesponsive, calcium-extruding memory T cells as a key feature of age dependent immune dysfunction. *Clin Immuno Immunopathol* 58:305–317, 1991.

24. Mocroft A, Youle M, Morcinek J, et al: Survival after diagnosis of AIDS: a prospective observational study of 2625 patients. *Br Med J* 314:409–413, 1997.

25. Nagel JE, Chopra RK, Powers DC, et al: Effect of age on the high-affinity interleukin-2 receptor of phytohemagglutinin stimulated peripheral blood lymphocytes. *Clin Exp Immunol* 75:286–291, 1989.

26. Masrullah I, Mazzeo RS: Age-related immuno-senescence in Fischer-344 rats: influence of exercise training. *J Appl Physiol* 73:1932–1938, 1992.

27. Newsholme E: Biochemical mechanisms to explain immunosuppression in well-trained and overtrained athletes. *Int J Sports Med* 15:S142–S147, 1994.

28. Nieman DC, Johanssen, LM, Arabatzis, K: Infectious episodes in runners before and after the Los Angeles Marathon. *J Sports Med Phys Fitness* 30:316–328, 1990.

29. Pyne DB: Regulation of neutrophils during exercise. *Sports Med* 17:245–258, 1994.

30. Rhind S, Shek PN, Shinkai S, et al: Effects of moderate endurance exercise and training on lymphocyte activation: in vitro lymphocyte proliferative response, IL-2 production, and IL-2 receptor expression. *Eur J Appl Physiol.* In press.

31. Sato T, Fuse A, Kuwata T: Enhancement by interferon of natural cytotoxic activities of lymphocytes from human cord blood and peripheral blood of aged persons. *Cell Immunol* 45:458–463, 1979.

32. Shek PN, Sabiston BH, Buguet A, et al: Strenuous exercise and immunological changes. A multiple time-point analysis of leukocyte subsets, CD4/CD8 ratio and immunoglobulin production and NK cell responses. *Int J Sports Med* 16:466–474, 1995.

33. Shephard RJ: Exercise in the prevention and treatment of cancer: An update. *Sports Med* 15:258–280, 1993.

34. Shephard RJ. *Physical Activity, Training and the Immune Response.* Carmel, IN: Cooper Publications, 1997.

35. Shephard RJ, Shek PN: Exercise, aging and immune function. *Int J Sports Med* 16:1–6, 1995.

36. Shephard RJ, Shek PN: Cancer, immune function, and physical activity. *Can J Appl Physiol* 20:1–25, 1995.

37. Shephard RJ, Kavanagh T, Mertens DJ: Personal health benefits of Masters athletic competition. *Br J Sports Med* 29:35–40, 1995.

38. Shinkai S, Kohno H, Kimura T, et al: Physical activity and immunosenescence in men. *Med Sci Sports Exerc* 27:1516–1526, 1995.

39. Smith JA, Telford RD, Mason IB, et al: Exercise training and neutrophil microbicidal activity. *Int J Sports Med* 11:179–187, 1990.

40. U.S. Surgeon General. *Physical Activity and Health. A report of the Surgeon General.* Washington, D.C.: U.S. Dept. of Health & Human Services, 1996.

41. Woods JA, Davis M: Exercise, monocyte/macrophage function, and cancer. *Med Sci Sports Exerc* 26:147–156, 1994.

42. Wu AH, Paganini-Hill A, Ross RK, et al: Alcohol, physical activity and other risk factors for colorectal cancer: a prospective study. *Br J Cancer* 55:687–694, 1987.

43. Yoshikawa TT, Norman DC. Ageing and Infectious Diseases. In: M.S.J. Pathy (ed.). *Principles and Practice of Geriatric Medicine*, 2nd ed. Chichester: John Wiley, pp. 313–314, 1991.

1 Epidemiology, Examination, and Prevention of Injuries

Athletic Injury Reporting: Development of Universal Systems
Meeuswisse WH, Love EJ (Univ of Calgary, Alta, Canada)
Sports Med 24:184–204, 1997   1–1

Introduction.—Many different athletic injury reporting systems have been established. These systems vary widely in the ways they define and report injury, making it difficult to make advances in understanding the epidemiology of athletic injury. The current state of athletic injury reporting systems in North America was reviewed.

Reporting Systems.—Some athletic injury reporting systems focus on a specific type of injury, some on a specific sport, and some on a specific population of athletes. However, their design, or method of collecting data, is what places limits on the interpretation and application of data. The case series approach is the least complex—data can be collected easily in a variety of settings. However, this design does not include the information on uninjured athletes or exposure to possible injury needed to demonstrate causal associations. The cohort design approach enrolls a cohort of athletes at baseline and follows them forward in time. This allows researchers to assess differences between injured and uninjured athletes, permits measurement of injury rates and estimation of injury risk, and provides sufficient data to make causal inferences. Exposure to potential injury can be estimated or measured; the former approach has its limitations but is easier to apply than the latter.

Methodologic Issues.—Several different issues can affect the reporting of athletic injuries. The definition of injury used can have a major effect on the pattern of injury reported. Severity may be measured by time loss or activity restriction, which also affects the injuries reported. Completeness of reporting is affected by the design and injury definition used. Different techniques to determine the "denominator" of athletic exposure can be used. These issues all depend on the design of the injury reporting system.

The design has a major impact on how the data are interpreted and applied.

Recommendations.—Clearly specifying the design of the reporting system and the data collection methods used will help to maximize comparison of data between systems. The definition of a reportable event—an "injury"—should be precise. For each reported injury, outcome data should be given if available; this will permit an injury definition to be applied at the time of data analysis. The injury reporting system should also acknowledge its own limitations or sources of data error. Further advances in system design will be needed to meet the goal of predicting and preventing athletic injuries.

▶ The authors have compiled a comprehensive catalogue of current injury reporting systems operational in the United States. Their position that "progression of thinking in athletic injury epidemiology is currently hindered by the wide disparity in the definition and reporting of injury" is well taken. However, interestingly they point out that "it is unlikely that one universal system will fit all the needs of injury reporting in all populations and settings." This comprehensive account is recommended reading for interested individuals.

J.S. Torg, M.D.

Principles of Epidemiology for the Orthopaedic Surgeon
Szabo RM (Univ of California, Davis)
J Bone Joint Surg Am 80-A:111–120, 1998   1–2

Introduction.—The basis of epidemiologic research is the systematic collection of observations related to the phenomenon of interest in a defined population. While epidemiologists study the occurrence of disease in defined populations, orthopedists are concerned primarily with individual patients. Orthopedists must now go beyond the individual and consider their practices in terms of the effectiveness on the lives entrusted to them, because of the changing profile of the health care delivery system. Epidemiology is the basic-science foundation of public health and is viewed as the study of the distribution and societal determinants of the health status of populations. The epidemiologic concepts that are important to the study of musculoskeletal were reviewed.

Observations.—The fundamental units of data are formed by observations and measurements. Accuracy, precision, reliability, and validity are the 4 terms used to describe the quality of the data. If a test measures what it purports to measure, a test is considered valid in epidemiologic terms. It is necessary to define a disease before it can be studied. Groups of individuals are compared quantitatively with respect to some framework of time in epidemiologic studies. Statistical dependence or the concept of an association between a factor and a disease is fundamental to ascribe the factor as a possible cause. The relative risk and odds ratio are the 2 most frequently used measures of association. A 2-by-2 table is often used to facilitate the calculation of these measures.

Inference.—The etiology of disease is a major concern for contemporary epidemiologists. An event that alone or with other elements produces a sequence of other events is a cause that results in an effect. One's viewpoint may influence the primary causal contingency. Philosophical theories are entertained by epidemiologists. The first criterion used in causal inference in epidemiology is the probability that an association exists. When a result is found in many studies, despite different circumstances, research designs, or time periods, it is said to be consistent. As the observations studied by epidemiologists are subject to random fluctuations, statistical inference is part of the basis of epidemiology. The calculation of a test statistic and some theoretical assumptions are used for the significance test. Two types of error associated with the significance test are rejecting a null hypothesis when a rare event has occurred, referred to as a true null hypothesis, and a false null hypothesis when the calculated test statistic is not significant. Estimation is also used in statistical inference.

Conclusions.—An incorrect estimation of the association between an exposure and the risk of a disease can occur with bias. A distortion in an effect measure is confounding. A factor that changes the magnitude of an effect measure is an effect modifier. A distortion in the estimation of an effect resulting from systematic differences in characteristics between individuals is selection bias. There are 3 types of observational studies: cross-sectional, case-control, and cohort. If sufficient attention is paid to alternative explanations and if there is recognition of the central role that epidemiologic principles play, the quality of orthopedic studies and literature will improve.

▶ The author defines epidemiologic research as the systematic collection of observations related to the occurrence of disease or other health-related conditions or events in defined populations. He states that "these data are then subjected to quantification, which includes the measurement of random variables, the estimation of population parameters, and the statistical testing of hypotheses." Of course, this represents half a loaf. It has been my experience over the years that there is a complete lack of appreciation by the orthopedic community with regard to the fact that the bottom-line principle of epidemiology is injury or disease prevention. The approach of the American Academy of Orthopedic Surgery in this area has been to publish pamphlets admonishing older women not to fall, and children not to become injured. One can only conclude from this inane approach that injury prevention is certainly not a top priority issue, in all likelihood, because it's not cost-effective. Perhaps some day responsible members of the orthopedic community will do more than pay lip service to injury prevention by supporting programs that identify etiologic variables, initiate appropriate activity or environmental modifications, and measure the effects vis a vis injury prevention. The background and circumstances resulting in intercollegiate and high school rule changes banning "spearing" and the use of the top of the helmet as initial point of contact in tackle football with the subsequent reduction in the occurrence of cervical quadriplegia serves as the model for this goal.[1]

J.S. Torg, M.D.

Reference

1. Torg JS, Vesco JJ, O'Neal MJ, et al: The epidemiologic pathologic biomechanical and cinemagraphic analysis of football induced cervical spine trauma. *Am J Sports Med* 18:50–57, 1990.

Trends in the Incidence and Cause of Sport-related Mandibular Fractures: A Retrospective Analysis
Emshoff R, Schöning H, Röthler G, et al (Univ of Innsbruck, Austria)
J Oral Maxillofac Surg 55:585–591, 1997   1–3

Background.—To make realistic recommendations for preventive measures and requirements for oral and maxillofacial surgery training programs, it is important to know the cause and incidence of facial injuries. Several countries report that traffic accidents, assaults, and falls are the most common causes of maxillofacial fractures, and it has been reported that the number of sports-related maxillofacial injuries is increasing.

Methods.—The medical records of all patients with mandibular fractures during a 10-year period were reviewed. All patients were treated at the Department of Oral and Maxillofacial Surgery, University of Innsbruck, Austria. Records were evaluated for age; sex; cause, date, and place of trauma; anatomic site of fracture; and associated maxillofacial and nonmaxillofacial injuries.

Results.—The most common cause of mandibular fractures was sports, making up 31.5% of the sample group. Traffic accidents accounted for 27.2% and falls accounted for 20.8%. The annual incidence of sports-related mandibular fractures was 28.6% from 1984–1988 and 34.5% from 1989 to 1993. Skiing accounted for 55.3% of all sports-related mandibular fractures, cycling accounted for 25.4%, and soccer accounted for 8.9%. The incidence of cycling-related mandibular fractures increased 19.3% from the 1984–1988 period to the 1989–1993 period. Skiing-related mandibular fractures decreased by 19.5% during the same time periods. The male-to-female ratio of mandibular fractures was 2.5:1.0, but the percentage of females was increasing. There was a high rate of associated injuries in cycling-related accidents. The rate of facial lacerations, tooth fractures, tooth luxations, and orbital fractures in cycling-related accidents was significantly higher than in skiing-related accidents. In soccer-related mandibular fractures, mucosal lacerations, tooth luxations, and cerebral concussions were the only associated injuries.

Discussion.—The 31.5% incidence of sports-related mandibular fractures in this study is substantially higher than the reported 1.4% to 5.4% incidence in the literature. The geographical location of Innsbruck and its extensive recreation and sports facilities may account for this difference.

These findings support the recommendation that skiers and cyclists wear safety helmets that cover the chin. Prevention programs and measures are needed to help decrease the rate of dentoalveolar trauma in individuals involved in skiing and cycling accidents.

▶ The inability to present these data in terms of injury rates precludes a precise definition of the extent of the problem of sports-related mandibular fractures. However, the incidence of associated orofacial and craniocerebral injuries is impressive. Clearly, the need for awareness and implementation of preventative measures is established.

J.S. Torg, M.D.

Profile of Dance Injuries in a Broadway Show: A Discussion of Issues in Dance Medicine Epidemiology
Bronner S, Brownstein B (SOAR Research, New York)
J Orthop Sports Phys Ther 26:87–94, 1997   1–4

Introduction.—Theatrical dance is defined as choreography presented on an ongoing basis. The epidemiology and etiology of dance injuries specific to theatrical dance performed during a Broadway show has been evaluated in only one retrospective trial. A description of dance injuries encountered in a Broadway show during a defined period of performance was described, and factors influencing these injuries were discussed.

Methods.—The injury rate for a cast of 36 (6 actors, 30 dancers) from a Broadway venture called "The Red Shoes" was followed for the 7-week run (56 performances). The age range of the 11 male and 19 female dancers was 19–38 years. Dancers averaged 44–54 hours of dancing and 8 performances each week. Injury was defined as time lost from performing.

Results.—None of the 6 actors sustained injuries during the 7-week period. In 1,680 individual performances, dancers had 9 major injuries that resulted in 82 missed performances and 35 partial performances. Three minor injuries resulted in 22 partial performances. The overall, major, and minor injury rates were 40%, 30%, and 10%, respectively. In any given performance, 4.9% of dancers missed the performance and 3.4% danced partial performances because of major injuries. The most common injuries were in the ankle-foot region. Seventy-six percent and 74% of missed and partial performances, respectively, were because of injury to the foot-ankle region. One male dancer required surgery for relief of ankle impingement. The lumbopelvic region was the second most frequently injured area (34%), followed by the knee and calf regions (8%).

Conclusion.—This is the first report of injury in a Broadway show using theatrical dance. It is commonly assumed that dancing the same repertoire would cause a higher incidence of injury. Injury rates were lower than those of ballet companies and other Broadway shows. The predominance of foot and ankle injuries in this trial was similar to patterns observed in ballet companies.

▶ This article raises a number of questions with regard to dance injuries as they occur in the theater. The authors point out that there is no standardized definition of injury, artistic and choreography styles vary, length of the season varies, and there are considerable differences in performance levels. They further point out that unlike a professional sports team, many dancers have no off season, no organized conditioning or strengthening programs, and no in-house medical supervision and care.

J.S. Torg, M.D.

Injuries Involving Off-road Cycling

Rivara FP, Thompson DC, Thompson RS, et al (Univ of Washington, Seattle; Group Health Cooperative of Puget Sound, Seattle)
J Fam Pract 44:481–485, 1997   1–5

Introduction.—In the United States, off-road bicycles, otherwise known as mountain bikes, have become increasingly popular. Bicyclists ride these bikes on various types of unpaved surfaces such as ski slopes, dirt roads, hiking trails, and other rough terrain. In 1992, sales of off-road bikes accounted for 62% of the bicycle market, and, in 1996, off-road cyclists had full Olympic medal competition. Injuries in the sport are frequent. The pattern of injuries to off-road cyclists was examined as part of a larger study of bicycle injuries and helmet use because of the tremendous growth of off-road biking and the potential importance of the injuries incurred.

Methods.—There were 3,390 injured riders who participated in this 2-year study of prospectively examined bicycle-related injuries. Medical examiners' patients and hospitalized patients were included in the study. Crash and rider characteristics and injury type and severity were provided through detailed questionnaires and abstraction of all medical records.

Results.—There were 127 (3.7%) who were injured riding "off road" of all the injured cyclists. The age was 20–30 years for 73% of the off-road cyclists, and 86.6% were male. Compared to 49.5% of the other cyclists, helmet use was 80.3% for off-road cyclists. For off-road cyclists, the number of head and face injuries was 40% of the number incurred by the other cyclists. Severe injuries were found in 4% of off-road cyclists and 6.3% were hospitalized. Severe injuries were found in 6.8% of the other cyclists and 9.4% were hospitalized.

Conclusion.—Head and face injuries are less likely to be found among off-road cyclists than other cyclists, and the majority of off-road bicycling injuries are minor. Helmets are more likely to be worn by off-road cyclists. Helmet use was found to be associated with a 65% reduction in injuries in another study.

▶ The findings of this study are similar to that of Kronisch et al., who also report a low injury rate and relatively benign injuries occurring in off-road bicycle racing. Rivara attributes the low injury rate in off-road cycling to the somewhat slower speeds and the unlikeliness of encountering a moving motor vehicle. It should be noted that in this group of 127 cyclists, 14 sustained head injuries, 1 of which resulted in death.

J.S. Torg, M.D.

Reference

1. Kronisch RL, Chow TK, Simon LM, et al: Acute injuries in off-road bicycle racing. *Am J Sports Med* 24:88–93, 1996.

Skiing Injuries in Children, Adolescents, and Adults
Deibert MC, Aronsson DD, Johnson RJ, et al (Univ of Vermont, Burlington)
J Bone Joint Surg Am 80-A:25–32, 1998   1–6

Introduction.—One of the most popular winter sports in the world is alpine, or downhill skiing, and it is known to have a high risk of injury. A reduction in the rate of injury has occurred with efforts to increase the safety of skiing by improving the ski-boot–binding system and by educating skiers. The overall rates of injury in children, adolescents, and adults participating in alpine skiing were documented. In each age group, the most common injuries were determined and to determine whether changes in equipment had an effect on the frequency or pattern of injury, short-term and long-term trends were analyzed.

Methods.—During a 22-year period, the rate of injuries was documented among skiers at the Sugarbush North and South areas. There were 5,758 injuries among 2,073,165 skiers in 1 cohort, 20,162 injuries among 3,641,041 skiers in another cohort, and 8,023 injuries among 2,480,096 skiers in a third group analyzed. The injured skiers were also compared to 2,083 non-injured skiers selected at random from the lift lines to ask them questions about their equipment The injured and noninjured skiers were divided into 3 groups: children, aged 1–10 years; adolescents, aged 11–16 years; and adults, older than 16 years.

Results.—There were 2.79 injuries per 1,000 skier days, with 2.69 injuries in adults, 2.93 injuries in adolescents, and 4.27 injuries in children. In children, the most common injury was a contusion of the knee. In adolescents, the most common injury was a sprain of the ulnar collateral ligament of the thumb. In adults, the most common injury was a grade III sprain of the anterior cruciate ligament. The frequency of tibial fractures decreased 10% in children and the incidence of fractures of the upper extremity increased 8%, according to the short-term trends analyses. In adults, the long-term trends showed that there was an 89% decrease in the rate of tibial fractures, whereas there was a 280% increase in injuries of the anterior cruciate ligament. From the beginning of the study to the end of the study, comprising 22 years, the overall rate of injury decreased 43%, with a 58% decrease in children, a 45% decrease in adolescents, and a 42% decrease in adults.

Conclusion.—The rate of injury will be decreased by the use of properly functioning modern equipment, particularly in children. Some skiers sustained injury of the anterior cruciate ligament as a result of the phantom-foot mechanism, because modern skis transmit torques to the knee that cannot be prevented by the ski-boot–binding system.

▶ This exhaustive epidemiologic study conducted over a 22-year period substantiates the findings of most of the other literature pertaining to the subject matter. Specifically, with regard to alpine skiing, injury rates are down in general, leg and ankle fractures have decreased, anterior cruciate ligament injuries have increased, and high binding-release values contribute to these injuries. Conspicuously absent from both the data and analysis were cervical spine and closed head injuries. Based on anecdotal reports, it is my impression that closed head and cervical spine injuries, because of the potential for disastrous sequelae, are really the major problems confronting this particular activity. The statement that "a large helmet may increase the risk of injury of the cervical spine" is not supported by any creditable data that I am aware of.

J.S. Torg, M.D.

Injuries to Elite Rowers Over a 10-Yr Period

Hickey GJ, Fricker PA, McDonald WA (Australian Inst of Sport, Canberra, Australia)
Med Sci Sports Exerc 29:1567–1572, 1997   1–7

Introduction.—Rowing is thought to have a low risk of major injury, but few studies of rowing injuries have been published. To determine the pattern of injuries sustained by elite rowers, researchers retrospectively analyzed the medical records of all rowers at the Australian Institute of Sport (AIS) from 1985 to 1994.

Methods.—All significant injuries sustained by AIS rowers are recorded and classified according to the time, location, and cause of injury and whether the injury is acute or chronic. Four sports physicians treated the majority of injuries during the study period.

Results.—There were 84 female and 88 male rowers on scholarship at the AIS during the 10-year period. Female rowers sustained 204 injuries, for an incidence of 1 injury per 7.6 months or 1.58 injuries per 12 months on scholarship. Fifty-seven of their injuries were acute and 147 were chronic. Among the male rowers, 116 injuries (35 acute and 81 chronic) were recorded. Their incidence of injuries was 1 per 14.2 months or 0.85 per 12 months on scholarship. For both men and women, injuries occurred most often in the summer months. The chest was the site of most injuries (22.6%) in female rowers, whereas the lumbar spine accounted for the greatest percentage of injuries (25.0%) in male rowers. Rib stress fractures were more common in women (15 cases) than in men (2 cases). Low back pain was common in both groups, and the majority of low back injuries were chronic.

Conclusion.—None of these rowers sustained life-threatening injuries during training or competition, and only 1 rower had to retire from rowing because of injury. One male and 4 female rowers required surgery. Overall, the risk of injury is not great among elite rowers. Most injuries are chronic, and most injured rowers can return to their sport.

▶ This article is one of the few in the literature dealing with the epidemiology of rowing injuries. The injuries were categorized according to time, location, and cause of injury and whether injury was acute or chronic. No attempt was made to categorize the injuries in terms of severity. However, despite this omission, it is concluded that "while there is a risk of injury in elite rowers, this risk is not great and the risk of major injury is very small." Also, the authors were unable to accurately quantify time loss because the "medical records often lacked precise information . . ." Despite this deficiency, the article concludes that the injuries "usually do not require prolonged periods away from rowing, and most often result in complete recovery." Thus, because of the deficiency in the study design, the conclusions are not substantiated by the data.

J.S. Torg, M.D.

Injuries in the Sport of Luge: Epidemiology and Analysis
Cummings RS Jr, Shurland AT, Prodoehl JA, et al (Univ of Pennsylvania, Philadelphia; Sports Med Clinic, Lake Placid, NY)
Am J Sports Med 25:508–513, 1997   1–8

Objective.—In luge, the athlete lies supine on a small sled, which is propelled down an iced track at speeds of ≥70 mph. Luge has a reputation as a dangerous sport, but there has been very little research into the associated injuries. In the past 2 decades, the United States has made major progress in competitive luging. This study examined the morbidity associated with luging, including possible ways of making the sport safer.

Findings.—Using data from the U.S. Training Center Sports Medicine Clinic, the investigators identified all luging injuries reported between 1985 and 1992. A total of 407 injuries occurred to 1,043 athletes taking 57,244 runs at the Center's luge track. This corresponded to an injury rate of 7 per 1,000 runs, or 0.39 per athlete per year. For injuries causing the loss of at least 1 practice day, the rate was 0.04 per person per year. The neck was the most common site of injury, though 96% of these injuries were mild. Contusions accounted for 51% of injuries, and strains for 27%. The most characteristic injuries identified in the series were strains of the neck muscles and contusions of the extremities, particularly the hands. Overall, 89% of injuries were classified as minor, 9% as moderate, and 2% as major. The latter categories included a 2% incidence of concussions and a 3% incidence of fractures. Nearly two thirds of the injuries were crash related.

Conclusions.—Though it looks dangerous, luge appears to be a relatively safe sport. The overall rate of injuries is low, similar to that of recreational Alpine skiing. Though severe injuries are rare, when they occur they often affect the head. Some measures to prevent luging injuries are recommended, including increased attention to neck and back conditioning, better protection for the luger's hands, and improved sled design.

▶ This article appears to be the only epidemiologic analysis of luge injuries. Familiarity with the activity has resulted from television coverage of the Olympics. As is pointed out by the authors, the activity has a reputation for being dangerous. However, the injury rates appear to be compatible with that of recreational Alpine skiing. An unusual mechanism of injury is described whereby the high centrifugal forces generated can exceed 5,000 newtons (1,094 pounds force) on the head and cervical spine. Apparently this can be a cause of neck strain, and is referred to as "losing one's head."

J.S. Torg, M.D.

Snowboard Traumatology: An Epidemiological Study
Pigozzi F, Santori N, Di Salvo V, et al (ISEF–Higher Education Inst of Physical Education of Rome; San Pietro Fatebenefratelli Hosp, Rome)
Orthopedics 20:505–509, 1997   1–9

Objective.—Although the incidence of snowboarding injuries is similar to that of downhill skiing, the incidence of injury for beginners is much higher and the location and seriousness of the injuries are different. An evaluation was made of the epidemiology of snowboarding injuries in Italy and the links between snowboarding injuries and the type of ski boot, skier's fatigue, type of snow, type of slope, and level of preskiing physical preparation.

Methods.—From December 1989 to December 1994, there were 106 snowboarding injuries reported that were covered by insurance. Age, sex, cause of trauma, and level of skill were analyzed, and anatomical regions involved in the injury were recorded.

Results.—Most injuries (72.4%) occurred in the 20-to-35 age group, and 85.8% occurred in men. Whereas amateur skiers had the highest injury incidence (47.9%), skilled skiers accounted for 34.8% of injuries. Whereas 21.5% of snowboarders were injured when they collided with someone else, 78.5% of snowboarders were injured on their own. Approximately 45% of injuries were to an upper limb; 38.5% to a lower limb; and 16% to the head, abdomen, or spine. Types of injuries encompassed contusions (31.0%), fractures (30.0%), sprains (23.5%), complete dislocations (8.5%), other injuries (3.8%), and incomplete dislocations (2.8%). Rigid footwear was involved in 61.5% of injuries and soft footwear in 38.5%. Injuries were sustained in the regular position in 62.8% of patients and in the goofy position in 37.2%. Slope conditions were described good in 47.6% of injuries, icy in 31.4%, wet in 5.7%, and fresh snow in 15.3%. Patients said they were in good physical condition in 79.5% of injuries, had prepared with specific physical exercises in 13% of injuries, and had done no preparation in 13.7%. More than half of snowboarders (52%) claimed to have learned on their own, and 53.8% thought they were fairly skilled at snowboarding. Sixty percent of injuries occurred on a medium-difficulty slope. Fewer ligamentous injuries occurred to snowboarders than to skiers.

Conclusion.—Training, upper limb guards, and soft boots could lower the snowboarding injury rate considerably.

▶ This rather simple retrospective review of 106 snowboarding-related injuries reported for insurance coverage purposes yields several interesting observations. Noteworthy was the occurrence of 3 serious interabdominal problems which included a serious kidney contusion, ruptured spleen, and a penetrating perineum injury involving the rectum. Although the occurrence of snowboarding injuries appears to parallel that of downhill skiing, injury types are, apparently, quite different.

J.S. Torg, M.D.

A Population-based Survey of In-Line Skaters' Injuries and Skating Practices
Jaffe MS, Dijkers MP, Zametis M (Rehabilitation Inst of Michigan, Detroit)
Arch Phys Med Rehabil 78:1352–1357, 1997   1–10

Introduction.—In-line skating or rollerblading has grown tremendously in popularity in the United States, with an estimated participation of 25 million in-line skaters in 1995. Members of an in-line skating club were surveyed to examine interests and practices, use of protective gear, and injury patterns.

Methods.—A 2-page questionnaire was sent to more than 1,000 members of an in-line skating club. All but 25 active members lived in Michigan. The survey contained multiple choice questions and 1 write-in response question on the worst injury related to skating. A total of 435 questionnaires were returned, for a response rate of 43%.

Results.—Respondents had a mean age of 35 years; 56.7% were men and 43.3% were women. Most had been skating for at least 2 years. Men were more likely than women to consider themselves "advanced" skaters. With the exception of helmets, women tended to wear all types of protective gear more frequently than men. Wrist guards were worn by more skaters (72.5%) than other types of protective gear. A majority of skaters reported skating-related injuries, and men were more likely to be injured than women (86.5% vs. 72.0%). Common causes of "worst injury" were an unspecified fall (40.8%) and a road hazard (21.4%). Lower extremity injuries were reported by 66.7% and upper extremity injuries by 58.8%.

Most injuries were not serious; concussions were reported by only 2.1% of skaters and fractures by 5.5%.

Conclusion.—Many of those surveyed were able to in-line skate when prohibited from participating in another sport, suggesting that in-line skating can provide a safe form of aerobic exercise. Although minor injuries are common in this sport, the risk of serious injury during in-line skating can be reduced by lessons and the use of protective gear.

▶ The value of this study is the fact that it represents the first population-based study of in-line skating practices and injury patterns. Previous studies have reported data obtained on injured skaters who had presented themselves to hospital emergency departments. As with any mail survey, there are a number of problems with this study. The response rate was only 43%. Injury severities were not determined. As the authors point out, their methodology was less than optimal for demonstrating a causal relationship between injury and the wearing of protective gear.

Clearly, as demonstrated by Schieber et al.[1] and others, in-line skating is an at-risk activity. Although the authors conclude that further studies are necessary to determine whether equipment reduces the frequency and severity of injuries, the desirability of wearing wrist guards, elbow pads, knee pads, and helmets is, in my mind, unquestioned.

J.S. Torg, M.D.

Reference

1. Schieber RA, Branche-Dorsey CM, Ryan GW: Comparison of in-line skating injuries with roller skating and skate-boarding injuries. *JAMA* 271:1856–1858, 1994.

Lower Extremity Alignment and Risk of Overuse Injuries in Runners
Wen DY, Puffer JC, Schmalzried TP (Univ of California, Los Angeles; Los Angeles Orthopaedic Hosp)
Med Sci Sports Exerc 29:1291–1298, 1997   1–11

Background.—The effects of anatomical malalignment on risk of running injuries is unclear. The few prospective studies of the question have given conflicting results. The relationship between various lower extremity alignment characteristics on the risk of overuse injuries in marathon runners was retrospectively examined.

Methods.—Participants were 304 runners from a marathon training program. Their mean age was 41 years, mean running experience 7 years, and mean mileage per week was 12. Each runner underwent measurement of alignment parameters, including arch index (AI), heel valgus (HV), knee tubercle-sulcus angle (TSA), knee varus (KV), and leg-length difference (LLD). They also responded to a questionnaire seeking information on their training practices and injuries during the preceding 12 months. The data were analyzed to determine whether any of the anatomical characteristics were associated with risk of overuse injury, defined as a gradual-onset injury that led to modification of training.

Results.—Bivariate and multivariate analyses found few consistent associations between alignment measures and injury risk. Left AI was associated with hamstring injuries and right AI with shin injuries. Right HV was related to back injuries, left TSA to ankle injuries, KV to hip injuries, and LLD to back, ankle, and foot injuries. Significant associations were noted between training mileage and hamstring injuries, interval training and shin injuries, hard surfaces and back and thigh injuries, shoe use patterns and foot and overall injuries, and body mass index and heel injuries.

Conclusions.—Lower-extremity alignment does not appear to be an important risk factor for running injuries. This is so even after controlling for potential confounders. The findings in this relatively low-mileage cohort need to be confirmed in prospective studies.

▶ An interesting article, the conclusions of which appear to contradict current podiatric thinking. As with most studies dealing with the problems of the runner, the injury definition leaves much to be desired. That is, an injury defined as the patient admitting to "injury or pain" that stops or alters one's activity level is purely subjective. The observations would be more convincing had injury been defined in terms of anatomy, pathology, and severity.

J.S. Torg, M.D.

A Review of Selected Noncontact Anterior Cruciate Ligament Injuries in the National Football League
Scranton PE Jr, Whitesel JP, Powell JW, et al (Seattle; Kirkland, Wash; Med Sports Systems, Iowa City, Iowa; et al)
Foot Ankle Int 18:772–776, 1997   1–12

Objective.—Many different factors affect the risk of anterior cruciate ligament (ACL) injury in football. Understanding these factors may reduce the risk of noncontact ACL injuries. Shoe and surface factors associated with noncontact ACL injuries in the National Football League were analyzed.

Methods.—National Football League data on 61 noncontact ACL injuries occurring during 5 seasons were reviewed. Factors analyzed for each injury included shoe type, surface type, the use of shoe spats (protective taping), sport-related variables, and wet vs. dry surface. The injury rate per practice or game was calculated.

Results.—Two thirds of the injuries occurred while the athlete was wearing conventional cleats on natural grass; one third occurred on an artificial surface. About half of the injuries occurred during games, even though the players spent 5 times more exposure during practice. Ninety-five percent of the injuries occurred when the field was dry. The injury rate per team per session (games and practices) was 0.0054 for artificial turf vs.

0.0034 for natural grass. According to the incidence density ratio, artificial turf was associated with a 59% increase in the likelihood of ACL injury. Although injuries on grass were more likely to occur during games than practices, injuries on artificial turf were more likely to occur during practices.

Conclusions.—Although the risk of noncontact ACL football injuries appears to be higher on artificial turf than on grass, the picture is different once game vs. practice and type of shoe are considered. Injuries are more likely to occur on grass during games and on artificial turf during practice. The conventional 7-cleat shoe is probably a risk factor for ACL injuries. More research is needed to clarify the effects of wet vs. dry surface and of spatting a shoe.

▶ The statement of the authors that "identification of the conventional 7-cleat athletic shoe as a probable risk factor in noncontact ACL injuries will lead to further investigation regarding minimizing the risks of cleat catch on natural grass surfaces" has a familiar ring. In 1971,[1-3] on the basis of an extensive clinical study over several years in the Philadelphia Public High School and Catholic High School Football Leagues, "we concluded that the conventional football shoe with seven long cleats is a major factor responsible for the epidemic of knee injuries at all levels of organized football." We further recommended the conventional shoe be condemned and replaced by a soccer-type shoe with the following specifications: (1) synthetic molded sole, (2) minimum of 14 cleats per shoe, (3) minimum cleat diameter of one-half inch, and (4) minimum cleat tip length of three-eighths inch."[1-3] It is somewhat amusing to see these current authors assume credit for an observation that was made and published 25 years ago.

J.S. Torg, M.D.

References

1. Torg JS, Quadenfeld TC: Effective shoe type and cleat length on incidents and severity of knee injuries among high school football players. *Res Q* 42:203–211, 1971.
2. Torg JS, Quadenfeld TC: Knee and ankle injuries traced to shoes and cleats. *Physician Sportsmed* 1:39–43, 1973.
3. Torg JS, Quadenfeld TC, Landau S: Shoe surface interface and its relationship to football knee injuries. *Am J Sports Med* 2:261–269, 1974.

Traumatology: The Achilles Heel in the Rehabilitation of Cardiovascular Outpatients?
Unverdorben M, Neuner P, Kunkel B, et al (Ctr for Cardiovascular Diseases, Rotenburg/F, Germany; Community Hosp Bamberg, Germany)
Int J Sports Med 18:62–65, 1997   1–13

Introduction.—Safety concerns for outpatients in cardiovascular rehabilitation typically focus on sustained angina, myocardial infarction, cardiac arrest, and death. Data on trauma in sports groups involving cardiovascular outpatients do not exist. Patients at risk for certain types of trauma and situations most prone to injuries were identified retrospectively.

Methods.—Questionnaires regarding specific injuries were mailed to rehabilitation groups for cardiac outpatients. Patients were asked questions regarding demographics, type and extent of participation in sports, medical history, and types and consequences of cardiovascular symptoms or injuries. Medical records were reviewed for information regarding cardiovascular symptoms and major injuries.

Results.—Nine hundred and three questionnaires were returned. There were 123 injuries in 100 patients (11.1%). The injuries were equivalent to 1 per 2,200 exercise hours. Men had a higher incidence of injuries than women (11.8% vs. 7.3%). Most traumas were minor strains and abrasions and most were minor in severity (Figure 2). The severe injuries were: 15 ruptured tendons, muscles or ligaments (12.2% per 18,000 exercise hours); 14 bone fractures (11.4% per 19,300 exercise hours); and 1 loss of eyesight (0.8% per 270,000 exercise hours). Two slashes and the loss of eyesight were caused by broken eyeglasses. Injuries were severe in 35.7% of women and 28.1% of men. Most injuries occurred during games, 79% of which were ball games. The upper and lower limbs were most often injured. The lower extremities were the site of all ruptured muscles, tendons, and ligaments. The 14 fractures occurred in various bones.

Conclusion.—Injuries involving outpatients in cardiovascular rehabilitation are rare and about three-fourths are minor. Patients in this cohort should be instructed to avoid overexertion and to use non-breakable

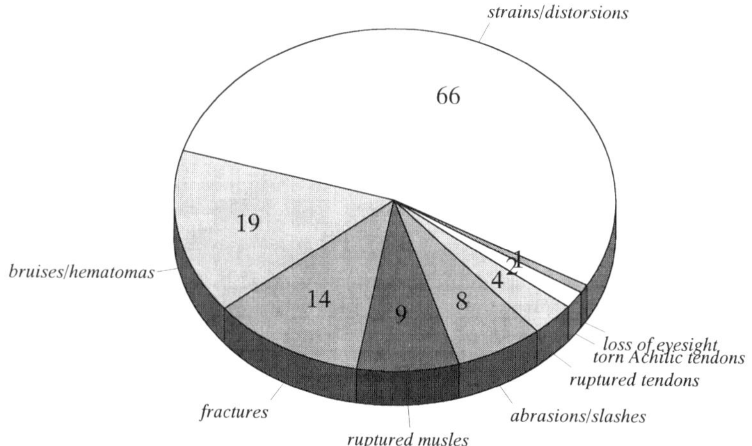

FIGURE 2.—Type of 123 traumas to the 100 injured patients. (Courtesy of Unverdorben M, Neuner P, Kunkel B, et al: Traumatology: The achilles heel in the rehabilitation of cardiac outpatients? *Int J Sports Med* 18:62–65, 1997.)

eyeglasses. Motor and technical skills and tactics should be taught, especially for patients participating in ball games.

▶ Some of the early reports of cardiac rehabilitation carried warnings that over-enthusiastic training of the middle-aged could lead to as many as a half of a group of exercisers being injured in the first 6 months of program participation. The present report provides a substantial database that reinforces the need for caution in the rate of progression of rehabilitation. The type A patient who is vulnerable to a coronary attack is also liable to be over-enthusiastic in subsequent rehabilitation. Many of the lesions reported in the present study—overstrains, distortions, bruises, and hematomas—may be thought of minor importance, although they can sometimes take a long time to heal in older people, and they can also have a negative impact on motivation. The present authors judge that the overall costs to the health system—1 medical consultation per 4,300 exercise hours, and 1 hospital admission per 54,000 exercise-hours—are acceptable. However, bone fractures in 11% of the patients, and particularly the loss of eyesight from broken spectacles in 1 patient, are warnings to those who organize programs for older people that exercise should be approached prudently.

R.J. Shephard, M.D., Ph.D., D.P.E.

Medical and Public Health Services at the 1996 Atlanta Olympic Games: An Overview
Brennan RJ, Keim ME, Sharp TW, et al (Ctrs for Disease Control and Prevention, Atlanta, Ga; Emory Univ, Atlanta, Ga; United States Marine Corps, Washington, DC, et al)
Med J Aust 167:595–598, 1997   1–14

Introduction.—The 1996 summer Olympic Games in Atlanta, the largest event in sporting history, required extensive preparation for medical and public health services. In addition to anticipated medical problems, officials had to be concerned about the possibility of a terrorist attack. These issues were reviewed to identify areas that might be improved by planners of the 2000 Sydney Olympic Games.

Medical Care.—The Atlanta Committee for the Olympic Games was responsible for providing medical and first aid services at all 35 Olympic sporting venues, the Olympic Village, and Centennial Olympic Park. Almost 700 physicians and 4,000 medical volunteers staffed the sites. Athletes and spectators were served by separate medical services and clinics. More than 30,000 individuals sought medical assistance and 10,723 were examined by physicians. One third of those seen by physicians had an injury. Many Olympic staff members and athletes from other countries sought routine dental and eye examinations. The number of emergency calls to Atlanta Fire Services increased by 16.2% over the usual number, but average response times did not increase. Extra radios were given to emergency medical personnel to ensure reliable communication among these workers, hospitals, and coordinating centers.

Public Health.—The state Division of Public Health coordinated public health services, addressing concerns regarding heat-related illness, infectious diseases, food and beverage safety, and environmental health. Surveillance systems were set up and rates of illness determined. To prevent heat-related illness, public health workers created an extensive media awareness campaign; placed water misters at crowded public sites; and gave out hats, fans, and sunscreen. Food inspectors were brought in from other areas of the United States to help prevent foodborne illness. A safe-sex campaign was designed to limit the spread of sexually transmitted diseases. Disaster planning considered the possibility of terrorists attacks, as well as natural disasters such as tornadoes. Involved in the planning were urban search and rescue teams, the Federal Bureau of Investigation, the United States Army and Navy, and the Centers for Disease Control. The bombing at Centennial Olympic Park demonstrated the difficulties of achieving a rapid disaster response despite extensive preparations.

Conclusion.—The sheer volume of visitors to an Olympic host city poses significant challenges to medical and public health services. Many agencies and service providers must be recruited to meet these challenges. Overall, the health promotion and prevention activities during the Atlanta Olympic Games were quite successful.

Hospital Use by Olympic Athletes During the 1996 Atlanta Olympic Games
Keim ME, Williams D (Emory Univ, Atlanta, Ga)
Med J Aust 167:603–605, 1997   1–15

Introduction.—The 1996 Olympic Games in Atlanta, which included more than 10,000 athletes from 197 countries, was the largest gathering of athletes for any event in history. Medical and dental care were provided by the Atlanta Committee for the Olympic Games. The site of primary care was the Polyclinic located at the Georgia Institute of Technology. Patients requiring outpatient emergency medical services and hospitalization were referred to Crawford Long Hospital of Emory University. The hospital records of Olympic athletes were reviewed to characterize their hospital use during the Games.

Hospital Preparation.—The hospital security force provided armed security for athletes. All members of the force were fully deputized to arrest and detain suspected law violators. Athletes who came to the emergency department were seen in private rooms with an armed sentry outside the door at all times, and access to their hospital rooms was restricted by armed security. Interpreting services were also provided.

Athletes Using the Hospital.—Forty-three Olympic athletes, 27 men and 16 women, were seen at Crawford Long Hospital between July 14 and August 7. Twenty-two were admitted, but none of the conditions were considered life-threatening. Sports-related injuries accounted for 31 of the 43 hospital presentations. Fifteen patients participated in 3 sports: boxing, wrestling, and track events (5 each). The most common primary diagnoses were concussion (4 cases) and ankle sprain (3 cases); cervical muscle sprain, degenerative disk disease, and Achilles tendon rupture accounted for 2 cases each. The longest hospital stay was 5 days, and no complications occurred during hospitalization. Except for a single appendectomy, all surgical procedures were orthopedic.

Conclusion.—Medical and surgical care of Olympic athletes required no extraordinary equipment or facilities. A number of special needs, however, should be considered for future Games: A continuous chain of security, an easily accessible translation service, ready availability of hospital-based clinicians, a small backup outpatient dispensary, and a hospital emergency contingency plan that includes response to an attack against athletes and is coordinated with the community response.

The Polyclinic at the 1996 Atlanta Olympic Village
Eaton SB, Woodfin BA, Askew JL, et al (Olympic Village, Atlanta, Ga)
Med J Aust 167:599–602, 1997   1–16

Introduction.—The Olympic Village Polyclinic at the 1966 Atlanta Games was designed to care for the more than 15,000 athletes, trainers, coaches, physicians, officials, and administrators living in the Olympic Village. In addition, almost 10,000 other personnel were eligible to receive emergency and routine services at the Polyclinic. Experiences at the 1996 Olympic Games were reviewed to provide useful information for medical care planners of future events.

Planning and Administration.—The planning committee had 25 members and began its work in 1992. Several members had been observers at the 1992 Olympic Games in Barcelona and the 1994 Winter Games at Lillehammer. The site of the Polyclinic was the Student Health Center at Georgia Institute of Technology. Volunteers made up 82% of the clerical and administrative staff during the Games. Administrative problems reported were inadequate incoming telephone and facsimile lines and the lack of a computerized filing system. Special services included physical and massage therapy and athletic training (housed in a separate facility), doping control rooms, and a gender verification program. In the future, gender testing might be more efficiently handled at the Accreditation Center rather than at a medical facility.

Clinical Services.—Dentistry, eye services, primary care, orthopedics, and emergency care were provided by the Polyclinic. A triage physician would have improved patient flow by making referrals to specialty care. Emergency care services would have benefitted from a nighttime clerical support person. Ancillary services—including a pharmacy, clinical laboratory services, and imaging services—successfully fulfilled their roles.

Discussion.—The Polyclinic operated 13 days before opening ceremonies and 3 days after closing ceremonies. The early start was helpful for testing equipment, familiarizing personnel with the system, and correcting supply deficiencies. An individual who was assigned logistic responsibility facilitated procurement of material by becoming familiar with the often complicated security provisions for moving supplies and equipment. Interaction with public health officers proved more important than originally anticipated.

▶ These 3 articles provide a fascinating account of the complexities involved in both the preparation and the implementation of medical coverage for all involved, both spectators and participants, at the 1996 Atlanta Olympic Games. Added to the anticipated medical problems of heat related injuries, foodborne and waterborne illnesses, and sexually transmitted diseases were preparedness planning for possible terrorist attack with conventional, chemical, biological or nuclear weapons.

Adding to these problems were the need for services covering doping control, gender verification, psychiatry/sports psychology, and disaster planning. Also involved was a 300-member United States Marine Chemical/Biological Incident Response Force. The Science and Technology Center at the Centers for Disease Control provided public health, emergency medical, toxicologic, and scientific consultation. Apparently, the only problem that arose occurred after the bombing in Centennial Olympic Park, when an excessive number of ambulances were dispatched before there was adequate assessment of the scene, potentially depleting emergency medical services to other areas of the city and contributing to vehicular congestion around the scene.

J.S. Torg, M.D.

Primary Care Sports Medicine in the Managed Care Environment: Coping in Today's Culture
Henehan M, Jones R (Stanford Univ, Palo Alto, Calif; Columbia San Jose Med Ctr, Calif; San Jose State Univ, Calif)
Physician Sportsmed 25:96–106, 1997   1–17

Objective.—Managed care is having a major impact on continuity of care, referral patterns, reimbursement, and access to testing. For the sports medicine physician, the managed care era poses some particular challenges. The effects of managed care on the sports medicine or primary care physician acting as a team physician are discussed.

Managed Care in Sports Medicine.—Sports medicine can be efficiently practiced when the patient, physician, and other providers are in the same managed care system. When they are not, problems may arise in getting authorization for desired tests, services, or referrals. Reimbursement issues may cause problems when the physician is expected to provide care for all athletes on a team. Even physicians who do not work with managed care entities may have to do so if they are to serve as a team physician. The medical needs of athletes, particularly elite athletes, may differ from those of other patients. The athlete's needs may conflict with what the insurance company allows, particularly in terms of the rapid diagnosis and aggressive management sometimes needed to minimize the impact of an injury on the athlete's career. Difficulties may arise related to fragmentation of care, limitations on referrals, cost constraints, liability issues, quality of care, and whether to choose a specialist or primary care designation.

Coping With Managed Care.—The physician can take several steps to deal with the problems raised by managed care in sports medicine practice. Physicians should familiarize themselves with the insurance plans, including what is covered and how referral systems work. Effective communication is essential, not only with athletes but also with coaches, trainers, parents, and insurance companies. The physician should sign on with as many plans as possible and find out which physicians are available for sports medicine referrals. A "referral specialist" may be designated from among the office staff, and, in large managed care plans, a sports medicine program can be initiated within the plan. If possible, the physician should require that all athletes join a plan in which he or she appreciates. The physician should learn to negotiate directly with insurance companies, including discussions of utilization review policies. Educating the reviewer about what a sports medicine primary care physician does may help to speed authorization for services. Forming alliances with other sports medicine physicians may strengthen the physician's position. Also, maintaining an identity as a primary care provider rather than a specialist helps the physician to function in the managed care environment.

Discussion.—Managed care is having a major impact on the practice of sports medicine, and will continue to do so for the foreseeable future. The primary care sports medicine primary care physician should understand the ways in which managed care influences his or her practice. This will help in forming coping strategies to deal with current and future challenges.

Patient Profile, Referral Sources, and Consultant Utilization in a Primary Care Sports Medicine Clinic
Butcher JD, Zukowski CW, Brannen SJ, et al (Dwight David Eisenhower Army Med Ctr, Ft Gordon, Ga; United States Naval Academy, Annapolis, Md; Uniformed Services Univ of Health Sciences, Bethesda, Md; et al)
J Fam Pract 43:556–560, 1996   1–18

Purpose.—At the same time managed care has encouraged the use of primary care physicians, the discipline of sports medicine has grown within primary care. The growing number of primary care sports medicine (PCSM) physicians vary widely in their practice, from practicing sports medicine part-time to serving as a team physician. Such physicians are increasingly incorporated into managed care organizations, though their optimal role in managed care remains to be defined. Using data from a primary care–based managed care system, this study specifically analyzed patient referrals to a sports medicine clinic.

Methods.—The data were drawn from a referral-based, freestanding primary care sports medicine clinic affiliated with a large managed care provider. The clinic included 3 part-time fellowship-trained PCSM physicians and 2 sports medicine fellows. The patients were all military beneficiaries who gained access to the clinic by referral from another health care provider. Patient referrals over a 10-month period were profiled, including not only diagnoses but also referral sources, diagnostic test utilization, and specialty referrals by the PCSM physicians.

Findings.—The analysis included a total of 1,857 patient contacts. Fifty-four percent of the patients were male, and their mean age was 34. More than half of visits were for follow-up of a previous problem or evaluation of a new injury. The new referrals came from a wide range of primary care physicians, including family practitioners, internists, pediatricians, and emergency physicians, and from specialist physicians. However, the greatest source of new referrals was the family practice clinic. Orthopedic injuries accounted for 95% of patient visits. The knee was injured in 27% of cases, the shoulder in 18%, the back in 14%, and the ankle in 10%. Diagnoses included tendinitis in 21% of patients, chronic anterior knee pain in 11%, and ligament sprains in 10%. Eight percent of patients were referred for specialized testing. However, most patients were managed at the clinic by PCSM physicians.

Conclusions.—Referrals to a managed care PCSM clinic were analyzed. The findings will be useful in defining the scope of practice for such clinics and for developing guidelines for orthopedic experience in primary care residency programs. Physicians practicing PCSM can provide an intermediate level of care for patients while maintaining their primary care specialty. Such dual practice is especially well suited for the primary care setting, where it can reduce the number of patients receiving nonsurgical care from orthopedic surgeons. Primary care sports medicine physicians and orthopedic surgeons should work synergistically, not in competition.

▶ As the saying goes, "It's a new ball game." The intrusion of managed care organizations into the team physician–athlete patient format is significant. Of course, the guiding principal is cost containment. And, of course, the question is: Will cost containment necessarily interfere with the needs of the athlete? These 2 articles suggest the answer to the problem is more extensive utilization of the primary care physician. Butcher et al. report a total of 1,857 patient contacts, 95.4% of which were for orthopedic injuries. Of these, 4.4% were referred for consultation with an orthopedic surgeon. The authors are further of the opinion that primary care physicians "offer an intermediate level of care in orthopedics while maintaining a practice in their primary care specialty." What is missing is an objective evaluation of the quality of orthopedic care being provided in this scenario.

J.S. Torg, M.D.

Field Splinting of Suspected Fractures: Preparation, Assessment, and Application

Meredith RM, Butcher JD (McDonald Army Community Hosp, Ft Eustis, Va; D D Eisenhower Army Med Ctr, Augusta, Ga)
Physician Sportsmed 25:29–32, 37–39, 1997   1–19

Introduction.—A careful initial evaluation and subsequent protection of the extremity are required for serious sports-related extremity injuries. The examiner must decide whether a splint is required after ruling out life-threatening injury and assessing neurovascular status. The physician must choose among a variety of preformed splints and materials. The type and severity of the injury as well as the need for radiographic imaging and specialty treatment must be determined.

Supplies.—Materials for splinting include fiberglass splinting tape, a wooden rigid splint, aluminum and foam splints, tape, prewrap, elastic bandages, an arm sling, wire splinting, and instant cold packs. Lower extremity splints include a rigid shoe, rocker-bottom boot, ankle stirrup brace, posterior splint, and straight knee immobilizer. Splints for upper extremity joints include the posterior elbow splint, Colles wrist splint, neutral wrist splint, and finger splints. Other splinting materials include a foam long leg splint, rigid arm splint, hare traction splint, Kendrick extrication device, Sager traction splint, and long spine board.

Assessment.—The need for radiographs is obvious for limb deformity, crepitation ecchymosis, or swelling. An open fracture is signaled by any defect in the overlying skin. Assessment of neurologic status includes evaluation of sensory and motor components by observing range of motion in joints or digits distal to the injury and light touch and 2-point discrimination. Palpating pulses distal to the injury is used to assess the vascular status of the injured limb.

Conclusion.—To avoid damage to the skin, splints should be well padded. The splint should immobilize the joints above and below the injury. Neurovascular status should be reassessed after the splint is applied. When no splint is available, a lower-leg injury can be protected by "buddy taping" the leg to the uninjured leg By wrapping an ice bag in the elastic bandage, the bag can be incorporated into the splint. Ice should not be applied for more than 10 minutes at a time. Proper splint principles, application, and preparation must be known by physicians because the need for assessing serious musculoskeletal injury in sports is common.

▶ The authors have described a variety of splints and splinting materials that may be used in emergency situations. Most athletic trainers on the university and professional levels also use a vacuum type of splint or a pneumatic type of splint. These splints (especially the pneumatic type) are relatively inexpensive and easy to use. They come in a variety of sizes, such as short- and long-leg splints. The knee immobilizer is also a very adaptable splint which can be used in a variety of situations. We have safely used ice for longer than 10 minutes at a time.

F.J. George, A.T.C., P.T.

The Physical Examination of the Glenohumeral Joint: Emphasis on the Stabilizing Structures
Wilk KE, Andrews JR, Arrigo CA (HealthSouth Rehabilitation Corp, Birmingham, Ala; Univ of Virginia, Charlottesville)
J Orthop Sports Phys Ther 25:380–388, 1997   1–20

Introduction.—Because of the normal amount of capsular laxity appreciated in most individuals during physical examination, examination of a patient whose history suggests subtle glenohumeral joint instability may make the diagnosis extremely difficult for the clinician. When attempting to determine the amount of normal acceptable ligamentous laxity compared with pathologic excessive laxity, clinicians may be challenged. Few scientific papers thoroughly describe the specific physical examinations that can be used to determine glenohumeral instability.

History and Examination.—A thorough and meticulous subjective history is an essential component of the physical examination and must include mechanisms of injury and/or dysfunction, level of disability, chief complaint, and aggravating movement. Patients with shoulder instability will usually be younger than 30 years of age; rotator cuff pathology is usually present in patients who are in their fourth or fifth decade. With some patients, the condition is readily perceived; other patients may report only vague shoulder pain.

Assessment.—Assessment of motion, static stability testing, muscle testing, and a neurologic assessment are necessary parts of the physical examination. Active and passive range of motion should be assessed. The patient should be asked to perform 4 active motions: elevation of the arms above the head, horizontal adduction/abduction, external rotation behind the head, and internal rotation behind the back. When passive motion is assessed, individuals with shoulder instability may frequently exhibit a spasm end feel or an empty end feel with no resistance met. When inferior stability is assessed, the anterior band of the inferior glenohumeral ligament is the primary restraint to inferior translation with the arm at 45 degrees of abduction. In the anterior dislocated shoulder, this portion of the capsule is a commonly injured area. Bilateral comparisons, end feel, reproduction of symptoms, and acquired appreciation of acceptable levels of laxity by the examiner are used to determine shoulder stability. The relocation test is a sensitive test of anterior instability in the overhead athlete in which the patient's arm is abducted to 90 degrees and fully externally rotated.

Anterior instability may be present if pain occurs anteriorly. The pain complaint can be reduced by relocating the humeral head within the glenoid (Fig 10). The jerk test can be used for determining posterior

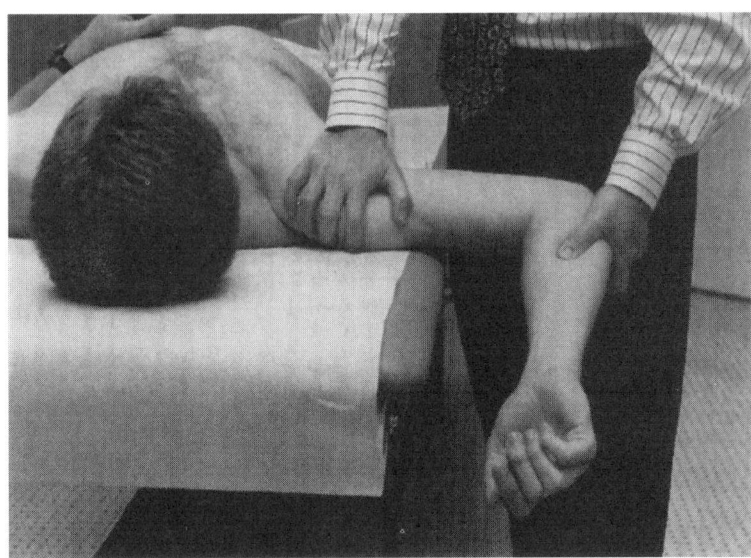

FIGURE 10.—The relocation test. The patient's arm is abducted to 90 degrees and fully external rotated. If pain occurs anteriorly, the humeral head is then relocated within the glenoid, which reduces the pain complaint. This may suggest anterior instability. (Courtesy of Wilk KE, Andrews JR, Arrigo CA: The physical examination of the glenohumeral joint: Emphasis on the stabilizing structures. *J Orthop Sports Phys Ther* 25(6):380–388, 1997.)

stability. The patient's arm is internal rotated and flexed to 90 degrees. The elbow is grasped to axially load the humerus in a proximal direction. The clinician moves the arm horizontally across the body. A sudden jerk is produced in many patients with recurrent posterior instability.

Conclusion.—The clinician must understand the various evaluation techniques to determine the passive stability of the glenohumeral joint and must practice the tests repeatedly so that they are performed correctly. The patient must be relaxed and comfortable for these types of hands-on examinations to be performed.

▶ An excellent article describing the evaluation of glenohumeral joint problems. The authors stress the importance of a subjective history, together with the assesment of motion, strength, and neurologic and shoulder stability testing maneuvers. They also point out the difficulty in performing these stability tests and emphasize that they must be practiced repeatedly before proficiency can be attained.

F.J. George, A.T.C., P.T.

Clinical Findings in Competitive Swimmers With Shoulder Pain

Bak K, Faunø P (Univ of Copenhagen; Aarhus Univ Hosp, Denmark)
Am J Sports Med 25:254–260, 1997   1–21

Introduction.—Shoulder pain is common among competitive swimmers, and the main cause appears to be a combination of overload and overuse. A clinical evaluation of a group of swimmers with histories of interfering shoulder pain was conducted to examine the biomechanical aspects of their pain.

Methods.—The study group consisted of 36 swimmers seen consecutively by 2 physicians during 1994 and 1995. All swimmers underwent detailed interviews and clinical examinations. Details of the history included localization of pain, presence of pain at night, presence of a snapping sensation from the shoulder during swimming, duration of symp-

TABLE 4.—Classification of Glenohumeral Subluxation and Associated Subacromial Impingement Modified after Jobe and Glousman

Group	Symptoms and findings

1: Pure impingement	1. Positive impingement sign
	2. Negative apprehension sign
	3. Grade 0 or 1 humeral head translation
	4. Arthroscopic
	  a) Stable examination
	  b) Undersurface cuff tear, subacromial bursitis
	  c) Labrum and glenohumeral ligaments normal

2: Anterior instability and associated impingement	1. Positive impingement sign
	2. Grade 2 or more humeral head translation
	3. Possible apprehension and relocation
	4. Arthroscopic
	  a) Unstable examination
	  b) Undersurface cuff tear
	  c) Labral damage
	  d) Humeral head chondromalacia
	  e) Subluxation of humeral head

3: Anterior instability and associated impingement (hyperelasticity)	1. Positive impingement sign
	2. Grade 2 or more humeral head translation
	3. Possible apprehension and relocation
	4. General joint hypermobility
	5. Arthroscopic
	  a) Unstable examination
	  b) Undersurface cuff tear
	  c) Attenuated but intact labrum
	  d) Glenohumeral ligament (capsular laxity)
	  e) Subluxation of humeral head over labrum

4: Pure anterior instability	1. Negative impingement sign
	2. Grade 2 or more humeral head translation
	3. Possible apprehension and relocation
	4. Arthroscopic
	  a) Unstable examination
	  b) Normal cuff?
	  c) Labral damage and capsular laxity
	  d) Humeral head chondromalacia and subluxation

(Courtesy of Bak K, Faunø P: Clinical findings in competitive swimmers with shoulder pain. *Am J Sports Med* 25:254–260, 1997.)

toms, and time absent from swimming. Degree of pain was assessed on a 4-point scale, ranging from pain only after heavy workouts to pain that prevented competitive swimming. Swimmers were tested for coracoacromial impingement, glenohumeral instability, scapulothoracic instability, and general joint hypermobility.

Results.—Twenty-two swimmers were women and 14 were men; the men were significantly older than the women and tended to have had a longer swimming experience. Shoulder pain was unilateral in 23 swimmers and bilateral in 13. The mean duration of pain was 59 weeks; duration was significantly longer in those with bilateral pain (mean 104 vs. 33 weeks). Shoulder pain was localized anteriorly or anterolaterally in 72% of swimmers. The degree of pain was I or II in 79% of shoulders. In 18%, pain was sufficiently disabling to interfere with performance, and in 2% pain made swimming impossible. Hawkins' test, positive in 39 of 49 painful shoulders, was more sensitive than Neer's test. Signs of impingement without excessive humeral head translation were present in 12 shoulders. Twenty-five shoulders had concomitant signs of impingement and increased glenohumeral translation. According to the classification of Jobe and Glousman, 12 shoulders had primary impingement, 25 secondary impingement, 8 impingement and general joint hypermobility, and 4 anterior instability without impingement (Table 4).

Conclusion.—Competitive swimmers with shoulder pain have a high prevalence of coracoacromial impingement with associated increased glenohumeral translation and positive apprehension. The predominant direction of shoulder laxity is anteroinferior. General joint hypermobility was present in only 22% of swimmers.

▶ This is basically a review article with supporting clinical data. The authors successfully differentiate among symptoms due to pure impingement, to anterior instability with associated impingement, to anterior instability, to impingement and laxity, and to pure anterior instability. They also point out that scapulohumeral instability is more common in symptomatic than in asymptomatic shoulders.

J.S. Torg, M.D.

The Evaluation and Treatment of the Injured Acromioclavicular Joint in Athletes

Lemos MJ (Lahey Hitchcock Med Ctr, Burlington, Mass)
Am J Sports Med 26:137–144, 1998   1–22

Introduction.—Acromioclavicular joint injuries are very common in athletes. However, they are easily confused with other types of shoulder injury. The last 20 years have seen major changes in our understanding and treatment of acromioclavicular joint injuries. The current management of acromioclavicular injuries in athletes was reviewed.

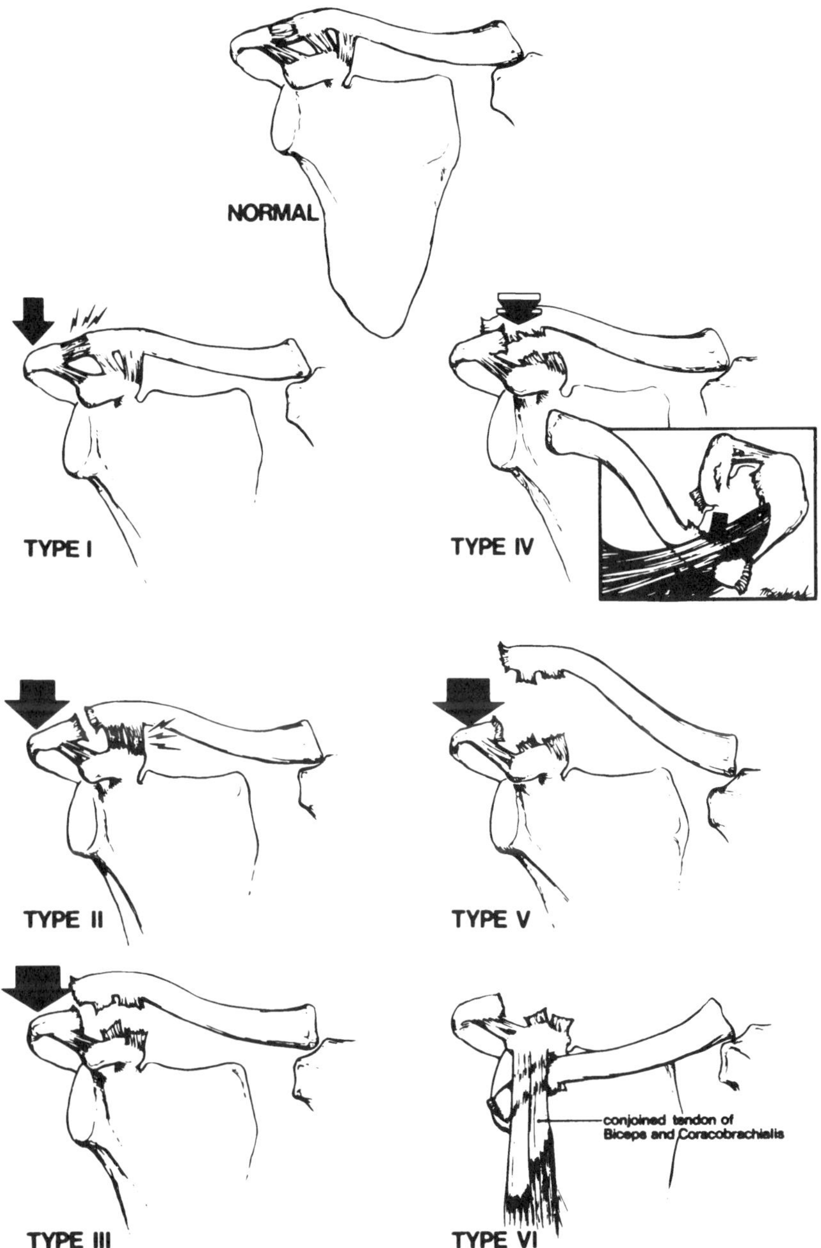

FIGURE 1.—Classification of injuries by type. From Lemos MJ: The evaluation and treatment of the injured acromioclavicular joint in athletes. *Am J Sports Med* 26:137–144, 1998. Courtesy of Rockwood CA Jr, Young DC: Disorders of the acromioclavicular joint, in Rockwood CA Jr, Matsen FA III [eds]: *The Shoulder*, vol 1. Philadelphia, WB Saunders, 1990, pp 413–476.)

Acromioclavicular Injuries.—The most frequent cause of acromioclavicular joint dislocation is direct trauma to the shoulder, typically a force applied to the acromion with the arm in adduction. These injuries may be classified into 6 types (Fig 1). Nonoperative treatment is indicated for type I and II injuries. There is debate as to the management of type III injuries, which have been managed both operatively and nonoperatively. However, the current trend is toward nonoperative treatment, with studies suggesting results at least as good as those of surgery. Currently, the author performs surgery for type III injuries for high-level pitchers or patients with open injuries, brachial plexus injury, or severe dislocations. Type IV through VI injuries are treated surgically.

Operative Management.—Five basic surgical techniques have been described for the treatment of dislocated acromioclavicular joints. One popular and simple option is pin fixation across the acromioclavicular joint. More recently, a hook plate technique has been used. Good results have been reported with dynamic muscle transfer, although this involves reconstructing a static constraint with dynamic tissues. Ligamentous reconstruction can be achieved by excision of the lateral end of the clavicle with transfer of the coracoacromial ligament. Fixation between the clavicle and coracoid can be achieved with either a Bosworth screw or synthetic augmentation. The latter technique is essential for adequate reduction of the clavicle relative to the acromion. This is currently the author's technique of choice, which is described in detail. For patients with acromioclavicular injury associated with coracoid fracture, open reduction and internal fixation is indicated. For athletes with chronic acromioclavicular dislocations and sprains, surgical options are available after nonoperative intervention has failed.

Summary.—The approach to acromioclavicular joint injuries has changed significantly over the years. There is a trend toward nonoperative management of these injuries, although surgery is recommended for some type III and all type IV, V, and VI injuries. Several surgical options have been described for management of the more severe acute injuries. For chronic injuries, surgery is considered if nonoperative treatment fails.

▶ This is a comprehensive Current Concepts article that includes 61 literature citations. The original article is recommended reading for the interested practitioner.

J.S. Torg, M.D.

Patellofemoral Pain: Let the Physical Exam Define Treatment
Post WR (West Virginia Univ, Morgantown)
Physician Sportsmed 26:68–78, 1998   1–23

Introduction.—Patellofemoral disorders often respond to nonoperative treatment. A systematic evaluation of the alignment of a patient's lower extremity, patellar mobility, muscle flexibility, strength, and coordination will help identify the causes of patellofemoral disorders. The assessment should also include soft-tissue and articular pain. The physician can make a specific diagnosis by combining this information with a careful history and appropriate radiographic studies.

Examination.—The physician will need to determine whether the source of pain involves the soft tissues or the patellofemoral articulation itself. A surgical finding that may represent areas of hyaline cartilage trauma or aberrant loading, but is not the cause of pain, is chrondomalacia, which should not be confused with a cause of anterior knee pain. Patellofemoral pain may also be caused by flexibility deficits in the hip external rotators, hamstrings, quadriceps, or gastrocnemius-soleus muscle groups. Patients with chronic pain often have significant prone quadriceps flexibility deficits and a home program of quadriceps stretching would produce dramatic improvement. Patients may also have iliotibial band tightness.

Rehabilitation.—Rehabilitation can involve strength training and muscle flexibility, orthoses, taping, analgesics, and therapy with heat and ice. Quadriceps strengthening is often recommended for patients with patellofemoral problems and the weight-bearing loads associated with closed-chain activities tend to be tolerated better in these patients than open-chain exercise. The rehabilitated strength and flexibility must often exceed the preinjury level for patients and athletes to return to their desired activity level, because their preinjury level was inadequate. Recurrence is likely when patients resume their activities when treatment features only rest and medication; thus, rehabilitation must include exercise.

Conclusion.—Patients must know what to expect from therapy, and change must be documented for managed care providers so that ongoing treatment may be justified. Improved diagnoses will help patients who are referred to different therapists to receive appropriate and consistent rehabilitation.

▶ The author stresses the importance of rehabilitation exercises for patients with patellofemoral pain. Structures with decreased flexibility must be stretched and weak structures must be strengthened. The timing of the contractions of the vastus medialis obliquus and vastus lateralis must be addressed as well as the use of orthoses.

F.J. George, A.T.C., P.T.

The Outcomes of Two Knee Scoring Questionnaires in a Normal Population
Demirdjian AM, Petrie SG, Guanche CA, et al (Louisiana State Univ, New Orleans)
Am J Sports Med 26:46–51, 1998   1–24

Objective.—Many different knee scoring scales are in current use, including the Noyes and Lysholm questionnaires. These instruments were developed from information on knees with preexisting pathologic conditions. Although they have never been standardized to normal knees, these scoring systems are commonly used for follow-up of patients undergoing knee surgery. There is debate over which questionnaire provides the most accurate assessment of outcome; both scales assume that a normal knee should achieve a perfect score of 100 points. The results of the Noyes and Lysholm questionnaires in a large population of normal knees were presented.

Methods.—Both the Noyes and Lysholm questionnaires were administered to 246 high school and collegiate team athletes. The sample was restricted to individuals with no history of surgery or injury to either knee, and no preexisting pathologic conditions of the knee. A total of 418 knees—from 253 male and 165 female athletes, average age 18 years—were available for analysis. The expectation was that the 95% confidence intervals of the mean scores achieved would include the maximal value of 100 points for each scale.

Results.—Average total Noyes score was 99.10 for male athletes and 97.82 for female athletes. Average Lysholm scores were 99.10 and 97.16, respectively. In each group, the calculated 95% confidence interval did not include the maximal value. On both instruments, the scores for female athletes were significantly lower than those of male athletes. Male athletes scored significantly less than 100 points on all categories of the Lysholm questionnaire except support and stair climbing. For female athletes, scores were significantly lower than the maximum in all categories except limping and thigh atrophy.

Conclusions.—The results of the Noyes and Lysholm knee scoring questionnaires in a highly selected "normal" population underscore the need for more accurate instruments for use in evaluating the outcomes of knee surgery. The authors propose a new approach to validating existing knee scores through the use of a reference values chart. This will produce a more accurate instrument that can be geared to specific patient populations. Differences in treatment outcomes based on subjective knee scoring systems should be interpreted with caution.

▶ This article clearly demonstrates the difficulty in evaluating subjective data from a "normal population" using questionnaires. It seems reasonable to assume that there would be even more disparity in data obtained from a population of individuals who were evaluated either after injury or after surgery. It appears that the major problems with the Noyes and Lysholm systems is combining objective with the subjective parameters. I agree with the authors that "perceived or claimed differences and treatment modalities that are based on such subjective knee scoring systems should be used with caution."

J.S. Torg, M.D.

Recognizing Posterior and Posterolateral Knee Instability
Shea JD (Springfield College, Springfield, Mass [tk])
Athletic Ther Today 2:30–34, 1997   1–25

Introduction.—The posterior cruciate ligament in the center of the knee is the axis around which the knee flexes, extends, and rotates. It is believed that knee instability can be classified according to the degree to which the posterior cruciate ligament is intact. Predraft physical examination of NFL players has shown a 2% incidence of posterior cruciate ligament deficiency among these players, and the players are often unaware of the injury. The most common causes of posterior cruciate ligament injury is sports and high-speed motor vehicle accidents.

Mechanism of Injury.—The most common mechanisms of injury to the posterior cruciate ligament are a direct blow to the tibial crest with the knee flexed at 70° to 90°, an extreme internal or external rotation, and hyperextension.

Symptoms.—Isolated injuries to the posterior cruciate ligament are often unnoticed at first. One should look carefully for lacerations or abrasions in the anterior tibial region. Individuals with chronic posterior cruciate ligament injury may have anterior and/or medial knee pain secondary to the increased medial compartment and patellofemoral contact forces. Instability associated with twisting or jumping may also be reported. Individuals with acute isolated posterolateral injury may have pain in the posterolateral knee. Peroneal nerve injury may be present and could lead to dysesthesia and leg and foot weakness. The individual may experience instability in positions of extension and some buckling of the knee into hyperextension. There may also be instability going up and down stairs.

Physical Examination.—One should not confuse posterior cruciate ligament laxity with anterior cruciate ligament laxity. The difficulty is in establishing the neutral point of tibiofemoral position. The posterior "sag" sign or gravity drawer test can help identify posterior cruciate ligament deficiency and posterior displacement of the tibia. Noyes et al. recommend the tibiofemoral rotation test in a supine position to evaluate external rotation of the tibia on the femur (Fig 2).[1] To differentiate posterolateral instability from anteromedial instability, the clinician should palpate the tibial plateaus to determine their positions in relation to the femoral condyles. Posterolateral instability is indicated by posterior movement of the lateral tibial plateau, and anteromedial instability is indicated by anterior movement of the medial plateau.

Discussion.—A knee with isolated posterior cruciate ligament injury will have minimum posterior translation at 30° of knee flexion and maximum posterior translation at 90° of knee flexion. There will be no change in varus stability or external rotation, but there will be a complete loss of coupled external rotation. A knee with isolated posterolateral corner injury will have maximum posterior translation at 30° of knee flexion and minimum posterior translation at 90° of knee flexion. At 30° of knee flexion, there will be significant increases in external rotation and coupled

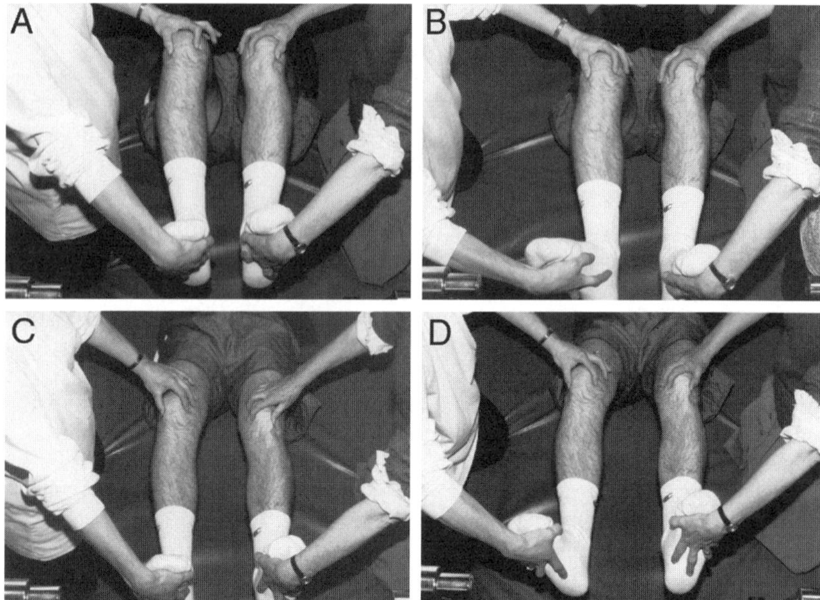

FIGURE 2.—The tibiofemoral rotation test. **A,** Position of the medial and lateral tibial plateaus relative to femoral condyles is assessed in the starting position of 90° of knee flexion and neutral tibial rotation. **B,** the examiner externally rotates the tibia, noting the amount of external rotation by comparing axis of medial border of the foot to axis of femur. Position of medial and lateral tibial plateaus is then compared to normal knee to detect anterior or posterior subluxation. **C and D,** Test is then repeated at 30° of knee flexion. (Courtesy of Shea JD: Recognizing posterior and posterolateral knee instability. *Athletic Ther Today* 2:30–34, 1997.)

external rotation. A knee with rupture to both the posterior cruciate ligament and posterolateral corner will have increased posterior translation, varus instability, and external rotation at all angles of knee flexion.

Reference

1. Noyes FR, Stowers FS, Grood ES, et al. Posterior subluxations of the medial and lateral tibiofemoral compartments: an in vitro ligament sectioning study in cadaveric knees. *Am J Sports Med* 21:407–414, 1993.

▶ The author describes the anatomy and function of the posterior cruciate ligament and the posterior lateral corner stabilizers of the knee. A series of stability tests and techniques are described to make a differential diagnosis of these injuries. The diagnosis of injuries to the posterior cruciate ligament are often missed or misdiagnosed. Forced hyperflexion of the knee joint may be the leading cause of this injury.

F.J. George, A.T.C., P.T.

Clinical Application of the Ottawa Ankle Rules for the Use of Radiography in Acute Ankle Injuries: An Independent Site Assessment
Verma S, Hamilton K, Hawkins HH, et al (Univ of Cincinnati, Ohio)
AJR 169:825–827, 1997   1–26

Introduction.—The second most commonly ordered musculoskeletal examination in the emergency department is the ankle radiographic series (cervical spine series is first). There are approximately 6 million ankle series performed each year in the United States and Canada costing more than $500 million annually. The yield of fractures requiring plaster immobilization is less than 15%. A doctor in Ottawa, Canada, created a set of criteria that would help determine when to order an ankle film to evaluate blunt trauma. Simple to use, the Ottawa ankle rules require assessment for point tenderness over the posterior edge of the medial or the lateral malleolus and assessment for the inability to bear weight immediately after the injury or for 4 steps in the emergency department. An ankle series is not performed when none of these criteria are positive. A previous prospective trial found these rules to be 100% sensitive for clinically significant ankle fractures, 50% specific, and decreased the number of ankle radiographs ordered by 28%. Whether these rules could be used by a broader group of emergency clinicians at a level-1 trauma center was determined.

Methods.—The Ottawa ankle rules were used on 926 patients who came to an emergency department with blunt ankle trauma during a 1-year period. The rules were used to determine the need for ordering ankle radiographs. The patients were between 18 and 55 years of age.

Results.—Ottawa ankle rule criteria for ordering radiographs of the ankle were met by 759 of 926 patients with blunt ankle trauma (Fig 1). A fracture was found in 152 of these patients. Ankle radiographs were deemed unnecessary in another 167 of the patients. For the purpose of detecting any missed fractures, 152 of these 167 patients (91%) were successfully followed up by telephone contact or medical records review. Two missed fractures were discovered, with plaster immobilization required for 1 of the patients. There was an overall sensitivity of 99% using the Ottawa ankle rules.

Conclusions.—The Ottawa ankle rules can adequately screen for ankle fractures when implemented at a level-1 trauma center.

► Interestingly, the authors admit that the Ottawa ankle rules are somewhat subjective, particularly when the patient insists on a study. To be questioned is the claim that its sensitivity was high, with only 1 fracture being missed. How do the authors know that more fractures were not missed in those individuals who did not have radiographs?

J.S. Torg, M.D.

ANKLE RADIOGRAPH ORDER FORM

Ordering   RN______________________________
or
MD______________________________

Ottawa clinical rules should not be applied if:

______Less than 18 or greater than 55 years old
______Injury occurred 10 or more days ago
______Return visit for same injury

An ankle radiographic series is only required if there is any pain in the <u>malleolar zone</u> and:

________Bone tenderness at A or B
________Inability to bear weight (4 steps) both
        immediately and in the emergency department
________Pain at base of fifth metatarsal (C)

Justification if ankle radiograph is required despite Ottawa clinical rules______

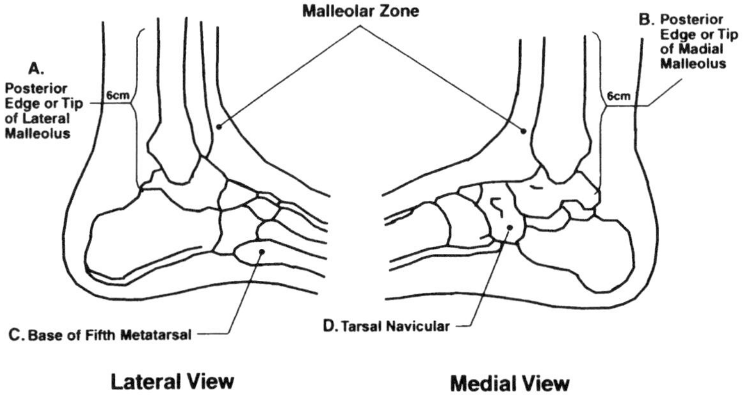

____

____

FIGURE 1.—Order form completed by physician or nurse in emergency department that incorporates Ottawa ankle rules with diagrams of ankles to determine need for obtaining radiographs of injured ankle. (Courtesy of Verma S, Hamilton K, Hawkins HH, et al: Clinical application of the Ottawa ankle rules for the use of radiography in acute ankle injuries: An independent site assessment. *AJR* 169:825–827, 1997.)

Implementation of the Ottawa Knee Rule for the Use of Radiography in Acute Knee Injuries
Stiell IG, Wells GA, Hoag RH, et al (Univ of Ottawa, Ont; Queensway-Carleton Hosp, Nepean, Ont; Univ of Toronto; et al)
JAMA 278:2075–2079, 1997   1–27

Objective.—More than 1 million adults annually in the United States and Canada have an acute knee injury. Because the accumulated cost of routine radiographs is high, the Ottawa Knee Rule was developed and validated as a clinical decision rule for radiography. The impact of implementing the Ottawa Knee Rule on actual use of radiography, waiting times, and direct medical charges was assessed.

Methods.—This nonrandomized, controlled clinical trial involved a before-and-after comparison of 3,907 nonpregnant adult patients with an acute knee injury, seen at 1 teaching and 1 community intervention hospital (using the Ottawa Knee Rule) or at 1 teaching and 1 community control hospital between July 1, 1994 and June 30, 1995 and between September 1, 1995 and August 31, 1996. The outcomes were the proportion of patients referred for knee radiographs, patient satisfaction with treatment, and charges.

Results.—In before and after periods, there was a 26.4% reduction in referrals for knee radiography in the intervention group (77.6% vs. 57.1%) compared to a 1.3% reduction in the control group (76.9% vs. 75.9%). At intervention hospitals, physicians interpreted the rule accurately for 97.7% of patients, with excellent interobserver agreement ($\kappa = 0.91$). In the after-intervention period, patients who did not have knee radiography spent significantly less time in the emergency department than patients undergoing radiography (85.7 minutes versus 118.8 minutes). When surveyed, 95.7% and 98.7% of these respective patients were satisfied with the care. Mean charges were significantly lower in the nonradiography group than in the radiography group ($80 vs. $183). All clinically important fractures were identified by the Ottawa Knee Rule for a sensitivity of 1.0 and a negative predictive value of 1.0.

Conclusion.—The Ottawa Knee Rule identified all important knee fractures while reducing radiographic utilization and medical costs significantly. The Rule is extremely sensitive and accurate.

Knee Tumors: Duration and Nature of Symptoms Prior to Investigation
Dickinson FL, Harper WM, Finlay DB (Leicester Royal Infirmary, England)
Br J Radiol 70:635–637, 1997   1–28

Purpose.—The knee is the most common site of musculoskeletal neoplasms. Current guidelines of the British Royal College of Radiologists do not call for routine radiographs in patients with knee pain without restricted movement or symptoms of locking. This study evaluated the number of knee tumors meeting the guidelines for radiologic evaluation.

Methods and Findings.—The 5-year review included 19 patients (age range, 11 to 86), with knee tumors ranging from adamantinoma and giant cell tumor to high-grade osteosarcoma. For most patients, knee symptoms were present for about 6 months before radiography was performed. This was so regardless of patient age or the grade of malignancy. Just 4 patients met the current guidelines for radiologic investigation. In these cases, the guidelines would not have been met had the patients not developed pathologic fracture or locking of the knee joint.

Conclusions.—Even in patients with a history of injury, the possibility of a knee tumor should be considered in the presence of persistent knee pain. Current guidelines for radiographic investigation should include an indication for persistent, unilateral knee pain lasting longer than 6 weeks. This should provide enough time for soft tissue injuries to resolve, and prevent delays in case of a more serious diagnosis.

▶ The Ottawa knee rule limits x-rays in the face of acute injury to patients 55 or older, or with isolated tenderness of the patella, or with tenderness of the fibula head, or with inability to flex the knee 90 degrees, or inability to bear weight. Stiell et al. conclude that widespread implementation of the Ottawa knee rule "could lead to important health care savings without jeopardizing patient care." Unfortunately, they do not precisely define what is an "acute" injury. It is important to note that the recommended criteria have not been applied to nor should be used in pediatric patients. Dickinson et al.'s observation that unilateral knee pain for longer than 6 weeks is an indication for imaging stands without question. We feel very strongly that persistent ill-defined pain in the vicinity of the knee joint requires an x-ray to rule out osseous tumors and an MRI to rule out soft tissue neoplasms. The busy sports medicine orthopedist is certain at some point to see a malignant knee tumor, and it should not be missed because of "radiologic guidelines or rules" or in the interest of cost containment.

J.S. Torg, M.D.

Near-infrared Spectroscopy for Monitoring of Tissue Oxygenation of Exercising Skeletal Muscle in a Chronic Compartment Syndrome Model
Breit GA, Gross JH, Watenpaugh DE, et al (Natl Aeronautics and Space Administration Ames Research Ctr, Moffett Field, Calif)
J Bone Joint Surg Am 79-A:838–843, 1997   1–29

Objective.—Dual-wave near-infrared spectroscopy may be an excellent tool for the noninvasive measurement of muscle ischemia resulting from high intramuscular pressure that occurs during exercise in chronic compartment syndrome. To simulate the hypoxia of muscle tissues secondary to the local ischemia occurring in chronic compression syndrome, external compression was applied around the legs of healthy volunteers. Near-infrared spectroscopy was used to monitor the oxygenation of the tibialis anterior muscle before and after exercise.

Methods.—A wide inflatable cuff was placed around the thighs of 10 healthy volunteers (3 women), aged 18–48 years, and gradually inflated to increase intramuscular pressure to 40 mm Hg during 14 minutes of plantar flexion and dorsiflexion of the ankle. A near-infrared probe placed over the tibialis anterior muscle of the dominant leg of each volunteer was used to measure intramuscular pressure with and without compression. Two sets of measurements were made at least 2 days apart. Baseline and minimum tissue oxygenation requirements of each volunteer were determined. The relationship between level of tissue oxygenation and subjective pain index was analyzed statistically.

Results.—Whereas during exercise with compression tissue oxygenation steadily declined at a rate of 1.4%/min, during exercise without compression, tissue oxygenation was essentially unchanged. During exercise with compression, hemoglobin concentration increased significantly after 2 minutes to 118% of the baseline level and remained there throughout the exercise. Without compression, hemoglobin values began to increase at 8 minutes into the exercise period and rose to levels comparable with those achieved with compression. After exercise with and without compression, hemoglobin levels rose, but the increase was significantly greater during recovery after compression (163% of baseline) than during recovery after no compression (140% of baseline). Volunteers exerted significantly lower maximum isometric torque with compression than without and reported significantly more pain with compression than without. Tissue oxygenation at the end of exercise with compression was significantly and inversely correlated with subjective pain index.

Conclusion.—Because near-infrared spectroscopy can detect a decrease in muscle oxygenation resulting from increased intramuscular pressure, it may be a useful noninvasive tool for diagnosing chronic compartment syndrome.

Intramuscular Deoxygenation During Exercise in Patients Who Have Chronic Anterior Compartment Syndrome of the Leg

Mohler LR, Styf JR, Pedowitz RA, et al (Univ of California, San Diego)
J Bone Joint Surg Am 79-A:844–849, 1997   1–30

Objective.—Pain from chronic compartment syndrome results from a decrease in blood flow to muscle and impaired oxygenation during exercise. Definitive diagnosis by measurement of intracompartmental pressure is invasive and can result in injury. Because near-infrared spectroscopy can detect changes in oxygen saturation of hemoglobin, its use as a diagnostic tool was evaluated in patients suspected of having chronic compartment syndrome of the leg.

Methods.—Between 1993 and 1995, 10 patients with chronic compartment syndrome of the leg, 8 patients with pain from other sources, and 10 healthy controls took part in an isokinetic exercise protocol during which intramuscular pressure was measured with a microcapillary infusion technique and relative oxygenation was monitored using a continuous dual wavelength near-infrared spectrometer that measured reflected light transmitted at 760 and 850 nm.

Results.—Patients exercised until they were in pain (an average of 8.2 minutes). Controls exercised for an average of 9.9 minutes. The mean work rates were 12.3 nm/min for patients with chronic compartment syndrome, 7.0 nm/min for patients without chronic compartment syndrome, and 9.1 nm/min for controls. Whereas mean resting pressures before exercise were similar between groups, after 2 minutes of exercise, mean resting pressure was significantly higher in patients with chronic compartment syndrome (55.4 mm Hg) than in patients with other pain (17.4 mm Hg) and in controls (16.9 mm Hg). After 30 seconds of exercise, relative oxygenation was significantly higher in patients with chronic compartment syndrome than in controls. During exercise, maximum relative oxygenation was significantly higher in patients with chronic compartment syndrome (−290 mV) than in patients with other pain (−190 mV) or in controls (−179 mV). Recovery of the baseline resting oxygenation level took significantly longer for patients with chronic compartment syndrome (184 seconds) than for patients with other pain (39 seconds) or for controls (33 seconds).

Conclusion.—Near-infrared spectroscopy is a useful tool for the noninvasive diagnosis of chronic compartment syndrome. Compared with normal individuals, patients with chronic compartment syndrome have significantly more deoxygenation during exercise and a significantly longer resting oxygenation recovery time, indicating an ischemic cause for the syndrome.

▶ The observation that near-infrared spectroscopy can detect the oxygenation of skeletal muscle presumably caused by elevated innermuscular pressure during exercise appears to have great potential for clinical application. That is, there certainly is a place for its use as a diagnostic tool for noninvasive detection of both acute and compartment syndrome. However, it appears that these observations should be correlated with determinations of intracompartmental pressures. For reasons unknown, this was not done in either study.

J.S. Torg, M.D.

Magnetic Resonance Imaging Assessment of the Rotator Cuff: Is It Really Accurate?
Wnorowski DC, Levinsohn EM, Chamberlain BC, et al (CNY Orthopedic Ctr, Syracuse, NY; Crouse Irving Mem Hosp, Syracuse, NY; Folsom, Calif; et al)
Arthroscopy 13:710–719, 1997
1–31

Background.—Magnetic resonance imaging is an accurate and increasingly popular technique for diagnostic assessment of the rotator cuff. However, the MRI findings of supraspinatus tendinopathy and rotator cuff tear remain unclear, as does the "normal" appearance of the rotator cuff. The diagnostic performance of rotator cuff MRI, compared with arthroscopy, was retrospectively assessed.

Methods.—Thirty-nine shoulders of 38 patients whose diagnostic work-up and treatment included MRI, as well as arthroscopy and subacromial bursal evaluation of the cuff, were studied. The sensitivity (SE), specificity (SP), positive predictive value (PPV), negative predictive value (NPV), and accuracy of MRI, compared with arthroscopy, were evaluated. The effects of MRI interpretation by community hospital radiologists vs. musculoskeletal radiologists were assessed as well.

Results.—When MRI scans were read by community hospital radiologists, diagnostic performance for all tears was: SE, 85%; SP, 52%; PPV, 50%; NPV, 87%; and accuracy, 64%. Corresponding values for partial tears were 0%, 68%, 0%, 82%, and 59%, respectively; values for complete tears were 56%, 73%, 36%, 86%, and 69%, respectively. When the scans were read by musculoskeletal radiologists, diagnostic performance for all tears was: SE, 71%; SP, 71%; PPV, 59%; NPV, 81%; and accuracy, 71%. Values for partial tears were 20%, 88%, 20%, 88%, and 79%, respectively; values for complete tears were 78%, 83%, 58%, 92%, and 82%, respectively.

Conclusions.—Compared with arthroscopy, MRI is not an accurate technique for diagnostic assessment of the rotator cuff. Rotator cuff MRI is most useful for its negative predictive value. It is of little help in the assessment of partial rotator cuff tears. For complete tears, accuracy is higher when the interpretation is made by an experienced orthopedic radiologist.

▶ With regard to MRI assessment of rotator cuff pathology, it is my view that the authors have somewhat overstated their case. It should be noted that the MRI studies reported were performed 4–8 years ago and primarily interpreted by a group of community hospital radiologists. Also, according to the authors, the majority of these cases were relatively difficult to diagnose and represented fewer than 20% of all patients seen by the authors who underwent arthroscopic shoulder surgery during this period. As they admit, "it is likely that we are still on the steep slope of the learning curve." Also, they recognize that "it may be argued that the interpretation by a single experienced radiologist with a specific set of criteria to evaluate rotator cuff signals would improve MRI accuracy." It has been my own experience that a technically satisfactory study interpreted by an experienced bone radiologist is highly accurate.

J.S. Torg, M.D.

Magnetic Resonance Imaging of the Shoulder

Herzog RJ (Philadelphia)
J Bone Joint Surg Am 79-A:934–953, 1997

1–32

Introduction.—An accurate clinical diagnosis is the foundation of successful patient care. In the diagnostic evaluation of patients who have a musculoskeletal disorder, radiographic imaging studies, such as plain radiography and CT, and radionuclide studies have played an important role. It is now possible to evaluate the soft-tissue structures of the body noninvasively with the advent of MRI. Defining the pathomorphological changes in a specific tissue, organ, or part of the body is the goal of any imaging study.

Magnetic Resonance Imaging.—To achieve a comprehensive evaluation of dysfunction of the shoulder, complete assessment of all the soft tissues and osseous structures of the shoulder girdle is mandatory. The spin-echo, gradient-echo, and short tau inversion recovery sequences are the MRI sequences typically used to evaluate the musculoskeletal system. The amount of information provided by these images has markedly increased. For each plane, the routine imaging examination of the shoulder, performed with a 1.5 tesla MRI system, is different (Table 1).

Considerations.—One of the largest tendinous structures in the body is the rotator cuff, which is prone to overload and failure. A spectrum of pathologic changes are represented in rotator cuff disease, including microscopic or macroscopic failure of fibers, tissue edema, hemorrhage, and fibrosis It is possible to depict all the osseous and soft-tissue structures that make up the coracoacromial arch with the direct multiplanar capabilities of MRI. One of the most frequent causes of musculoskeletal dysfunction related to sports activities is muscle injury. Muscle contusions may occur in the shoulder girdle, which is indicated by abnormal signal intensity and morphology of a muscle on MR images. To diagnose acute dislocation, imaging can confirm the presence of the dislocation, identify fractures and injuries, and evaluate the adequacy of reduction. The etiology of an irreducible dislocation may be evaluated with MRI. Patients who have symptoms or signs suggestive of recurrent subluxation or dislocation of the shoulder and who have inconclusive histories and physical examinations may benefit from MRI in the evaluation of instability. Additional applications are trauma, osteonecrosis, tumor, arthritis, and osteoarthrosis.

Conclusions.—The detection of isolated structural abnormalities is the focus of most imaging studies. The understanding of the dysfunction of the shoulder has been greatly increased with MRI because it can detect not only pathologic conditions that are precipitating symptoms, but also alterations in tissue resulting from chronic microtrauma or aging that do not precipitate symptoms. A closer working relationship among physicians who care for patients who have musculoskeletal disorders can enhance the efficacy of MRI. To compare the cost-effectiveness of the various imaging

TABLE 1.—Routine Protocol for Magnetic Resonance Imaging of the Shoulder

Plane*	Relaxation Time (msec)	Echo Time (msec)	No. of Excitations	Image Matrix	Thickness (mm)	Skip (mm)	Comments
Oblique coronal							Parallel to long axis of body of scapula, including soft tissues anterior and posterior to humeral head
1	2500	Dual-echo minimum/70	1	256 by 192	4	0.5	Classic multi-echo
Oblique sagittal							Perpendicular to long axis of scapula from base of coracoid through humeral head
1	1500	Minimum	1	256 by 192	4	0.5	
2	4000	Approximately 90	2	256 by 192	4, same location as 1	0.5	Fast spin echo-echo train length-8; fat-saturated band width, 32 kHz
Axial							From superior to acromioclavicular joint through glenoid and humeral neck
1	1500	Minimum	1	256 by 192	3	0.5	
2	4000	Approximately 90	2	256 by 192	3, same location as 1	0.5	Fast spin echo-echo train length-8; fat-saturated band width, 32 kHz

*1, made with the upper extremity in neutral or slight external rotation; 2, a field of view of 16 cm for all sequences. (Courtesy of Herzog RJ: Magnetic resonance imaging of the shoulder. *J Bone Joint Surg Am* 79-A:934–953, 1997.)

and diagnostic modalities used to evaluate the shoulder, prospective, controlled studies are still needed.

▶ This is an extremely comprehensive and well-written article authored by the recognized MRI maven. The interpretive value of shoulder MRI is explained on a pathophysiologic basis, and specific indications for use are well delineated. Importantly, the author makes the point that "an imaging study should be ordered only when its results will directly affect the management of a patient," and correct interpretation is dependent on both the quality of the study and experience of the musculoskeletal radiologist.

J.S. Torg, M.D.

Magnetic Resonance Imaging for the Evaluation of Acute Posterolateral Complex Injuries of the Knee
Ross G, Chapman AW, Newberg AR, et al (The New England Bone and Joint Inst; New England Baptist Hosp, Boston; United States Naval Academy, Annapolis, Md)
Am J Sports Med 25:444–448, 1997   1–33

Objective.—Posterolateral complex injuries of the knee are uncommon, usually occurring along with cruciate ligament injuries. Failure to recognize these injuries in the acute stage can lead to failed anterior eruciate ligament reconstruction. The clinical tests for posterolateral corner injury are poorly understood and sometimes difficult to perform. The acutely injured patient may be unable to perform such tests as the posterolateral drawer, passive external rotational, varus instability, posterior instability, Lachman, pivot, and reverse pivot shift tests. The value of MRI in assessing posterolateral complex injury was studied.

Methods.—The prospective study included 6 patients with clinical findings suggestive of posterolateral complex injury. All underwent preoperative imaging with standard MRI sequences, the results of which were correlated with the findings of examination under anesthesia or open lateral reconstruction.

Results.—The preoperative diagnosis—complete posterolateral complex injury in 5 patients and partial injury in 1—was confirmed in all cases. All patients had anterior cruciate ligament tears in addition, and 1 had a partial posterior cruciate ligament injury. The MRI scans accurately depicted the iliotibial band, which was seen to be avulsed from Gerdy's tubercle in 3 patients. The lack of joint effusion in knees with acute, complete tears was attributed to capsular tears, which were present at surgery in 4 patients. The MRI scans also permitted visualization of the arcuate complex, biceps femoris tendon, lateral capsule, iliotibial band, popliteal tendon, and lateral collateral ligament. All patients with complete posterolateral disruptions had a characteristic bone contusion of the anteromedial femoral condyle. This finding was absent in the patient with a partial posterolateral corner injury, who also showed no subluxation and a contained effusion.

Conclusions.—MRI can accurately depict lateral complex injuries of the knee. Certain features are characteristic of posterolateral complex injuries, particularly bone contusion involving the anterior aspect of the medial femoral condyle. Preoperative MRI scanning will help in early identification of posterolateral complex injuries, thus permitting timely surgical treatment.

▶ As pointed out in this article, chronic posterolateral complex injuries of the knee do not yield consistently good results with current reconstructive techniques. Therefore, it is imperative to identify the injury as early as possible. This, coupled with a variety of poorly understood and difficult clinical tests, emphasizes the value of using MRI to identify injuries to the posterolateral capsule, arcuate complex, biceps and popliteal tendons, and lateral collateral ligament. Also, as pointed out by the article, concomitant anterior cruciate ligament injuries are common, and failure to achieve successful reconstruction can result if the posterolateral component is not recognized and dealt with.

J.S. Torg, M.D.

The Natural History of Bone Bruises: A Prospective Study of Magnetic Resonance Imaging–detected Trabecular Microfractures in Patients With Isolated Medial Collateral Ligament Injuries
Miller MD, Osborne JR, Gordon WT, et al (United States Air Force Academy Hosp, Colo; Texas Orthopedic Hosp, Houston)
Am J Sports Med 26:15–19, 1998   1–34

Purpose.—Bone bruises—trabecular microfractures caused by trauma—are most commonly noted in the knee, often in association with anterior cruciate ligament injuries. However, little is known about the final outcome of these injuries. The authors have also observed bone bruises in association with isolated medial collateral ligament (MCL) injuries. The prevalence, natural history, and classification of bone bruises associated with MCL injuries were described.

Methods.—A total of 65 patients with isolated MCL injuries, identified by physical examination and imaging studies, were prospectively studied. On MRI, associated trabecular microfractures were present in 29 patients (45%). Follow-up MRI scans, available in 24 patients, were used to determine the ultimate fate of the bone bruises.

Findings.—From the MRI findings, the bone bruises were classified into 5 types based on their location and extent of injury, as illustrated in Figure 1. All bone bruises resolved completely with time. The healing process appeared to involve gradual diffusion of the bruise over a period of 2–4 months.

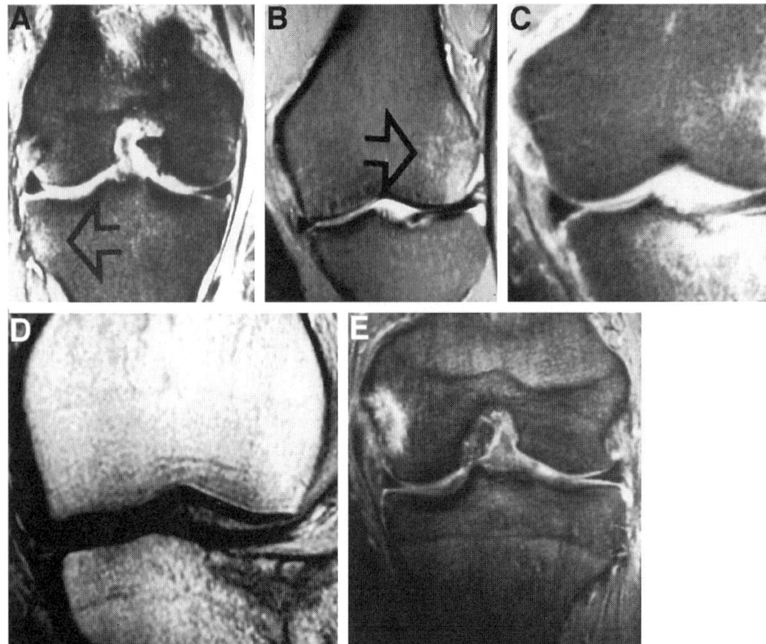

FIGURE 1.—Types of bone bruises. **A,** type I, lateral tibial plateau only. **B,** type II, lateral femoral condyle only. **C,** type III, lateral tibial plateau and lateral femoral condyle. **D,** type IV, lateral tibial plateau fracture. **E,** type V, other. (Courtesy of Miller MD, Osborne JR, Gordon WT, et al: The natural history of bone bruises: A prospective study of magnetic resonance imaging–detected trabecular microfractures in patients with isolated medial collateral ligament injuries. *Am J Sports Med* 26:15–19, 1998.)

Conclusions.—Patients with MCL injuries are less likely to have associated bone bruises than those with anterior cruciate ligament injuries. The MCL-associated injuries may have a better natural history because they are managed without surgery. Although not routinely indicated in MCL injuries, MRI may be useful in ensuring that these injuries are truly isolated before nonoperative treatment is started.

▶ This is a good article which demonstrates that increased signal observed on MR images in those patients with concomitant MCL injuries resolve. However, whether there are long-term sequelae involving the articular cartilage is the important question yet to be answered.

J.S. Torg, M.D.

Magnetic Resonance Imaging, Scintigraphy, and Arthroscopic Evaluation of Traumatic Hemarthrosis of the Knee
Adalberth T, Roos H, Laurén M, et al (Lund Univ, Sweden)
Am J Sports Med 25:231–237, 1997   1–35

Background.—Anterior cruciate ligament (ACL) injuries rarely occur as isolated entities. They are more commonly associated with injury to the lateral compartment than to the medial compartment. Also, tears of the lateral meniscus are more common than those of the medial meniscus. The current study was done to correlate MRI with arthroscopic findings for meniscal and ligament tears, the appearance of subchondral damage on MRI with scintigraphic uptake, and MRI with arthroscopic findings in the diagnosis of chondral injuries.

Methods and Findings.—Forty patients with traumatic knee hemarthrosis were assessed within 1 week after injury. Findings on MRI, scintigraphy, arthroscopic evaluation, radiography, and physical examination were noted. Eighty-five percent of the patients had anterior cruciate ligament injuries on arthroscopy. Eighty-three percent had associated meniscal tears. These findings were confirmed by MRI, especially when only meniscal tears requiring surgery were considered, with sensitivities of 94% and 83% for the lateral and medial meniscus, respectively. However, MRI had a specificity of only 29% and 27% for the lateral and medial menisci, respectively, with accuracies of 28% and 50%. Marrow edemas were noted in 80% of the patients on MRI, occurring mainly in the lateral compartment. Bone scan findings correlated well with MR findings of marrow edemas. Plain radiographs yielded normal findings in all but 1 patient.

Conclusions.—Magnetic resonance imaging adds no new information regarding the status of the anterior cruciate ligament compared with that gained by clinical examination. This imaging modality may be as good as arthroscopic assessment for diagnosing meniscal tears that require surgery.

Acutely Injured Knee: Effect of MR Imaging on Diagnostic and Therapeutic Decisions
Maurer EJ, Kaplan PA, Dussault RG, et al (Univ of Virginia, Charlottesville)
Radiology 204:799–805, 1997   1–36

Background.—The number of arthroscopic procedures performed in the United States increased by 145% in 1990. Several authorities feel there is a possible excess of such procedures. The current study determined the efficacy of knee MR imaging and its effects on the diagnosis and patient care.

Methods.—Eighty-four of 91 consecutive patients with acute knee injuries were included in the study. Two orthopedic knee surgeons prospectively completed imaging questionnaires for each patient before and after MR scans were obtained. Clinical diagnoses before and after MR imaging,

certainty about these diagnoses, other diagnostic testing, and subjective impressions of the value of MR imaging were documented.

Findings.—Pre- and post-MR imaging diagnoses were in agreement in 731 of 840 cases. Agreement was lowest for medial meniscal injuries, with significantly fewer such injuries suspected after MR imaging. For all diagnoses, clinical diagnostic certainty increased by a mean 14%. The increase in diagnostic certainty was highest for medial meniscal injuries, at 30%, followed by lateral meniscal injuries, at 21%. Treatment plans were changed for 41 patients, resulting in 37% fewer arthroscopic procedures.

Conclusions.—MR imaging affects the diagnosis and management of acute knee injury. With MR imaging, the number of arthroscopic procedures is reduced and diagnostic certainty is improved, aiding in management decisions.

Correlation of Arthroscopic and Clinical Examinations With Magnetic Resonance Imaging Findings of Injured Knees in Children and Adolescents

Stanitski CL (Children's Hosp of Michigan, Detroit)
Am J Sports Med 26:2–6, 1998
1–37

Background.—Magnetic resonance imaging has become a widely used technique for diagnosis of knee disorders. However, few studies have correlated the results of MRI with the clinical and arthroscopic findings, and there is very little information on these relationships in children. The clinical, MRI, and arthroscopic findings were correlated in a series of children and adolescents with knee injuries.

Methods.—Twenty-eight patients who underwent MRI followed by arthroscopic surgery of the knee were studied. Their average age was 14 years. The clinical and MRI diagnoses were compared with the arthroscopic findings, which were considered the standard for comparison. The analysis included meniscal, anterior cruciate ligament, and articular surface injuries.

Results.—There was total disagreement between the clinical and MRI findings in 75% of patients. In contrast, 78.5% of patients showed complete agreement between the clinical and arthroscopic findings. The accuracy of clinical evaluation was 96% for anterior cruciate ligament (ACL) injuries, 93% for meniscal injuries, and 89% for articular surface injuries. In contrast, there was total disagreement between the MRI and arthroscopic findings in 78.5% of patients. The accuracy of MRI was 89% for ACL injuries, 37.5% for meniscal injuries, and 79% for articular surface injuries. In addition to accuracy, positive and negative predictive values, sensitivity, and specificity were all greater with clinical examination than MRI.

Conclusions.—In the evaluation of injured knees in children and adolescents, clinical examination provides much better diagnostic information than MRI scanning. Little information useful for patient management is

provided by MRI, which has a high false-negative rate. In pediatric knee injuries, MRI should be used as an adjunct when the diagnosis is in question after clinical and radiographic assessment. The radiologist performing MRI should always be made aware of the clinical findings.

► These 3 articles are representative of conflicting viewpoints regarding the efficacy of magnetic resonance imaging in contributing to management decisions in those patients with acute injuries to the knee. It appears, however, that several basic observations can be culled from these reports. First, the routine use of magnetic resonance imaging in evaluating the acutely injured knee is not warranted. Second, in most instances, the history and physical examination performed by an experienced orthopedist should provide an accurate diagnosis. Third, in those instances where the diagnosis remains in question following a competent history and physical examination, MRI is indicated. Lastly, and, perhaps, most importantly, the study must be of acceptable technical quality and read by an experienced radiologist.

J.S. Torg, M.D.

Shin Splints: MR Appearance in a Preliminary Study

Anderson MW, Ugalde V, Batt M, et al (Univ of California, Sacramento; Queens Med Ctr, Nottingham, England)
Radiology 204:177–180, 1997   1–38

Background.—Shin splint syndrome is a term used to describe stress injuries involving the tibia. This activity-related pain typically involves diffuse tenderness along the posteromedial tibia in the middle to distal aspect. Plain radiographs often appear normal, but they may show longitudinal periosteal new bone formation along the distal tibia during later phases. Magnetic resonance imaging is a very sensitive method of detecting periosteal fluid and marrow edema or hemorrhage associated with fatigue damage in bone. Magnetic resonance imaging can show details of any soft-tissue involvement. The MRI appearance of activity-related lower leg pain and the relative involvement of bone and soft tissues were investigated.

Methods.—Clinical examination and MRI were performed in 19 patients with activity-related lower leg pain and tenderness along the posteromedial tibia. Plain radiographs were also obtained in 5 patients. Findings from MRI were compared to patient demographics, clinical findings, and plain radiographs.

Results.—Four patterns on MRI studies were identified: normal appearance in 7 patients, periosteal fluid only in 5 patients (Fig 1), abnormal marrow signal intensity in 5 patients (Fig 2), and stress fracture in 2 patients. There was a strong correlation between increased length of symptoms and a normal MRI image. Findings on plain radiographs were normal.

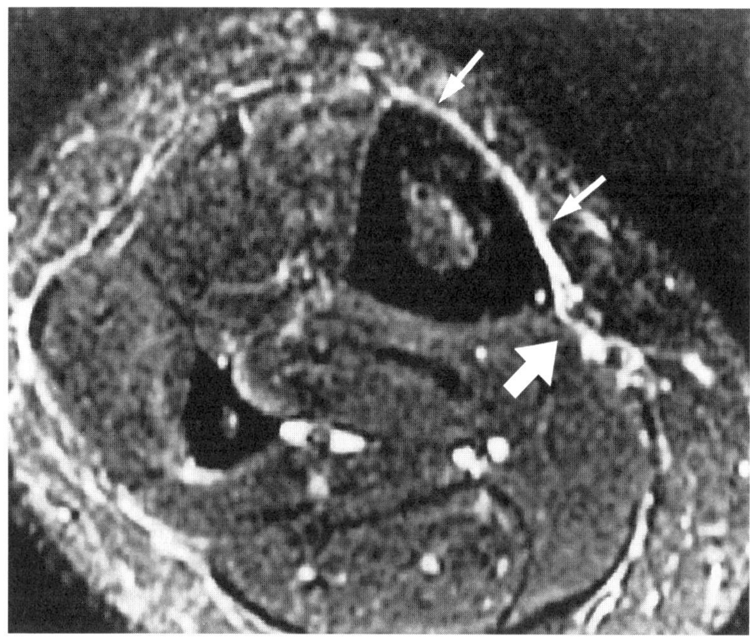

FIGURE 1.—Axial fast spin-echo, inversion-recovery image (3,200/57/140) in a 17-year-old female volleyball player with a 12-month history of shin splints. Note the thin rim of high signal intensity periosteal fluid tracking along the anterior margin of the tibia (*small arrows*) with extension along its posteromedial margin near the attachment of the soleus fascia (*large arrow*). (Courtesy of Anderson MW, Ugalde V, Batt M, et al: Shin splints: MR appearance in a preliminary study. *Radiology* 204:177–180, 1997. The Radiological Society of North America.)

Discussion.—A range of findings on MRI studies will be seen in patients with acute shin splints. This indicates that shin splints are part of a continuum of stress response in bone, although the distribution of periosteal fluid in some patients suggests that a traction periostitis along the insertion of the soleus fascia may also be involved. The strong association between chronic symptoms and a normal image indicates that MRI has little diagnostic value in individuals with this injury.

▶ The observations in this study help us understand more clearly the underlying pathology affecting those with pretibial pain euphemistically diagnosed as shin splints. The finding of normal appearing MRIs in those individuals with chronic symptoms is noteworthy. I'm not sure that I agree, however, that on the basis of the imaging findings, one can assume that stress fractures are necessarily the end point of the shin splint continuum. That is, "shin splints are part of the continuum of fatigue damage in bone." If this were so, why do those with chronic shin splints have normal MRI findings?

J.S. Torg, M.D.

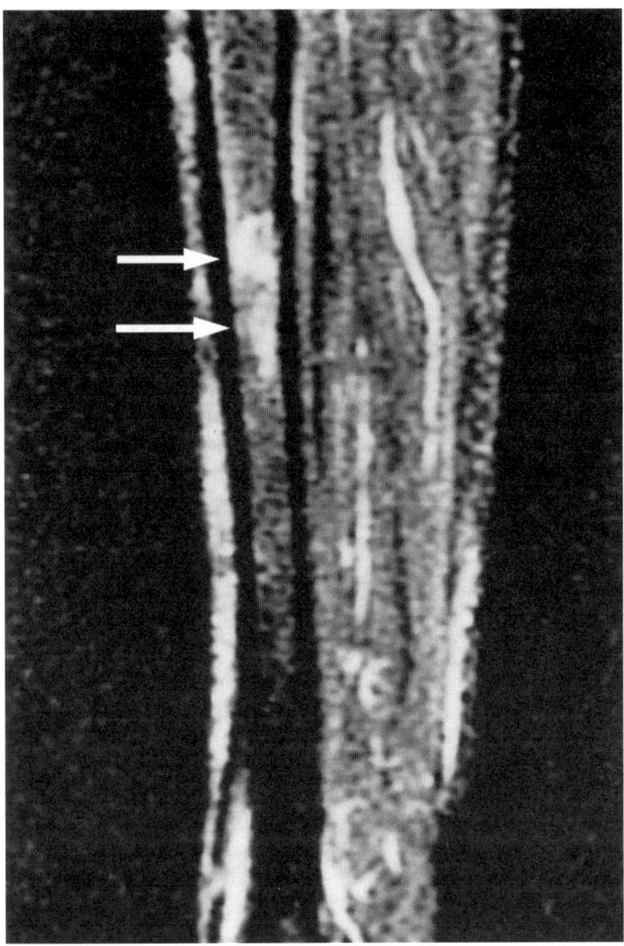

FIGURE 2.—Sagittal fast spin-echo, inversion-recovery image (3,000/54/140) in a 29-year-old female soccer player with a 2-month history of shin splints. Note the abnormal signal intensity within the marrow of the middle of the right tibia (*arrows*), which is compatible with edema or hemorrhage. (Courtesy of Anderson MW, Ugalde V, Batt M, et al: Shin splints: MR appearance in a preliminary study. *Radiology* 204:177–180, 1997. The Radiological Society of North America.)

Matrix Assessment of the Articular Cartilage Surface After Chondroplasty With the Holmium:YAG Laser

Lane JG, Amiel ME, Monosov AZ, et al (Univ of California San Diego, La Jolla)
Am J Sports Med 25:560–569, 1997   1–39

Background.—Articular defects in the joint surface can cause pain, clicking, restricted activity, and effusion. Currently, there is no acceptable method of smoothing the articular surface and stabilizing the edges of

chondral fissures to prevent further spreading of the fissures. It is difficult to débride articular cartilage back to a stable fragment because of the potential for removing excessive cartilage and denuding underlying bone. Blistering articular cartilage can only be treated by removing the full thickness of articular cartilage. The holmium:yttrium-aluminum-garnet (Ho:YAG) laser has been proposed as a means of creating a very smooth articular surface for chondroplasty on an area with a chondral fracture or chondromalacia, but there is concern about potential injury from the laser energy. It is unknown if long-term changes in articular cartilage and underlying subchondral bone occurs.

Methods.—Chondroplasty was performed in 30 rabbits using the Ho:YAG laser at an intensity of 0.8 J at a rate of 10 Hz. A sham procedure was also performed. The animals were sacrificed at 12 weeks, and repair of the articular cartilage was evaluated histologically and biochemically.

Results.—Histologic examination showed good correlation between the safranin O staining index of proteoglycan and biochemical results, indicating a decrease of proteoglycan in the repaired tissue after laser chondroplasty. There was extensive damage to the articular cartilage surface after laser application. The damage was gradually distributed along the radius from the central point of the laser beam application. Biochemical examination showed there was statistically less glycosaminoglycan in the repaired tissue than in sham-treated tissue. There was 8 to 10 times less sulfate incorporated into proteoglycans in laser-treated tissue than in sham-treated tissue. This indicated that cell viability was significantly less in treated tissue or that expression of proteoglycans was significantly reduced. In the subchondral area, there was a lack of osteocytes in lacunae of the bone tissue after laser application. Damage was seen in the architecture of the subchondral bone in the chondroplasty area and in the membranes of the blood vessels.

Discussion.—In this rabbit model, significant damage to articular cartilage occurred 12 weeks after chondroplasty with a Ho:YAG laser. The zone of thermal energy was large, with damage from the laser occurring to a depth of 1.6 mm, which is nearly 3 times the thickness of articular cartilage in a rabbit joint. After using the minimum amount of energy needed to create a chondroplasty in this rabbit model, significant damage was seen in the matrix and its cellular components. Long-term analysis of possible regeneration of the newly formed articular cartilage matrix repair and the vascularity of the subchondral area is needed.

▶ On the basis of several anecdotal reports, there is concern regarding the potential destructive collateral effects of arthroscopic laser procedures. Clearly, there are many factors involved that include type of laser, energy intensity, wavelength, and distance from source. It is generally recognized that the Ho:YAG laser admits energies at a wavelength that is highly absorbed by meniscal tissue and cartilage, thus delivering less energy to underlying bone. However, the neodymium:YAG laser admits light energy at a wave-length that is poorly absorbed by nonpigmented tissues such as meniscus and hyaline cartilage and presumably would have a more delete-

rious effect on underlying bone. This article seems to question this concept with regard to the relative safety of the Ho:YAG laser in arthroscopic procedures. The authors, however, do point out with regard to animal model and human conditions that "one should be cautious when comparing these 2 models."

J.S. Torg, M.D.

A New Biological Glue for the Cartilage-Cartilage Interfaces: Tissue Transglutaminase
Jürgensen K, Aeschlimann D, Cavin V, et al (Univ of Bern, Switzerland)
J Bone Joint Surg Am 79-A:185–193, 1997   1–40

Introduction.—Fixation of lesions involving articular cartilage is very difficult. The cartilage matrix has an anti-adhesiveness quality that is attributed to its high proteoglycan content. A large family of enzymes that catalyze the calcium-dependent formation of bonds between proteins are the transglutaminases. Various differentiated cartilages express tissue transglutaminase, a monomeric globular protein with a molecular mass of about 77 kd. In the treatment of cartilaginous lesions, the effectiveness of tissue transglutaminase as a biological glue was examined. The capacity of tissue transglutaminase to increase the adhesive strength at a cartilage-cartilage interface was tested using in vitro model.

Methods.—Fresh adult bovine shoulder joints were used to prepare full-thickness cartilage-bone cylinders. To provide a plane surface, the superficial half of the hyaline cartilage was removed. On the freshly cut surface of one cylinder, tissue transglutaminase was applied. A calcium-chloride solution was applied to the other surface to act as an activating agent. Under defined humidity conditions, the apposed cartilage surfaces were placed one on top of the other for 10 minutes with an 88–g weight applied to the upper cylinder. A measured force was applied on the upper cylinder until that cylinder was displaced from the lower one. The force recorded here was used as a measure of the adhesive strength found at the cartilage-cartilage interface.

Results.—With an increasing concentration of tissue transglutamines (0.25–2.75 mg/mL), the adhesive strength increased linearly. By increasing the duration of incubation, the adhesive strength was enhanced, but the level of humidity did not influence adhesive strength. When the cartilage surfaces had been pretreated with condroitinase AC or hyaluronidase to remove glycosaminoglycan chains of proteoglycans, which are largely responsible for the intrinsic anti-adhesive properties of cartilage, the adhesive strength was improved by as much as 40%.

Conclusion.—Serious problems are posed for the orthopedic surgon with the mechanical fixation of cartilage fragments in diarthrodial joints and the fixation and immobilization of cartilage transplant materials or biodegradable matrices containing chondrogenic cells. The adhesive strength achieved with the use of Tissucol, a commercially available fibrin

sealant, was less than that achieved with use of tissue transglutaminase at the cartilage-cartilage interface. For practical application in clinical orthopedics, transglutaminase has great promise. It is possible to produce this material in large quantities with the use of recombinant DNA technology because it has a relatively simple single-polypeptide-chain structure. To improve the repertoire for the treatment of chondral lesions, this material offers new possibilities as a biological adhesive.

▶ To be emphasized, as pointed out by the authors, is that "the data related to the adhesive strength achieved with the use of tissue transglutaminase are very encouraging, but long-term in vivo experiments are needed to establish whether it will be of real value as a biological glue in orthopedic procedures." It would appear, however, despite problems pertaining to the necessary adhesive strength and the question of the availability of the enzyme in large enough quantities at high enough concentrations, that "tissue transglutaminase holds great promise for future applications in the treatment of chondral lesions."

J.S. Torg, M.D.

Proprioceptive Neuromuscular Facilitation Techniques in Sports Medicine: A Reassessment

Surburg PR, Schrader JW (Indiana Univ, Bloomington)
J Athletic Train 32:34–39, 1997   1–41

Background.—Proprioceptive neuromuscular facilitation (PNF) techniques involve diagonal, spiral-patterned movements against resistance through a full range of motion. The pattern is chosen to enhance a targeted muscle group. The diagonal spiral pattern is key in PNF, serving as a basis for various techniques. There are 2 basic patterns, named by ending position, per direction.

Methods.—The subjects, 131 athletic trainers who used PNF, were surveyed at a 1993 conference to determine the techniques they found effective for specific body areas. The survey, congruent with a 1981 study, included questions about application of 9 PNF techniques and about the most successful treatments with PNF techniques.

Results.—The PNF techniques are most often used with the knee (31%), shoulder (30%), and hip (28%), much as in 1981, except for increased use in ankle rehabilitation (27%). Contract-relax and hold-relax remain the most frequently used techniques, but contract-relax-contract and hold-relax-contract, not studied in 1981, are now often used for elbow, wrist, hip, and knee. Trainers in 1981 did not report use of PNF in muscle reeducation, whereas they did in this survey.

Conclusions.—The PNF techniques feature movement in all 3 body planes, consistent with current emphasis on multiplanar exercises for athletic injuries. Although important, strength and range of motion are only part of rehabilitation; neurologic and neuromuscular enhancements

are also important, because proprioceptive and kinesthetic deficits are seen with many injury types. Athletic trainers now use PNF techniques in the reeducation phase of injury treatment.

▶ Proprioceptive neuromuscular facilitation techniques have been used to improve flexibility and in rehabilitation programs for injured athletes. With proper instruction and supervision, athletes can use these techniques with a partner, in both their warm-up and cool-down regimens. As the authors state, these techniques can easily be incorporated into functional rehabilitation and conditioning programs.

F.J. George, A.T.C., P.T.

A Model Lightning Safety Policy for Athletics
Bennett BL (College of William and Mary, Williamsburg, Va)
J Athletic Train 32:251–253, 1997   1–42

Introduction.—In the development of an athletic training policy manual, a policy on lightning safety is often overlooked. Each year, lightning kills more people than any other weather phenomenon—up to 600 people in the United States—and leaving many hundreds injured. At The College of William and Mary where more than half of sports are practiced outdoors, a model policy on lightning safety for athletic trainers was presented.

Policy.—Education and prevention are the keys to lightning safety. The weather report should be checked each day before a practice or event. Signs of nearby thunderstorm development should be watched by the coaching/athletic training staff. To estimate how far away lightning activity is occurring, the "flash-to-bang" method is the most convenient; it involves counting the seconds between seeing the flash of lightning and hearing the bang of thunder. To determine how far away in miles lightning is occurring, divide this number by five. All outdoor and swimming pool athletic activities should stop if the "flash-to-bang" interval approaches 30 seconds.

More Policy.—One should not take shelter under tall trees, light or flag poles, metal fences, standing pools of water, or open fields. If, within a reasonable distance, there is no safe shelter, one should crouch with only the feet touching the ground and the arms wrapped around the knees to minimize the body's surface area. As quickly as possible, safe shelter should be located. After the last sound of thunder or flash of lightning, 30 minutes should pass before resumption of athletic activity. The telephone should not be used because people have been struck by lightning and killed while using a hand-line telephone. In reviving lightning strike victims, CPR is a safe method.

Conclusion.—Someone should be assigned responsibility for deciding to leave a field or event. Criteria should be established for leaving the field. A

safe shelter should be defined. Safety guidelines should be developed. To return to play, criteria should be developed.

▶ Establishing a lightning safety policy is important for all athletic departments. The author outlines the basics of this policy as being (1) establishing responsibility for making the call to leave the field; (2) explaining the "flash-to-bang" method; (3) selecting criteria that will be used; (4) defining and listing locations of safe shelters; (5) developing lightning safety guidelines; and (6) establishing criteria for return to play. A study by Walsh et al. "demonstrated the lack of lightning safety policy in the 48 surveyed universities and the need for a systematic plan of action to make fields safer for all who are involved in outdoor sport activities."[1]

F.J. George, A.T.C., P.T.

Reference

1. Walsh KM, Hanley MJ, Graner SJ, et al: A survey of lightning policy in selected Division 1 colleges: *J Athletic Train* 32:206–210, 1997.

The Efficiency of Tools Used to Retract a Football Helmet Face Mask
Knox KE, Kleiner DM (Decatur Mem Hosp, Ill; Univ of North Florida, Jacksonville)
J Athletic Train 32:211–215, 1997   1–43

Introduction.—In the management of an injured football player with a suspected spinal injury, the current practice is not to remove the football helmet, but only to remove or retract the face mask to gain access to the athlete's airway. Of primary importance is reducing movement of the athlete's head and neck to avoid further damage to the cervical spine. Little research has been conducted to determine the amount of movement generated using various tools to retract a football helmet face mask. Several popular tools for retracting a football helmet face mask were evaluated in terms of time that it takes to remove the loop straps, the resulting amount of head movement, and ratings of satisfaction.

Methods.—There were 5 certified athletic trainers, 5 emergency medical technicians, and 5 student athletic trainers who retracted a face mask using a Phillips screwdriver, a Trainer's Angel, and an anvil pruner. A force platform was used to measure movement, and a stopwatch was used to measure time. Total time and radial area were used to calculate efficiency. The participants rated their satisfaction.

Results.—The time to retract the face mask using the 3 tools did not differ. The Trainer's Angel caused significantly greater movement than the anvil pruner or screwdriver. There was higher satisfaction among the participants with the anvil pruner than with the Trainer's Angel or screwdriver. There was no difference in time or rating of satisfaction between the certified athletic trainers, emergency medical technicians, or student athletic trainers. In terms of movement, the certified athletic trainers produced

the most movement and student athletic trainers produced the least movement.

Conclusions.—It is important to learn and practice the skill of face mask retraction. It is still recommended to remove the face mask and not the entire helmet. More research should be conducted regarding how to remove a face mask.

▶ If removing a face mask from a football helmet can be difficult in a laboratory situation, imagine how difficult it will be in an emergency. Athletic trainers must have the proper equipment readily available for face mask removal, and they must practice this skill before every season. This study indicates that a modified, spring-loaded anvil pruner is the easiest tool to use and will cause the least amount of head movement.

F.J. George, A.T.C., P.T.

Playing With Metal: Fracture Impacts and Contact Sport
Evans NA, Evans RON (Morriston Hosp, Swansea, UK)
Br J Sports Med 31:319–321, 1997   1–44

Introduction.—Injured athletes with fractures are usually anxious to return to their contact sport, but there are no guidelines to help determine when, particularly if the fracture was fixed with a metal implant. It is not known whether the implant should be left in situ or removed before resuming sporting activities. Acting as a stress riser, the retained implant may place the adjacent bone at risk of a further fracture. Removal of the implant mandates a prolonged absence from contact sports while bone density is restored, which results in a long period of unemployment for the professional athlete. The outcome of athletes returning to contact sports with indwelling fracture implants was assessed.

Methods.—Fifteen athletes from 6 professional rugby union teams who returned to competitive rugby with retained fracture implants during a 7-year period were retrospectively studied. One player had a fracture alongside a radius plate after 2 years of playing and which healed 4 weeks after cast immobilization, resulting in 12 weeks of missed competitive action (Fig 1).

Results.—Within 1–12 months after fracture fixation, the players resumed their preinjury level of contact sport. The location of the fracture and the type of implant used in fixation, as well as the recommendation of the surgeon, were the factors involved in the amount of time until resumption of playing. There was range of 6 months to 6 years of playing time with asymptomatic fracture implants in situ. If implant removal was advised before participating in contact sports, the time delay was more. Elective implant removal can be planned for the off-season, which would allow 3–4 months for the residual screw holes to heal. Complications in relation to the retained implant were found in 2 athletes. The other 13 athletes played without symptoms for up to 6 years.

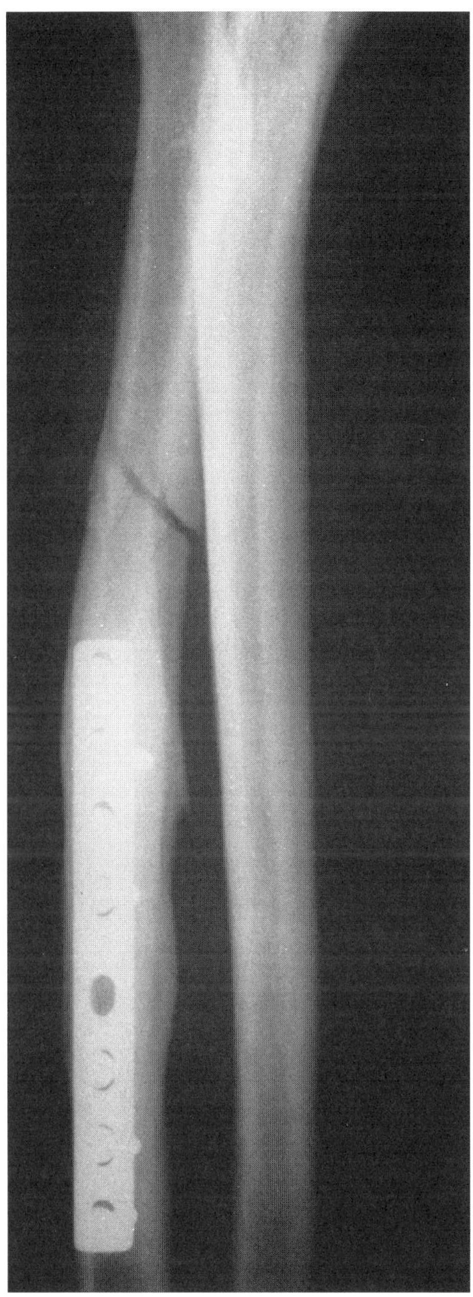

FIGURE 1.—Fracture of proximal radius adjacent to AO (3.5 mm) dynamic compression plate. (Courtesy of Evans NA, Evans RON: Playing with metal: Fracture implants and contact sport. *Br J Sports Med* 31:319–321, 1997.)

Conclusions.—In selected athletes, an early return to contact sports is possible. By avoiding the extended delay associated with implant removal, players disrupt their competitive participation only minimally and prevent prolonged financial losses.

▶ On the basis of experience with 15 individuals who returned to collision activities with fracture-fixating devices in situ, the authors conclude that "early return to contact sports is feasible in selected cases." However, they have failed to define what they mean by "selected cases." It would appear that decisions with regard to return must be individualized, with a variety of factors taken into consideration. Specifically, the nature of the fracture, presence of localized osteopenia, role of stress risers, activity level, and willingness on the part of the patient to assume risk must all be considered. Although this paper is the only one that I am familiar with dealing with the subject matter, it is certainly not definitive.

J.S. Torg, M.D.

Treatment of Acute Fractures With a Collagen-Calcium Phosphate Graft Material
Chapman MW, Bucholz R, Cornell C (Univ of California, Sacramento; Univ of Texas, Dallas; Hosp for Special Surgery, New York)
J Bone Joint Surg Am 79-A:495–502, 1997   1–45

Background.—Autogenous bone is recognized as a superior graft material for filling traumatic defects or repair of segmental bone losses, although it does have certain limitations. The autogenous bone may be of poor quality or there may not be enough available. Obtaining an autogenous graft may cause serious morbidity at the donor site and add 20 minutes or more to the operative time. Also, the patient may be draped and positioned in a manner that makes it difficult to obtain a graft if the need is determined during the operation. This study evaluates material shown to be effective in bridging segmental defects of long bones in rats and dogs.

Methods.—To compare the safety and efficacy of 2 graft materials for fractures of long bones, a prospective, randomized clinical trial of 213 patients at 18 medical centers was conducted. The 2 graft materials were autogenous bone graft from the iliac crest and a composite material of purified bovine collagen, a biphasic calcium-phosphate ceramic, and autogenous marrow. Healing and complications were monitored. There were 249 fractures in the 213 patients. Follow-up was at least 24 months.

Results.—There were no significant differences in rates of union or functional measures between the 2 groups. The rate of complications was similar in both groups, except that patients treated with autogenous graft had a higher rate of infection. Twelve patients who received the synthetic graft had a positive antibody titer to bovine collagen. Seven of these 12 patients had an intradermal challenge with bovine collagen; 1 patient had a positive skin response, but no complications with healing of the fracture.

Discussion.—These results indicate that this composite graft material is safe and effective for traumatic defects of long bones. Use of the composite graft material shortens operative time and lowers the risk associated with obtaining an autogenous graft from the iliac crest. Various types of injuries, operative techniques, and postoperative regimens were used to represent the range of bone grafting practices actually used for acute fractures.

▶ The authors point out that autogenous graft provides immediate structural support, osteoconductive scaffolding, and osteogenic stimulus. The synthetic graft material does not fulfill the first of these roles, that is, immediate structural support. However, it does appear that the material has a place in the management of selected fractures.

J.S. Torg, M.D.

Preventing Throwing Injuries to the Shoulder
Barker S, Barker A (California State Univ, Chico)
Athletic Ther Today 2:14–17, 1997   1–46

Objective.—Early-season throwing injuries are common in throwing athletes—especially, but not exclusively, pitchers. These injuries result mainly from the decreased intensity and frequency of throwing in the off-season; as such, they can be prevented by an off-season exercise program. The authors outlined an effective off-season exercise program to prevent early-season injuries in throwing athletes.

Off-Season Exercise Program.—Instead of "overuse" injuries, early-season throwing injuries might better be classified as "underprepared" injuries. They occur because the athlete's off-season workout is not skill specific or progressively demanding. The authors propose an off-season exercise program consisting of slide board use and progressive throwing to strengthen the muscles and stabilize the joints. Three basic slide board exercises are used to strengthen the shoulder girdle. The first is glenohumeral flexion/extension. While kneeling perpendicular to the slide board with pads on the hands and the arms fully extended, the athlete flexes the shoulder on 1 side while extending the other shoulder. Reciprocal motion is continued for 10-second sets. The second exercise, glenohumeral horizontal abduction/adduction, uses the same starting position. With the arms fully extended, the athlete performs simultaneous horizontal abduction and adduction. Again, the exercise continues for 10-second sets. For glenohumeral circumduction, the athlete performs simultaneous circular shoulder movements, both clockwise and counterclockwise, with the arms fully extended.

Progressive throwing exercise begins with a warm-up. The athlete should "warm up to throw," not "throw to warm up"; increased heart rate, body temperature, respiratory rate, and blood flow should be achieved before the athlete starts to throw. Throwing should start with easy catches at a distance of 60 to 90 ft, with the number of throws varying

as the arm warms up. After warming up, the athlete progressively increases the distance thrown by backing up a few steps after each throw. This continues until the athlete reaches maximum throwing distance, which is maintained for the rest of the workout. The ball is thrown from a fairly high release point with an arch trajectory. As a rule, 60% of throws should be made at the maximum distance. The result should be equally divided between the progressive and cool-down phases. After 3 to 4 weeks, as it becomes easier to throw at maximum distance, the athlete can begin making more intense, line-drive throws.

Discussion.—This off-season exercise program can help to prevent early-season injuries in throwing athletes. The combination of slide-board exercises and progressive throwing incorporates overall muscle strengthening and joint stability, permitting the athlete to start the season in good condition.

▶ The authors state that "Throwing injuries related to dramatic increases in intensity and frequency of throwing can be reduced with an adequate off-season program." They classify these injuries as being "underprepared" rather than "overuse" injuries. They have described good off-season and "long throwing" programs. They also stress the importance of general body warmup before throwing begins.

F.J. George, A.F.C., P.T.

Hazard of Deceptive Advertising of Athletic Footwear
Robbins S, Waked E (McGill Univ, Montreal)
Br J Sports Med 31:299–303, 1997   1–47

Introduction.—Although athletic footwear is extensively advertised, with many claims of its ability to cushion impact via sole materials, no type of athletic footwear has even been shown to protect well against injuries. Researchers tested the hypothesis that deceptive advertising creates a false sense of security among users of expensive athletic shoes.

Methods.—Study participants were 15 healthy young men with a mean age of 31 years, a mean body mass of 75 kg, and a mean height of 175 cm. All participated actively in sports and leisure activities and had no conditions that would affect walking, running, or balance. They were provided with identical sole interface materials, but fabric was used to encase the sole so that participants could not identify the material. Participants were told that 1 type of sole material was quite expensive and had superior impact absorption and protection (deceptive message), another was cheap and associated with frequent injuries (warning message), and a third was a new material that had not been tested for impact absorption (neutral message). An experimental setup was used to record ground reaction forces for 10 barefoot footfalls (Fig 1).

Results.—The advertising claims that study participants heard affected their footfall impact. Impact was greatest (121% body weight) when

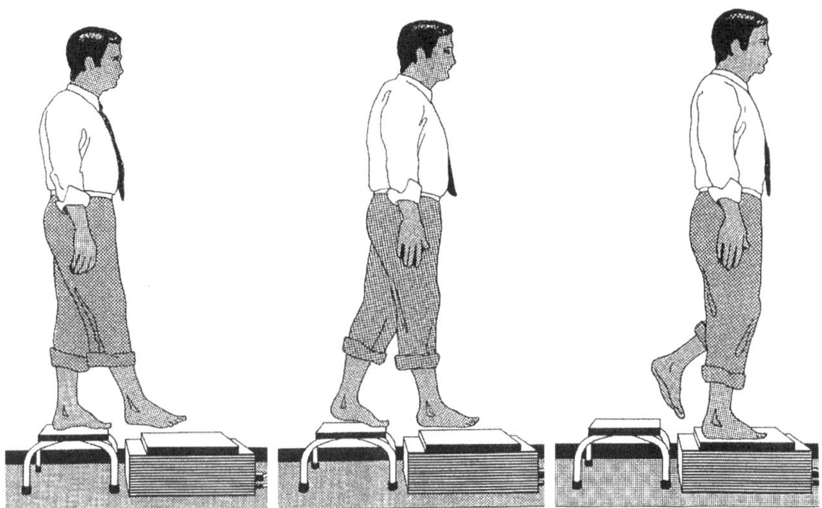

FIGURE 1.—Schematic representation of experimental setup for dynamic footfall testing. Subject stepped down onto force moment platform, which was either bare or covered by athletic shoe sole material. He balanced on 1 foot after foot contact with platform. Subjects were barefoot with gaze straight and arms to sides. (Courtesy of Robbins S, Waked E: Hazard of deceptive advertising of athletic footwear. *Br J Sports Med* 31:299–303, 1997.)

subjects believed they were stepping onto an expensive sole material that provided superior impact absorption and protection. The lowest impacts occurred when subjects stepped onto a bare platform (108% body weight) or onto the material described as cheap and having poor impact absorption (110% body weight). The impact when stepping onto a sole material described as new but untested was 117% body weight. Differences in footfall impact grew with repetition, increasing with the deceptive message and significantly decreasing with the warning message.

Conclusion.—Deceptive advertising that claims a protective benefit for expensive athletic shoes may lead to a higher frequency of injuries when such shoes are worn. Individuals wearing shoes with false claims may become less cautious, thereby increasing their footfall impact and chance of injury.

▶ This is an interesting, although quasiscientific, analysis of the effects of running shoes on injury. The 123% greater injury frequency quoted in the article for those wearing expensive athlete shoes is not substantiated by data. The statement that "There are no data supporting the notion that athletic footwear are capable of protecting against injury through cushioning of impact" is questioned. Not the least of the limitations of the study is what to this observer appears to be a dubious testing protocol. However, if nothing more, this study raises an interesting question regarding both advertising and athletic footwear.

J.S. Torg, M.D.

Prevention of Infectious Disease Transmission in Sports
Mast EE, Goodman RA (Centers for Disease Control and Prevention, Atlanta, Ga)
Sports Med 24:1–7, 1997   1–48

Introduction.—Because a variety of infectious diseases can be transmitted among athletes, it is important that coaches, team physicians, and trainers be aware of modes of transmission and preventive measures that can be taken. Subjects discussed in this article included hygiene and infection control practices; vaccination; and the education of officials, coaches, trainers, and athletes.

Modes of Transmission.—Infectious diseases can be transmitted by person-to-person contact, particularly in sports such as wrestling. Skin injuries—such as cuts, abrasions, and bruises—may facilitate transmission. Outbreaks of viral infections, including herpes simplex virus, have been reported among wrestlers and rugby players. Other skin and mucous membrane infections have resulted from person-to-person contact, including staphylococcal and streptococcal skin infections and fungal infections. Although the risk of HIV or hepatitis B virus transmission during sports is quite low, the prevention of blood contact is important. A gathering of large groups of athletes and spectators in a confined environment increases the potential for transmission of infectious diseases by airborne/droplet spread.

Prevention of Disease Transmission in Sports.—Measures for preventing infectious diseases include general hygiene practices, prompt treatment of athletes with infectious diseases, vaccination, and the prevention of exposure to blood. Athletes who engage in sports with extensive skin-to-skin contact should be examined for skin wounds and excluded from matches or practices when lesions cannot be securely covered. All athletes should be vaccinated against communicable diseases. Special precautions need to be taken to prevent exposure to blood during athletic competition, and athletic trainers should use disposable gloves when treating athletes who are bleeding profusely.

Conclusion.—Coaches, athletes, trainers, and officials should be aware of the potential for infectious diseases to be transmitted during sports activities. Information required includes the basic principles of hygiene and first aid infection control, approaches for the prevention of sexually transmitted diseases, and knowledge of the risks associated with nonmedical uses of injectable steroids and other drugs.

▶ This is a creditable report from the Centers for Disease Control and Prevention that deals with common infection problems. It includes a recommended vaccination schedule for adolescents and young adults and is based on a bibliography of 55 citations. It presents a minimum core of knowledge with which every team physician and athletic trainer should be familiar.

J.S. Torg, M.D.

2 Injuries to Head, Neck, Torso, and Arms

Neuropsychological Functioning and Recovery After Mild Head Injury in Collegiate Athletes
Macciocchi SN, Barth JT, Alves W, et al (Univ of Virginia, Charlottesville; Pew Found, Philadelphia)
Neurosurgery 39:510–514, 1996   2–1

Introduction.—Mild head injuries are usually associated with few symptoms and a quick recovery. However, some patients report multiple symptoms, which can continue for a long time. This variation has led to discussion of the causes of neuropsychologic symptoms after mild cerebral trauma. Contributing to the difficulty of this debate has been the methodologic differences between studies. Using National Collegiate Athletic Association injury data, this study prospectively assessed neuropsychologic symptoms occurring after mild head injury in football players.

Methods.—The analysis included 183 Division A collegiate football players with single, mild head injuries, identified from a group of 2,300 players from 10 universities. The patients underwent a battery of neuropsychologic assessments, including the Paced Auditory Serial Addition Test, the Digit Symbol Test, and the Trail Making Test, as well as a symptom checklist. These tests were administered at 24 hr, 5 days, 10 days, and 12 wks after the injury. The same assessments were performed in a group of 48 student controls matched for sex, age, and education. The presence and duration of postconcussive symptoms and neurocognitive impairment were analyzed.

Results.—The injured athletes had lower test scores and more symptoms than did controls when assessed at the time of injury. By 5 days the impairment had resolved for most injured athletes. By 10 days the patients and controls were equivalent on all test measures. In the injured players, significant improvement occurred between 24 hr and 5 days and between 5 and 10 days.

Conclusions.—Football players sustaining single, uncomplicated, mild head injuries have limited neuropsychologic impairment. However, the symptoms are usually quick to resolve, with few prolonged sequelae. It is unknown whether football injuries are truly analogous to vehicular accidents or other causes of mild head injury. However, the neurocognitive impairment, headaches, and dizziness encountered in this group of patients is similar to that reported in other populations.

▶ To my knowledge, this study represents the only comprehensive prospective study of cerebral concussions occurring in the athlete. The definition of mild traumatic brain injury is "physiologic disruption of brain function with <30 min of unconsciousness, memory impairment, and/or alteration in consciousness." Also, the study included only those individuals experiencing their first concussive episode and not those with recurrent episodes. The conclusion of the authors that "we can be reasonably certain that most football players sustaining a mild head injury recover quickly without apparent residual neurocognitive impairment or symptoms" is reassuring. However, this study does not answer the question with regard to the individual with recurrent concussive episodes, and, to my knowledge, there is no creditable data dealing with this problem.

J.S. Torg, M.D.

Concussive Convulsions: Incidence in Sport and Treatment Recommendations
McCrory PR, Berkovic SF (Univ of Melbourne, Heidelberg, Australia)
Sports Med 25:131–136, 1998   2–2

Introduction.—Concussive convulsions (CCs) occur immediately after a concussive brain injury. The convulsive movements, which may be transient or can last up to 3 minutes, follow a brief tonic stiffening. Although widely assumed to be a form of posttraumatic epileptic seizure, CCs are nonepileptic and have a universally good outcome. The etiology, incidence, diagnosis, management, and outcome of CCs was discussed.

Incidence and Etiology.—In Australian Rules football, the rate of CC is estimated to be 1 convulsive episode for every 70 cases of concussion. The overall incidence rate is unknown for other sports. No association has been found between CC in collision sport and structural brain injury, ongoing epilepsy, or epileptiform electroencephalographic abnormalities. Concussive convulsions are considered a distinct entity somewhat akin to a convulsive syncope. The concussion may initiate a transient decerebration, resulting in convulsive movements.

Diagnosis.—Episodes of CC follow a typical pattern, and after the collision the player recovers with behavioral and neuropsychological features indistinguishable from those of mild concussion. Differential diagnoses include convulsive syncope and idiopathic generalized epilepsy. Medical assessment is essential in all cases because of the possibility that the convulsive episode represents true postraumatic epilepsy. Individuals with CC have normal electroencephalographic, CT, and MRI findings.

Treatment and Outcome.—The convulsive episode should be managed expectantly with appropriate first aid measures, including airway management. When the convulsion subsides, care should focus on the concussive injury. Outcome is universally good, and players have returned to their sport within 2 weeks, free of any change in functional performance.

Conclusion.—A team physician needs to be aware of CC so that players are not given a misdiagnosis of posttraumatic epilepsy and treated inappropriately. Players can be reassured that CCs are benign and not associated with a risk of epilepsy.

▶ This article makes several important observations. First, athletes who sustain CCs can be reassured that the episode is benign and not associated with long-term epilepsy. Also, specific pharmacotherapy is not required and management should be concerned with the concussion problem.

J.S. Torg, M.D.

Incidence of Fever in the Rehabilitation Phase Following Brain Injury
Clinchot DM, Otis S, Colachis SC III (Ohio State Univ, Columbus)
Am J Phys Med Rehabil 76:323–327, 1997   2–3

Introduction.—Fever occurring in the acute phase of recovery after brain injury is in most cases caused by infectious agents. A diagnosis of central fever is made when no cause is identified. The incidence and causes of fever in the rehabilitation phase after brain injury were analyzed in this study.

Methods.—Data were gathered from a retrospective review of 286 consecutive admissions to a brain injury rehabilitation unit. Items recorded included demographic information, length of time since injury, rehabilitation length of stay, injury category and severity, and details of the fever events. Fever was defined as any core temperature higher than 37.7°C (99.9°F).

Results.—Patients were divided into the following 3 groups: (1) traumatic brain injuries (79%), (2) anoxic brain injuries (12%), and (3) brain injuries resulting from aneurysmal subarachnoid hemorrhage (SAH) (9%). The injuries were classified as severe in 60% of traumatic cases, 67% of aneurysmal SAH cases, and 50% of anoxic cases. The average length of acute hospital stay was 35.4 days in the traumatic group, 45.4 days in the aneurysmal SAH group, and 67 days in the anoxic group. Average length of rehabilitation stay was 38.4 days, 45.1 days, and 38.4 days, respectively.

Overall, 24% of patients experienced fevers, and each group had similar occurrence rates. Fever among patients with anoxic brain injury occurred most often in those who had cardiac arrest, and approximately one third of the fevers in anoxic injuries were caused by urinary tract infection.

Thirty fever events were found in 34.6% of patients with aneurysms; 46% of their fevers were attributed to atelectasis or pneumonia. Fever events of unknown cause were found only in the traumatic brain injury (7%) and aneurysmal SAH (8%) groups. No fever of unknown cause was higher than 38.0°C (100.4°F).

Conclusion.—In this group of patients with brain injuries of various types, the incidence of explained fever events was far higher than that of unexplained fever events. Because most cases of fever after brain injury result from treatable conditions, these conditions should be excluded before a diagnosis of central fever is considered.

▶ Fever following brain injury is sometimes attributed to a dysfunction of thermoregulatory centers in the hypothalamus. Clinchot et al found that about 24% of patients developed fever after brain injury, but this was almost always the result of some type of infection, rather than of hypothalamic dysfunction. Even in patients with traumatic and aneurysmal injuries, there was almost always some explanation other than hypothalamic dysfunction. It is thus important to search for a treatable cause, rather than accepting a diagnosis of hypothalamic dysfunction, if fever develops during the course of rehabilitation following brain injury.

R.J. Shephard, M.D., Ph.D.

Cervical Cord Neurapraxia: Classification, Pathomechanics, Morbidity, and Management Guidelines
Torg JS, Corcoran TA, Thibault LE, et al (Allegheny Univ, Philadelphia; Hosp for Special Surgery, New York)
J Neurosurg 87:843–850, 1997   2–4

Background.—Cervical cord neurapraxia (CCN) is a distinct clinical condition characterized by narrowing of the anteroposterior diameter of the cervical canal. The typical patient is an athlete with an acute but transient neurologic episode of cervical cord origin. Symptoms include sensory changes, with or without motor changes, in both arms, both legs, both arms and legs, or the arm and leg on one side. The episodes can last from 15 min to 48 hr. The authors have reported the radiographic findings of CCN, but not the MRI findings. A series of 100 cases of CCN were analyzed to develop a classification system, propose a new computerized measurement technique for MRI, and assess the relationship of the cervical cord to the canal.

Methods.—The patients were 109 males and 1 female, average age 21. All episodes of CCN occurred during sports participation, 87% were football related. Follow-up data (average, 3.3 yr), were available for 105 patients. The clinical and imaging data were analyzed in detail to gain a clearer understanding of the condition, assess the associated risk for permanent neurologic injury, identify factors associated with recurrent episodes of CCN, and propose clearer management guidelines. The MRI

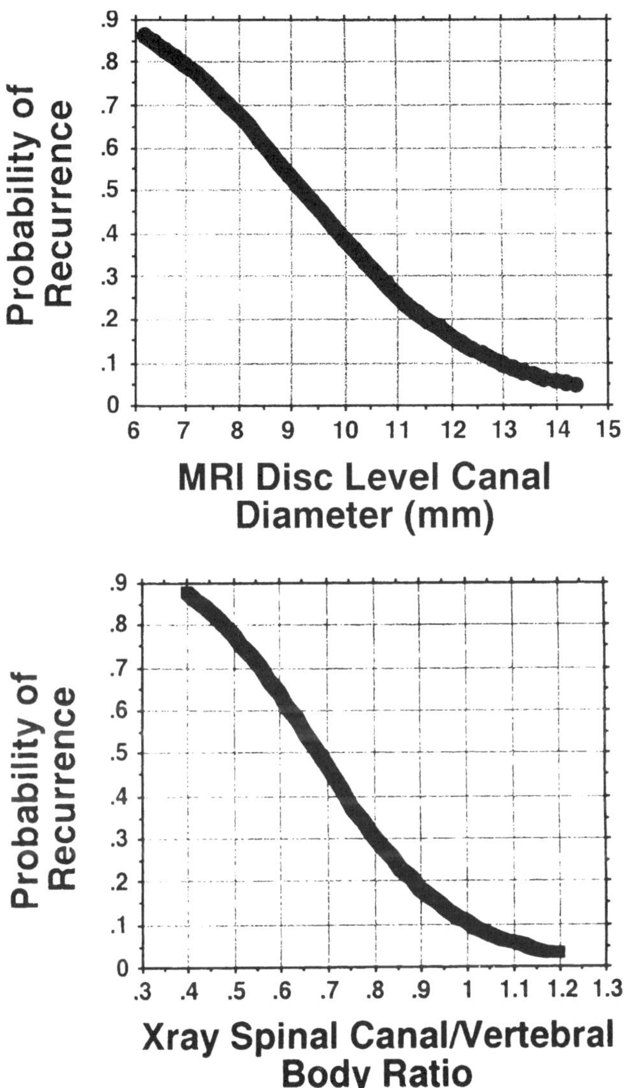

FIGURE 2.—Graphs developed using logistic regression analysis in which the risk of recurrence can be plotted as a function of the disc-level diameter measured on MRI (*top*) and the spinal cord/vertebral body ratio calculated on the basis of x-ray films (*bottom*). The construction of these plots is based on the result that increased risk of recurrence is inversely correlated with canal diameter. Future CCN patients can be counseled regarding their individual risk of recurrence based on the particular size of their spinal canal. (Courtesy of Torg JS, Corcoran TA, Thibault LE, et al: Cervical cord neurapraxia: Classification, pathomechanics, morbidity, and management guidelines. *J Neurosurg* 87:843–850, 1997.)

images were digitized to provide insight into the relationship of the spinal cord and intravertebral disk to the bony cervical canal.

Results.—The findings suggested that CCN was causally related to narrowing of the sagittal diameter of the cervical canal in the adult spine.

There were no cases of permanent neurologic damage resulting from CCN. Sixty percent of patients returned to sports competition, and none of these experienced any permanent morbidity. However, CCN recurred in 56% of patients who returned to sports; the recurrence rate was particularly high for football players. Other factors related to recurrence risk were a smaller spinal canal/vertebral body ratio, a smaller disk-level canal diameter, and less space available for the spinal cord. The classification of the CCN episode and the imaging findings had no influence on the risk for recurrence.

Conclusions.—This experience shows that CCN is a transient neurologic condition. Athletes with uncomplicated CCN can return to competition with no increased risk for permanent neurologic damage. The occurrence of CCN appears to be related to congenital or degenerative narrowing of the sagittal diameter of the cervical canal. Most patients can return to their sport, though there is a high risk for recurrent CCN. This risk is strongly and inversely related to the sagittal canal diameter. Spinal canal measurements will be a useful aid to physicians counseling their patients as to future CCN risk (Fig 2).

▶ This article clearly establishes that individuals without spinal instability who experience an episode of CCN can return to contact sport activities without increased risk of permanent neurologic injury. It further documents that the real problem is recurrent episodes of cord signs and symptoms. However, the data do enable the physician to counsel patients with regard to their individual risk of occurrence based on either the MRI disk level, canal diameter, or canal/vertebral body ratio.

J.S. Torg, M.D.

Management Guidelines for Participation in Collision Activities With Congenital, Developmental, or Postinjury Lesions Involving the Cervical Spine

Torg JS, Ramsey-Emrhein JA (Allegheny Univ, Philadelphia; Dickinson College, Carlisle, Pa)
Sports Med Arthro Rev 5:226–242, 1997   2–5

Background.—Many different injuries to the cervical spine and associated structures can occur as a result of sports participation. Although much has been written about the diagnosis and treatment of these problems, there are no accepted guidelines regarding the return to collision activities. Available information was reviewed to guide the clinician in making decisions about returning to sports activities by patients with congenital or developmental problems or injury to the cervical spine.

Methods.—The guidelines were based on information on more than 1,200 cervical spine lesions reported to the National Football Head & Neck Injury Registry, a thorough review of the literature, and knowledge of the mechanisms of injury. For each congenital, developmental, or posttraumatic condition, return to collision activities was classified as presenting no contraindication, a relative contraindication, or an absolute contraindication.

Congenital Conditions.—The findings suggested that odontoid agenesis, odontoid hypoplasia, and os odontoideum are absolute contraindications to contact sport participation. The same is true for atlanto-occipital fusion, whether isolated or combined with other abnormalities. Klippel-Feil anomaly is an absolute contraindication for type I and some type II lesions. However, for type II lesions involving fusion of 1 or 2 interspaces at C3 or below in a patient with full cervical range of motion, this anomaly presents no contraindication.

Developmental Conditions.—Several studies have addressed the problem of developmental stenosis of the cervical spine associated with neurapraxia. For an asymptomatic patient with a canal/vertebral body ratio of 0.8 or less, this condition presents no contraindication. However, depending on the symptoms and associated conditions or neurologic findings, cervical spine stenosis constitutes a relative-to-absolute contraindication. Spear tackler's spine is an absolute contraindication to football and other collision activities. However, spina bifida occulta is an incidental finding that should not preclude participation.

Posttraumatic Conditions.—Injuries causing occipital or atlantoaxial instability are potentially serious. Anytime the transverse and/or alar ligament is disrupted, it is an absolute contraindication to collision activity. The same is true for any form of atlantoaxial rotary fixation, fractures of the upper cervical segment, and C1–C2 fusion. In the middle and lower cervical spine, ligamentous injuries constitute an absolute contraindication if there is more than 3.5 mm of horizontal displacement of 1 vertebra in relation to another, or more than 11 degrees of rotation compared with either adjacent vertebra. Lesser degrees of displacement and rotation are relative contraindications, depending on other patient factors. Acute fracture of the vertebral body in the middle and lower cervical spine is an absolute contraindication. Healed fractures are also a contraindication if there is any pain, neurologic abnormality, or limitation of motion.

Discussion.—Guidelines for participation in collision activities for athletes with various abnormalities of the cervical spine are presented. In addition to congenital, developmental, and posttraumatic lesions, guidelines for patients with intervertebral disk injury and those with a history of cervical spine fusion are provided. The guidelines are subject to future modification and should consider other patient-related factors.

▶ Presented are the only published management guidelines for return to collision activities in individuals with problems involving the cervical spine. The original article is a recommended reference for the interested reader.

J.S. Torg, M.D.

Pneumomediastinum in a Surf Lifesaver

Fallon KE, Foster K (Australian Inst of Sport, Canberra)
Br J Sports Med 30:359–360, 1996   2–6

Introduction.—An unusual case of pneumomediastinum was seen in a young asthmatic surf lifesaver is described.

Case Report.—Man, 20, a professional lifeguard and competitive surf club swimmer, was seem with a 4-hour history of sore throat. He had a history of mild asthma. The previous day he had trained for a surf belt race, in which a snug belt is wrapped around the swimmer's abdomen and affixed to a rope fed through the hands of 4 lifesavers on the beach. The event is a race that simulates the rescue of a drowning victim. The patient mentioned that the rope had not been fed fast enough and he had strained against it and been forced to swim underwater for long periods. The patient's throat was normal and he was not dyspneic. Lung and heart sounds were normal. Subcutaneous emphysema was detected in the neck and upper chest. Chest radiography revealed pneumomediastinum and subcutaneous emphysema. The patient was treated expectantly. The emphysema resolved within 3 days. Chest radiographs showed no abnormalities at 2-week follow-up.

Discussion.—Pneumomediastinum is relatively rare, primarily occurring in young males. The most common symptoms are chest pain, dyspnea, and neck pain and the most common physical sign is subcutaneous emphysema, especially in the neck region. Treatment is expectant; resolution is rapid and complications are rare.

▶ This practical report expands the spectrum of pneumomediastinum in athletes and includes a brief yet comprehensive review. Likely causal factors were asthma, straining against a surf belt, and underwater swimming. An informative account of pneumomediastinum in a weightlifter has recently appeared.[1] We have reviewed cases in weightlifters[2] and after shoulder arthroscopy.[3] Pulmonary barotrauma in football players was reviewed last year[4] and the first report of pulmonary contusion in a football player appeared in 1997.[5]

E.R. Eichner, M.D.

References

1. Jones SL, Fred HL: Sudden retrosternal pain in a young weight lifter. *Hosp Practice* 32:152–159, 1997.
2. 1996 Year Book of Sports Medicine, pp' 210–211.
3. 1993 Year Book of Sports Medicine, pp' 50–51.
4. 1997 Year Book of Sports Medicine, pp' 106–107.
5. Meese MA, Sebastianelli WJ: Pulmonary contusion secondary to blunt trauma in a collegiate football player. *Clin J Sport Med* 7:309–310, 1997.

Lumbar Spondylolysis: A Study of Natural Progression in Athletes
Congeni J, McCulloch J, Swanson K (Sports Medicine Ctr, Akron, Ohio; Northeastern Ohio Univs, Akron)
Am J Sports Med 25:248–253, 1997   2–7

Objective.—Spondylolysis is a relatively common injury in young athletes, occurring with an incidence of 47%, compared with an incidence of 5% in adults. Computed tomography scans were used to follow the natural progression of subtle fractures, not visible on plain radiographs, and to characterize and follow up these stress fractures of the pars interarticularis.

Methods.—Between 1990 and 1994, 40 young athletes (9 female), aged 12 to 20, with negative findings on plain radiographs and CT scans performed 10 weeks after a diagnosis of spondylolysis, received a lumbar CT scan and a reverse-gantry angled CT scan at Children's Hospital Medical Center of Akron (Fig 1 Fig 3, Fig 6). Two to 4 weeks after diagnosis, all patients had received 4 weeks of rehabilitation that included treatment with a nonrigid brace and trunk flexion and flexibility and

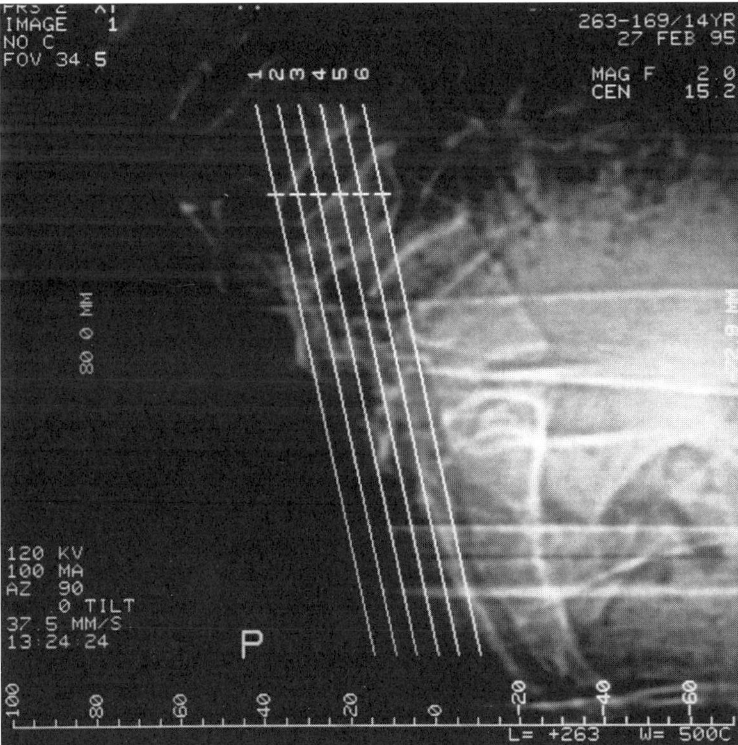

FIGURE 1.—Computed tomography scan made using the reverse-gantry angle technique. (Courtesy of Congeni J, McCulloch J, Swanson K: Lumbar spondylolysis: A study of natural progression in athletes. *Am J Sports Med* 25:248–253, 1997).

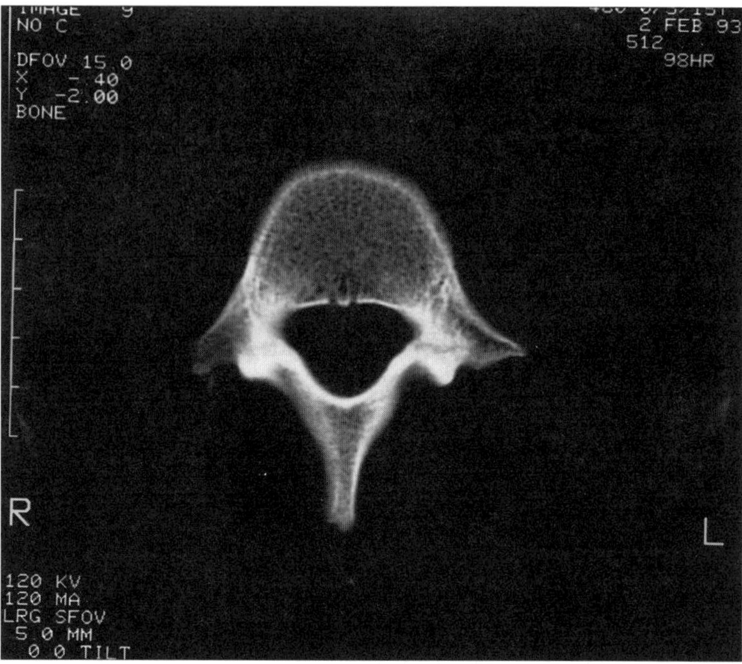

FIGURE 3.—Stress reaction of the pars interarticularis without complete fracture. (Courtesy of Congeni J, McCulloch J, Swanson K: Lumbar spondylolysis: A study of natural progression in athletes. *Am J Sports Med* 25:248–253, 1997).

strengthening exercises, and all were encouraged to undertake cross-training in nonextension activities and to avoid hyperextension activities. At 6 to 8 weeks after diagnosis, athletes were given functional progress activities to prepare them for return to their competitive activities at 8 weeks. Athletes were surveyed about painful flare-ups, any sports limitations, and athletic activity before and after injury.

Results.—Patients were divided into those with chronic, nonhealing fractures (Group A, n = 18), those with healed or healing acute fractures (Group B, n = 16), and those with no complete fractures (Group C, n = 6). Duration of symptoms ranged from less than 3 weeks to more than 6 months. Fourteen Group A patients and 8 Group B patients had bilateral fractures.

Conclusion.—CT scans, particularly with reverse-gantry angle, are useful in verifying the diagnosis of spondylolysis in young athletes with back pain and normal plain radiographs. Aggressive physical therapy for 6 to 8 weeks that avoids hyperextension exercises is helpful in facilitating the return to competitive activities. Whereas acute fractures should be treated with a brace and restricted activity, chronic fractures should be treated symptomatically and braced only if necessary.

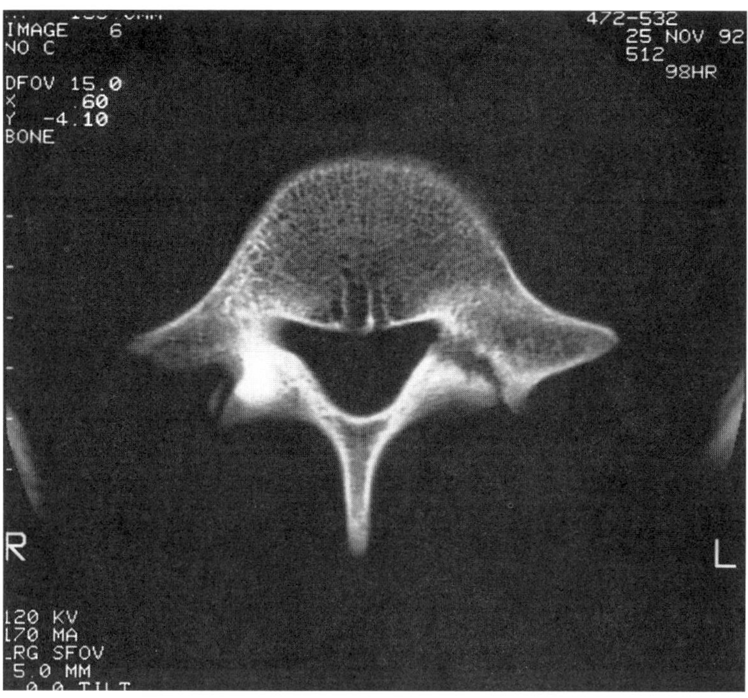

FIGURE 6.—This scan shows healing of the pars lesion. (Courtesy of Congeni J, McCulloch J, Swanson K: Lumbar spondylolysis: A study of natural progression in athletes. *Am J Sports Med* 25:248–253, 1997).

▶ This is an excellent article clearly delineating the important role that computed tomography scans using reverse-gantry angled technique can play in diagnosis and management of this common and potentially troublesome problem. The original article is recommended for the interested reader.

J.S. Torg, M.D.

Subcapsular Liver Hematomas Caused by Bar Ends in Mountain-Bike Crashes

Nehoda H, Hochleitner BW (Univ Hosp of Innsbruck, Austria)
Lancet 351:342, 1998   2–8

Background.—Mountain biking is an increasingly popular sport. The authors have noted a number of patients with liver trauma related to mountain biking. They review their experience with this type of injury, which they attribute to a handlebar modification used by mountain bikers.

Patients.—Fifty-two patients were treated in a trauma department for mountain bike injuries over a 2-year period. Eight patients had subcapsular liver hematoma caused by a fall, in each case resulting from the handlebars being driven into the right side of the abdomen. The patients' average age was 27. Their symptoms included abdominal pain with right upper quadrant tenderness. Head injuries and other injuries were present as well. All patients were initially monitored in the ICU, followed by gradual mobilization. All hematomas resolved within 3 months.

Discussion.—A series of subcapsular liver hematomas in mountain bikers is presented. The authors believe these injuries are related to the use of bar ends on the handlebars, which mountain bikers use as an aid to climbing. Physicians should be alert for liver injuries caused by mountain bike accidents. To avoid such injuries, bikers should use forward-inclining and foam-covered bar ends.

▶ The authors have made a worthwhile observation with regard to patients with abdominal pain following a mountain bike mishap.

J.S. Torg, M.D.

Pelvic Stress Injuries: The Relationship Between Osteitis Pubis (Symphysis Pubis Stress Injury) and Sacroiliac Abnormalities in Athletes

Major NM, Helms CA (Duke Univ, Durham, NC)
Skeletal Radiol 26:711–717, 1997   2–9

Background.—Osteitis pubis is a painful, often debilitating condition of the symphysis pubis believed to result primarily from pelvic infection, usually seen in elderly men after prostate surgery and in women after bladder, neck, and urethral surgery. Osteitis pubis has also been reported

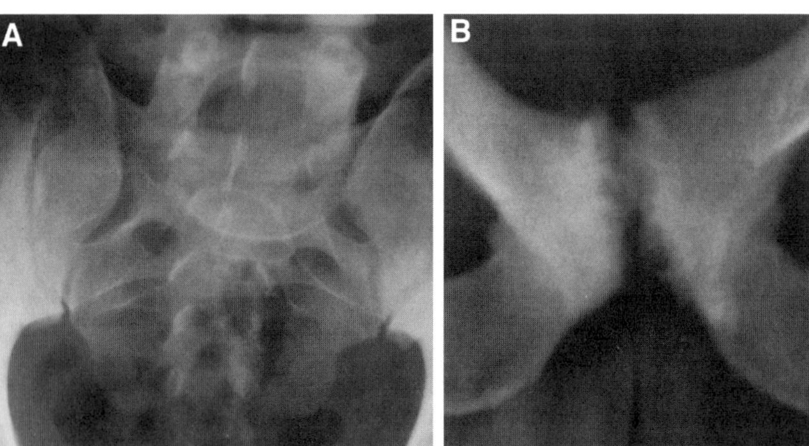

FIGURE 5.—A 26-year-old male basketball player with pubic symphysis pain and left sciatica. **A,** erosions and sclerosis are present on both sides of the symphysis consistent with stress changes, **B,** in addition, the sacroiliac joints show bilateral sclerosis and erosions slightly more prominent on the left side. (Courtesy of Major NM, Helms CA: Pelvis stress injuries: The relationship between osteitis pubis (symphysis pubis stress injury) and sacroiliac abnormalities in athletes. *Skeletal Radiol* 26:711–717, 1997.)

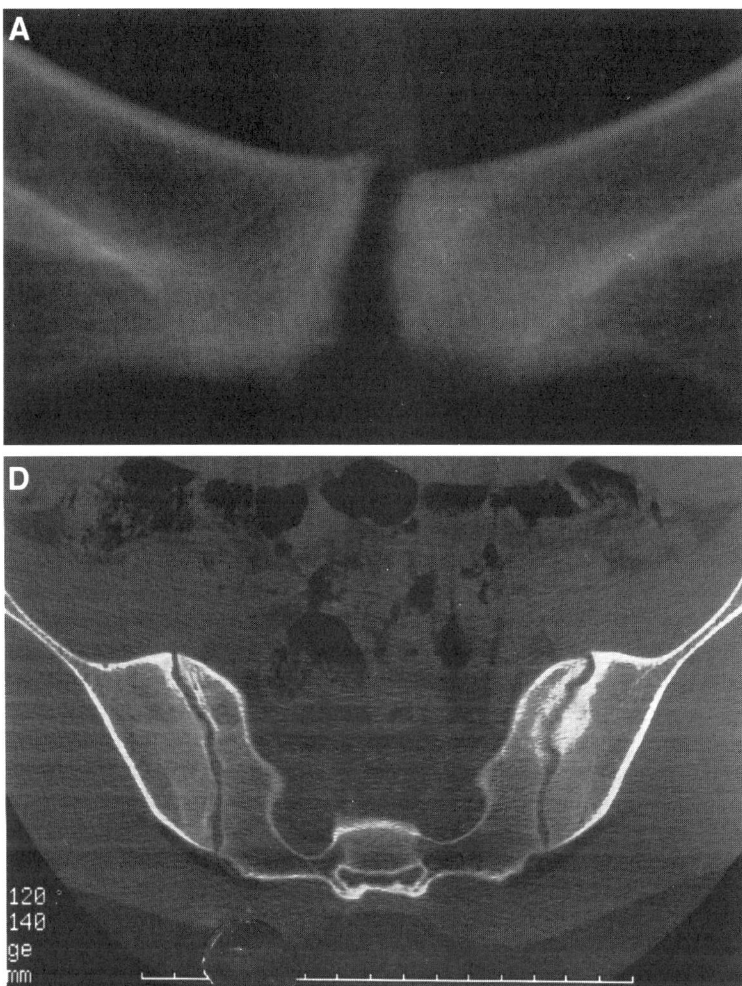

FIGURE 9.—This female 22-year-old college varsity basketball player was playing about 3–4 hours of full-court basketball per day and complained of left sciatica. **A,** the plain film shows increased sclerosis primarily on the left side of the joint with subtle erosions bilaterally; **D,** the CT scan through the sacroiliac joints shows to better advantage the increased sclerosis and erosions involving the left joint. (Courtesy of Major NM, Helms CA: Pelvis stress injuries: The relationship between osteitis pubis (symphysis pubis stress injury) and sacroiliac abnormalities in athletes. *Skeletal Radiol* 26:711–717, 1997.)

in athletes, but is associated with symphysis pubis stress injury more than pelvic infection in this population. Symphysis pubis stress injury has been reported in long-distance runners; soccer, cricket, hockey, and basketball players; and individuals who participate in indoor track events and road walking.

Methods.—There were 9 male and 2 female athletes who participated in long-distance running, soccer, and basketball. The average patient age was about 37 years. The patients complained of pubic symphysis pain, sciatica, groin pain, or a combination of these. Plain radiographs were obtained in all patients, and CT, MRI, and a bone scan were also performed in some patients. Anteroposterior plain radiographs of the pelvis were also obtained in 20 individuals without back or pubic pain.

Results.—On plain radiographs, all athletes had evidence of sclerosis, erosions, or offset at the pubic symphysis (Fig 5). Four patients had avulsion of cortical bone at the insertion site of the gracilis tendon. Four patients had sacroiliac joint abnormalities such as sclerosis, erosions, and osteophytes; 1 patient had bilateral sacroiliac changes (Fig 9). In 2 patients, normal sacroiliac joints were seen on plain films, but increased radionuclide uptake bilaterally at the sacroiliac joints was noted on a bone scan. In 1 patient, sacroiliac abnormalities were seen on plain films and CT scans, and abnormal signal at both sacroiliac joints and the pubic symphysis was seen on MRI scans. One patient with sciatica had a sacral stress fracture detected by CT. In the control group, 6 individuals older than 55 years had mild sclerosis of the symphysis, but there was no evidence of sacroiliac abnormalities on plain radiographs.

Discussion.—In these athletes, stress injuries of the pubic symphysis were associated with degenerative changes in the sacroiliac joint or a sacral stress fracture. This may result from abnormal stresses across the pelvic ring structure that cause a second abnormality in the pelvic ring. Abnormalities in the sacrum are not detected with conventional imaging. Individuals with pubis symphysis stress injury typically have gradually increasing discomfort or pain in the pubic area, one or both groins (adductor areas), and around the lower rectus abdominis muscle. There may an acute episode after forced abduction at the hip, forced hip rotation, kicking, or a fall. There is increasing evidence that fractures of the pubic rami are associated with fractures or ligamentous injuries in or around the posterior arch of the pelvic ring.

▶ The authors describe what I believe is a previously unrecorded observation. The article is concise and nicely illustrated. The statement that "there is growing evidence that fractures of the pubic rami are almost invariably associated with fractures or ligamentous injuries in or about the posterior arch of the pelvic ring" is actually well-recognized and easily explained. From a mechanical standpoint it is impossible to have an isolated fracture of a rigid ring. That is, 2 fractures will occur in the ring. It would appear that the association of a symphysis pubis stress injury and sacroiliac abnormalities in the athlete is similarly explained.

J.S. Torg, M.D.

Major Pelvic Injuries in Equestrian Sports

O'Farrell DA, Irshad F, Thorns BS, et al (Meath Hosp, Dublin)
Br J Sports Med 31:249–251, 1997   2–10

Introduction.—Horse-riding accidents can result in major life-threatening fractures. A group of riders who sustained pelvic and acetabular fractures was reviewed for the nature of the accident, injuries, treatment, and follow-up.

Methods.—Between 1987 and 1995, 205 patients with pelvic and acetabular fractures were treated by operation at the study institution. The 9 patients who were injured during horse-racing or horse-riding activities were asked to complete a questionnaire related to their level of riding experience, level of training of the horse, circumstances of the accident, and type of protective riding equipment used.

Results.—The mean age of the riders at the time of injury was 46 years. One was a professional jockey and the others were very experienced amateurs. Six had been previously involved in minor horse riding accidents. The horse fell on the rider in 5 cases; 4 riders were thrown clear and fell to the ground. The injury consisted of complete disruption of the pelvic ring involving symphyseal diastasis and sacroiliac joint separation in 5 cases. A pelvic external fixator was applied soon after admission to stabilize the pelvis and reduce blood loss. Seven to 10 days later, patients underwent open reduction and internal fixation of the sacroiliac joint and pubic symphysis. Two of the remaining patients had fractures of the ilium and 2 had fractures of the acetabulum; all 4 were managed surgically with open reduction and internal fixation. The mean hospital stay was 24 days. Only 1 of the horses was untrained at the time of the accident. All riders were wearing helmets, but none wore body protectors. At a mean follow up of 17 months, 5 patients had returned to riding and 4 believed that they would be unable to ride again.

Discussion.—Up to 15% of horse-riding accidents require hospitalization. Most deaths result from head injuries. Crush injury is likely to occur when the horse falls on the rider, whereas fractures of the acetabulum are common when the rider is thrown forcibly to the ground.

▶ Described are 2 basic injury mechanisms resulting in major pelvic injuries in equestrian sports. In those cases where the horse falls onto the rider, there results a crush injury to the pelvis. This injury involves complete disruption of the pelvic ring with symphyseal diathesis and sacroiliac joint separation, referred to as an "open book" pelvic injury. In those injuries in which the rider is thrown clear of the horse, fractures of the acetabulum and/or femoral head dislocation occurs. The 9 injuries reported all occurred in experienced riders, leaving the authors to conclude that lack of riding experience was not a contributory factor. However, Silver and Perry[1] reported that a third of serious spinal injuries caused by falls from horses were associated with inadequate rider experience. In addition to wearing a helmet, the authors recommend that equestrians wear a "body protector" but provide no data supporting its effectiveness.

J.S. Torg, M.D.

Reference

1. Silver JR, Perry JM: Hazards of horse riding as a popular sport. *Br J Sports Med* 25:101–110, 1991.

Suprascapular Neuropathy: Results of Non-operative Treatment
Martin SD, Warren RF, Martin TL, et al (New York Hosp-Cornell Univ)
J Bone Joint Surg Am 79-A:1159–1165, 1997   2–11

Introduction.—If left untreated, suprascapular neuropathy can cause prolonged and disabling shoulder pain. Both operative and nonoperative treatment approaches have been described, with most authors favoring the former. The results of nonoperative treatment for suprascapular neuropathy were reviewed.

Methods.—The 15 patients were 13 males and 2 females, whose average age was 35 years. The patients complained of pain in the posterolateral aspect of the shoulder, exacerbated with activity. They also had shoulder weakness, particularly when performing overhead activities. Electrodiagnostic studies were performed to confirm the clinical diagnosis of suprascapular neuropathy. All patients received a minimum of 6 months of physical therapy, with the aim of increasing strength in the rotator cuff muscles, the deltoid muscle, and the periscapular muscles. The patients were followed up for an average of nearly 4 years; the most recent evaluation included electrodiagnostic studies and dynamic isokinetic testing.

Results.—Three patients had persistent shoulder symptoms leading to surgery, which produced an excellent result in 1 patient, a good result in 1, and a poor result in 1. Of the remaining 12 patients, 5 had an excellent result and 7 a good result with nonoperative therapy. Follow-up electromyography showed abnormal results in 6 of 13 patients, including 4 patients in whom nonoperative treatment was successful. Patients with good results of nonoperative treatment showed subtle deficits on isokinetic testing, compared with the normal side.

Conclusions.—This retrospective study demonstrates good results with nonoperative treatment for suprascapular neuropathy. Although there may be some residual muscle atrophy and weakness, they do not interfere with normal shoulder function. Nonoperative treatment appears to be indicated for patients whose symptoms are not being caused by a space-occupying lesion. If symptoms persist, surgery is indicated.

▶ An interesting article reporting on what appears to be a relatively uncommon problem. Because of the small numbers involved, it is not possible to demonstrate a significant difference between the operative and nonoperative groups. Thus, statistically speaking, the data do not support the conclusion that "nonoperative treatment of suprascapular neuropathy is indicated if a space-occupying lesion is not the cause of the condition."

J.S. Torg, M.D.

Management of Shoulder Dysfunction With an Alternative Model of Orthopaedic Physical Therapy Intervention: A Case Report
Holmes CF, Fletcher JP, Blaschak MJ, et al (Univ of Central Arkansas, Conway; Northern Illinois Univ, DeKalb; Univ of Texas, San Antonio)
J Orthop Sports Phys Ther 26:347–354, 1997   2–12

Introduction.—Multiple sessions in physical therapy are often required to manage patients with musculoskeletal problems, and the therapy involves multiple treatment modalities. An alternative treatment approach which includes minimal use of palliative interventions initially, may be possible for a patient diagnosed with shoulder impingement and adhesive capsulitis. The emphasis is on establishing a home program. As a basis or rationale for this treatment approach, patient compliance is reviewed.

Case report.—Woman, 53, with impingement syndrome and adhesive capsulitis began a comprehensive program of patient education and home exercise. The following exercises were part of her program: Codman's exercises using clockwise, counterclockwise and left-right movements with the weight of the extremity; bilateral shoulder retraction exercises; and left shoulder internal and external rotation in standing position, using red Theraband (Fig 4). She later had active shoulder flexion and extension exercises added to her routine. Over a period of about 10 and a half weeks, she was seen 6 times. At 1 month after the last treatment she was followed up by telephone. After 1 year, she was re-examined.

Results.—After 1 year, no abnormalities were seen. Compliance with the home program was reported by the patient for 6 months after the last visit. For this patient, this model of care was successful.

Conclusion.—The development of an internal locus of control may have contributed to the success of this treatment approach by allowing the patient to be as actively involved as possible in treating her condition. When one considers current reimbursement systems, this approach is timely. However, every patient with this diagnosis may not have similar success with this graduated treatment model.

▶ Shoulder impingement syndrome is a common malady in middle-aged patients, and its treatment requires long-term physical therapy and exercise therapy consisting of both flexibility and strengthening exercises. However, extensive visits to a therapist may be expensive and time-consuming for the average patient. This study examined a treatment model which included intensive patient education and home program therapeutic exercise for up to 1 year following the last visit to physical therapy. Unfortunately, the study included only 1 patient. For this patient the program was successful and

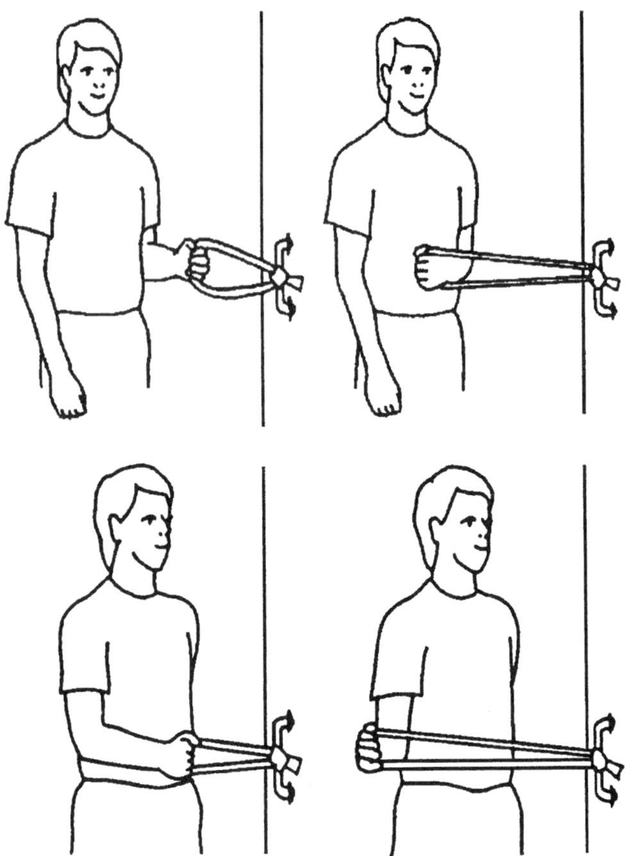

FIGURE 4.—Shoulder internal and external rotation exercise. (Courtesy of Holmes CF, Fletcher JP, Blaschak MJ, et al: Management of shoulder dysfunction with an alternative model of orthopedic physical therapy intervention: A case report. *J Orthop Sports Phys Ther* 26:347–354, 1997. Reprinted with permission from PTEX Systems software, version 2.71, copyright 1992.)

resulted in improved shoulder function, but the approach may not be successful with all patients, depending on their ability to work on their own and to follow a prescribed program. However, the home program does hold some promise for placing the responsibility for treatment of a chronic injury with the patient. Patients then have control of their treatment outcome, and success is dependent only on their own commitment to rehabilitation. This home treatment model will undoubtedly be used much more frequently in future care of such chronic conditions.

M.J.L. Alexander, Ph.D.

A Correlation Between Shoulder Laxity and Interfering Pain in Competitive Swimmers

McMaster WC, Roberts A, Stoddard T (Univ of California, Irvine, Orange)
Am J Sports Med 26:83–86, 1998   2–13

Objective.—Shoulder pain in swimmers can have a negative effect on performance. If the pain is the result of shoulder laxity, there should be a correlation between shoulder pain and laxity scores. Shoulder pain in national and elite swimmers was investigated for correlation with shoulder laxity scores weighted for clinical signs of instability.

Methods.—Clinical examinations were performed on both shoulders of 40 swimmers (13 women), aged 14 to 24 years, using 5 standard clinical testing maneuvers. Shoulder scores were analyzed against results of pain questionnaires completed by the swimmers.

Results.—There were 28 shoulders at risk in 14 swimmers (35%) reporting unilateral pain (5 patients) pain or bilateral pain (9 patients). Scores were higher in swimmers with interfering pain.

Conclusion.—There was a significant correlation between interfering shoulder pain and clinical examination score. Maneuvers that contribute to laxity should be identified. Training capacity should be maintained to avoid significant detraining in endurance athletes.

▶ The authors have confirmed the commonly accepted concept that there is a correlation between shoulder pain and shoulder laxity. On the basis of this, a series of training adaptations are suggested. However, no data are presented to substantiate their efficacy. The authors point out that they have "tested a remedial exercise protocol to ameliorate the rotator cuff strength ratio shifts that occur in swimmers and found that this can be helpful in symptomatic athletes but may not be universally effective." Clearly, the next step is to document a program or programs that will meet what the authors believe to be "the most important goal for the medical management of the swimming athlete" which "should be maintaining training capacity."

J.S. Torg, M.D.

Laser-assisted Shoulder Surgery

Nottage WM (Orthopaedic Med Associates Inc, Laguna Hills, Calif)
Arthroscopy 13:635–638, 1997   2–14

Background.—The use of lasers in arthroscopic surgery has been controversial since its introduction in the early 1980s. The ongoing debate over the use of laser or thermal energy in arthroscopic shoulder surgery was reviewed.

Lasers in Shoulder Arthroscopy.—On the positive side, laser use offers coagulation and tissue vaporization. On the negative side are concerns about cost, complications, and the lack of evidence showing that laser techniques are superior to current mechanical techniques. The holmium-

2.1 laser has been used for ablation of hypertrophic synovium and for various procedures in the subacromial space and glenohumeral joint, including débridement of labral lesions, release of the coracoacromial ligament, and chondroplasty. Recent studies have reported good results with 2.1 nm holmium:yttrium, aluminum, and garnet arthroscopic laser surgery of the shoulder. However, comparisons with conventional techniques are still needed. "Laser-assisted capsular shift" refers to the use of lasers to shrink the capsular tissue of the shoulder in patients with glenohumeral instability. This technique produces a change in the morphological characteristics of the shoulder capsule, depending on the laser used, the time of exposure, and the heat intensity. However, so far there is no specific feedback mechanism by which the surgeon can measure heat exposure and temperature, and thus control the amount of collagen shrinkage produced. More basic science and clinical research of this application are needed. Radiofrequency instruments have been developed as an alternative to lasers for heating tissues.

Discussion.—There have been several promising studies of laser-assisted shoulder surgery, including laser-assisted capsular shrinkage. However, until concerns about cost, safety, and relative efficacy can be addressed, these procedures must be considered investigational. Orthopedic surgeons are reassured that, until further evidence is available, they are not compromising patient care by not using laser techniques in shoulder arthroscopy.

Tissue Shrinkage With the Holmium: Yttrium Aluminum Garnet Laser: A Postoperative Assessment of Tissue Length, Stiffness, and Structure
Schaefer SL, Ciarelli MJ, Arnoczky SP, et al (Michigan State Univ, East Lansing)
Am J Sports Med 25:841–848, 1997   2–15

Introduction.—The effect of laser energy on joint-associated connective tissue has not been thoroughly assessed. Significant shrinkage of rabbit joint capsular tissue and reduced capsular stiffness have been observed in vitro after application of nonablative laser energy. There are no known in vivo trials evaluating the laser's effect on joint-associated connective tissue. A rabbit patellar tendon model was used to evaluate the effect of laser energy on the length, stiffness, and connective tissue structure.

Methods.—A calculated dose of holmium:yttrium-aluminum-garnet laser energy (300 J/cm^2) was delivered to 1 randomly-selected patellar tendon in 13 adult New Zealand White rabbits. The contralateral patellar tendon acted as control. Standard lateral radiographs were taken with radiopaque markers, placed in the patella and tibial tuberosity, to measure patellar tendon length. These measurements were taken before and 4 and 8 weeks after laser application. Limbs were not immobilized after surgery. Tendons were harvested at 0 weeks in 7 rabbits and 8 weeks in 6 rabbits.

Tendons were examined for tensile stiffness, cross-sectional area, histologic changes, and electron microscopic appearance.

Results.—Significant tendon shrinkage was observed after application of the calculated laser energy dose. Tendon length increased significantly beyond the immediate postlaser length at 4-week follow-up, and beyond its original length at 8-week follow-up. The lased tendons were significantly less stiff and had significantly greater cross-sectional areas at 8-week follow-up, compared to those of controls. A generalized fibroblastic response and marked increase in cellularity were observed throughout the entire lased tendon. The normal bimodal pattern of large- and small-diameter collagen fibers was changed to a unimodal pattern, with predominantly small-diameter fibers in the lased tendons.

Conclusion.—The observed tissue alterations in lased tendons indicate that the biologic response of connective tissue to laser energy causes additional compromise in tissue integrity, beyond that attributed to the initial physical effects of the laser. Physicians seeking rehabilitative approaches must consider these changes.

▶ Laser energy is currently being used by some orthopedic surgeons to effect, by arthroscopic application, shrinkage of the glenohumeral capsule in patients with recurrent subluxation/dislocation. The procedure has been euphemistically referred to as "laser assisted capsular shift." However, as pointed out by Nottage, "application of laser energy to produce capsular shrinkage must be considered investigational because the ultimate fate of the tissue remains unknown." Schaefer, et al., using the rabbit patella tendon model, demonstrate that "after initial shrinking, laser-modified connective tissues demonstrate a loss of tensile stiffness and can stretch out beyond pre-shrinkage lengths when exposed to normal physiologic loads." It appears that clinical studies designed to evaluate the effectiveness of laser-induced capsular shrinkage for glenohumeral instability will require long-term comparison with current open and arthroscopic mechanical stabilizations.

J.S. Torg, M.D.

Arthroscopic Transglenoid Multiple Suture Repair: 2 to 8 Year Results in 150 Shoulders
Torchia ME, Caspari RB, Asselmeier MA, et al (Mayo Clinic, Rochester, Minn; Orthopaedic Research of Virginia, Richmond; Glen Ellyn Clinic, Ill; et al)
Arthroscopy 13:609–619, 1997   2–16

Objective.—There is growing interest in the arthroscopic assessment and treatment of glenohumeral instability. However, most reports to date have included small numbers of patients or short-term follow-up. This makes it difficult to compare the results with those of open capsular repair, or to identify factors associated with outcome. A large experience with arthroscopic repair of chronic anterior shoulder instability was reviewed, including the influence of patient and surgical variables on the risk of recurrent instability.

Methods.—The experience included 150 shoulders and 147 patients with chronic anterior instability. One hundred four patients were men and 43 were women, with a mean age of 29 years. Most patients had a chief complaint of instability. All patients underwent arthroscopic repair by the transglenoid multiple suture technique; all procedures were performed by a single surgeon. All patients had at least 2 years' follow-up (mean 4 years). The effects of multiple variables on the probability of recurrent instability over time were assessed by survival analysis.

Results.—Redislocation occurred during follow-up in 7% of shoulders operated on. In another 9% of shoulders, there was at least 1 episode consistent with recurrent subluxation. On survival analysis, the 5-year probability of recurrent instability was 18%, with nearly half of failures occurring more than 2 years postoperatively. Multivariate analysis suggested that the probability of failure was significantly related to type of pathology (Bankart lesion) and patient age (younger patients). The failure rate was also somewhat higher for patients with generalized ligamentous laxity and for those involved in collision activities. Thirteen patients required revision surgery. At last follow-up, the results were classified as excellent in 80% of shoulders, good in 3%, fair in 5%, and poor in 12%, according to the Bankart scale.

Conclusions.—The transglenoid multiple suture technique of arthroscopic repair of chronic anterior shoulder instability appears to be effective in restoring stability in the shoulder. However, it is less effective in shoulders with a Bankart lesion and in patients younger than 25 years. Flexibility is an important advantage, as the technique can be used to treat both capsular detachment and capsular laxity via standard portals with use of simple instruments.

Arthroscopic Reconstruction of Traumatic Anterior Instability of the Shoulder: The Caspari Technique
Savoie FH III, Miller CD, Field LD (Mississippi Sports Medicine & Orthopaedic Ctr, Jackson; Kansas Orthopaedic Ctr, Wichita)
Arthroscopy 13:201–209, 1997   2–17

Introduction.—In traumatic anterior instability of the shoulder, the key lesion is found in the anterior inferior glenohumeral ligament, which is the primary static restraint to anterior translation of the humeral head. Several different techniques for arthroscopic treatment of this condition have been reported, with success rates ranging from 54% to 100%. An experience with arthroscopic treatment of traumatic anterior instability of the shoulder was reported, including an analysis of factors affecting the results of treatment.

Methods.—The 3-year experience included 163 consecutive patients with traumatic anterior instability of the shoulder. The patients were 125 males and 38 females, with an average age of 27 years. The average duration of instability symptoms was 13 months, with an average of 11 dislocations per patient. Average preoperative Bankart score was 15. The reconstructions were all done using the suture punch technique of Caspari and Savoie. Key features of this procedure included anterior portal placement, adequate debridement and release of the capsulolabral complex, abrasion of the glenoid neck, placement of multiple sutures in an antero-posterior-to-posteroinferior direction, placement of a Beath pin, and use of the thick fascia on the medial scapular border to tie the sutures. Three- to 6-year follow-up data were available on 161 patients.

Results.—The overall postoperative Bankart score was 89. Ninety-one percent of patients had satisfactory results, including 76% of patients younger than 18 years, 91% of college-age patients, and 98% of adults older than 22 years. Good results were achieved in 31 patients who were high school or collegiate throwing athletes. The risk of failure was unaffected by the number of dislocations or the duration of symptoms of instability. Although all patients complained of discomfort from the posterior suture knot, this resolved spontaneously in most cases. There were no problems with nerve atrophy or infraspinatus atrophy.

Conclusions.—In patients with traumatic anterior instability of the shoulder, the arthroscopic reconstruction technique of Caspari and Savoie appears to give good results. However, the success rate of the procedure is affected by age. For adults age 22 years, the results are equivalent to those of open surgery. However, the procedure fails in 1 of 4 patients younger than 18, and so is not indicated in this age group. Good results are obtained in throwing athletes.

▶ These 2 articles (Abstracts 2–17 and 2–16) clearly demonstrate that the success of arthroscopic transglenoid multiple suture repair for traumatic anterior instability of the shoulder correlates with the age of the patient. This, of course, is important information when dealing with younger patients. The limitation of both studies, however, is that there are no control groups either with or without open surgical intervention.

J.S. Torg, M.D.

Bankart Repair for Anterior Instability of the Shoulder: Long-term Outcome

Gill TJ, Micheli LJ, Gebhard F, et al (Children's Hosp, Boston)
J Bone Joint Surg Am 79-A:850–857, 1997   2–18

Objective.—Whereas the Bankart procedure is the treatment of choice for traumatic instability of the shoulder, there have been no studies of long-term outcome. Long-term outcome of the Bankart procedure was examined, and a system was developed for rating results of operative procedures for instability of the shoulder.

Methods.—Charts of 56 patients (17 females), aged 16 to 42 years at surgery, with 60 shoulders treated by the Bankart procedure were reviewed. Patients were examined for range of motion, stability, and strength of the shoulder compared with that of the contralateral shoulder, according to American Shoulder and Elbow Surgeons standards. The patients were asked to complete a questionnaire on the history of shoulder instability; level of participation in sports before and after surgery; preoperative and postoperative pain levels; the need for reduction after dislocation; and current functional level at home, at work, and during sports. Patients were also asked to rate their satisfaction with the surgery. The patients were followed for an average of 11.9 years.

Results.—At follow-up, the operated shoulder had lost an average of 12 degrees of external rotation (P less than 0.0001). Twenty nine shoulders had pain, mostly mild, during strenuous activity, and 55 patients had returned to their previous occupations. Three patients had an isolated dislocation. Overall functional scores were 4.7 out of 5 points. A 100-point shoulder rating system was developed that allocated 50 points to function, 20 to motion, 20 to stability, and 10 to pain. Overall results were rated excellent by 43 patients, good by 9, fair by 3, and poor by 1. Fifty-four patients said they would have the procedure again.

Conclusion.—Most patients were satisfied with the functional results of the Bankart procedure and would be willing to have the procedure again. The rating system developed to assess shoulder function was based on those goals patients believed were most important.

▶ The authors present a most creditable long-term outcome evaluation of the Bankart repair for anterior glenohumeral instability. Excluded from the study were those patients with multidirectional instability or revision of a previous failed procedure. To be questioned is whether the success of the procedure can be determined by merely reporting a redislocation rate of 5%. In my view, of equal importance is the resubluxation rate, as well as subjective instability experiences. This was not done in this report.

J.S. Torg, M.D.

Instability of the Shoulder: Complex Problems and Failed Repairs: Part I. Relevant Biomechanics, Multidirectional Instability, and Severe Loss of Glenoid and Humeral Bone
Flatow EL, Warner JJP (New York Orthopaedic Hosp; Univ of Pittsburgh, Pa)
J Bone Joint Surg Am 80-A:122–140, 1998   2–19

Introduction.—Recurrent locked anterior glenohumeral dislocation is the main problem in glenohumeral instability, and many operations yield successful results in eliminating such a dislocation. The needs of active, athletic individuals, however, require higher standards for the success of operative reconstruction that is, the maintenance of full motion and strength and the restoration of stability. The evaluation and management of patients with multidirectional instability, major loss of bone from the glenoid, or a large humeral impression fracture were reviewed. Each of these problems increases the level of complexity of operative reconstruction.

Biomechanics of Shoulder.—Several factors are involved in evaluating a shoulder, including the static stabilizers, such as the articular anatomy, the capsuloligamentous structures, and laxity compared with instability. Dynamic stabilizers that should be understood are the rotator cuff, the long head of the biceps brachi, negative intra-articular pressure, and scapulothoracic motion. Isolated lesions and combined conditions must be identified. Recurrent anterior subluxation or dislocation is the most common form of shoulder instability. Symptomatic glenohumeral instability in more than one direction, such as anteriorly, inferiorly, and posteriorly, is known as multidirection instability. A discrete injury may initiate symptoms, such as repetitive stress on the shoulder from athletic activities or work-related events. Anterior instability is associated with pain in the overhead, abducted, and externally rotated position. Posterior instability is suggested with discomfort with the arm in forward elevation and internal rotation. Pain and paresthesias when carrying heavy objects may be symptoms of inferior instability.

Operation.—Reduction of capsular volume on all sides of the capsule by thickening and overlapping the anterior aspect of the capsule is the most widely used reconstruction for an anterior approach. Balancing the capsular tension on all sides is the goal of treatment. Careful and frequent postoperative follow-up is necessary. For a posterior approach, a variety of skin incisions are used. Patients wear a brace with the shoulder in neutral or slight extension and in slight external rotation after the operation. In several studies, treatment of multidirectional instability with a capsular shift reconstruction has been successful. Humeral impression fractures and loss of glenoid bone are considerably more complex in reconstructions.

Conclusions.—An operation is not necessary for most patients with glenohumeral instability. Most patients with posttraumatic unidirectional anterior instability who need surgery do well after anatomical capsular reconstruction and repair of an associated Bankart avulsion, if one is present. A more complex reconstruction is needed when a patient has severe capsular redundancy or marked loss of glenoid or humeral bone. Biomechanics of the shoulder, operative techniques, and postoperative rehabilitation must be understood to lead to a gratifying result.

▶ This article deals with the relevant biomechanics of multidirectional instability, and severe loss of glenoid and humeral bone. The authors point out that in those patients with severe capsular redundancy or marked loss of glenoid or humeral bone, a more complex reconstruction is required. Apparently implementation of appropriate operative techniques predicated on the biomechanics of the glenohumeral joint can usually lead to a gratifying result. The original article is recommended reading for those performing shoulder surgery.

J.S. Torg, M.D.

Assessment of Failed Arthroscopic Anterior Labral Repairs: Findings at Open Surgery

Mologne TS, McBride MT, Lapoint JM (Naval Med Ctr, San Diego, Calif)
Am J Sports Med 25:813–817, 1997   2–20

Background.—Arthroscopic techniques have recently been used to repair traumatic anterior glenohumeral instability. Twenty patients with postoperative instability after arthroscopic Bankart repair were examined at open Bankart stabilization to determine the cause of persistent instability.

Study Design.—A retrospective review of patients who underwent open shoulder stabilization procedures between 1990 and 1995 detected 19 male and 1 female patient who had previously had an arthroscopic stabilization procedure. At the time of the arthroscopic stabilization procedure, 15 patients had recurrent dislocations and 5 had recurrent subluxations. The arthroscopic procedure was performed with transglenoid sutures in 10 patients, 8-mm Suretac devices in 7, G-II Mitek Suture Anchors in 2, and an arthroscopic Dyonics screw in 1. Five patients recalled an injury before recurrence of instability. The average time from the arthroscopic procedure to the open procedure was 17.9 months.

Findings.—Of the 20 patients in the study group, 12 had healed Bankart lesions and 8 had persistent lesions. Fifteen had attenuated and redundant anterior capsules. Seven of 9 patients with postarthroscopic dislocation had persistent Bankart lesions, whereas only 1 of 11 with subluxation had a persistent Bankart lesion. The presence of a persistent Bankart lesion was correlated with postarthroscopic dislocation. All 11 patients with postarthroscopic recurrent subluxation had redundant anterior capsules.

Conclusion.—Twenty patients who had undergone open shoulder stabilization for recurrent instability after arthroscopic shoulder stabilization were reviewed to evaluate their capsulolabral lesions. The presence of a persistent Bankart lesion was significantly correlated with postarthroscopic dislocation, whereas the presence of persistent capsular laxity was significantly correlated with postarthroscopic subluxation. Failure to successfully treat either the Bankart lesion or capsular laxity arthroscopically may lead to persistent postoperative instability.

Two- to Five-Year Followup of Arthroscopic Bankart Reconstruction Using a Suture Anchor Technique

Koss S, Richmond JC, Woodward JS Jr (Tufts Univ, Boston; New England Med Ctr Hosp, Boston)
Am J Sports Med 25:809–812, 1997   2–21

Background.—A Bankart lesion—separation of the inferior glenohumeral ligament–anterior labral complex from the glenoid rim—is found in the majority of traumatic anterior shoulder dislocations. The most common repair technique is the open Bankart procedure, although shoulder arthroscopic techniques are now being used. Results of an arthroscopic procedure used to repair anterior shoulder instability were described.

Methods.—From 1990 to 1993, arthroscopic Bankart reconstruction was performed on 27 patients with recurrent anterior shoulder instability. The average number of shoulder dislocations before surgery in this study group was 5. The surgical technique consisted of arthroscopic placement of suture anchors along the anteroinferior glenoid, which were used to repair the capsulolabral detachment. Of the 27 patients in this series, 20 returned for a follow-up visit 26–64 months after surgery. This consisted of a physical examination, pain and function questionnaires, and radiographs. Two patients were interviewed by telephone. Five patients in whom the procedure was unsuccessful had undergone open surgical stabilization.

Results.—The average Bankart rating score in this study group was 88, with 70% having good-to-excellent results and 30% having fair-to-poor results. The average UCLA shoulder function score was 32. The average loss of external rotation in abduction was 1 degree. The procedure failed in 8 patients who had recurrence of shoulder instability. In 7 of the failures, there were repeat traumatic events. Multivariate analysis indicated that success was correlated with fewer shoulder dislocations before repair.

Conclusion.—After arthroscopic Bankart reconstruction using a Mitek suture anchor technique, a follow-up of 2 to 5 years revealed a 30% failure rate with recurrent shoulder instability. In 7 of these 8 failures, there was repeat trauma. Because of this high failure rate, this arthroscopic stabilization technique is not recommended for patients who plan to return to contact sports. It should be considered for patients who value maintenance of external rotation or improved cosmetic results.

▶ These 2 articles establish additional criteria for implementation of arthroscopic stabilization of the unstable glenohumeral joint. Mologne et al. emphasize the importance of successfully managing a Bankart lesion for capsular laxity to prevent postoperative instability. Koss et al. point out that postoperative dislocations occur more frequently in those who had multiple preoperative dislocations. They also advise that the technique be limited to patients not returning to contact sports.

J.S. Torg, M.D.

Operative Treatment of Irreparable Rupture of the Subscapularis
Wirth MA, Rockwood CA Jr (Univ of Texas, San Antonio)
J Bone Joint Surg Am 79-A:722–731, 1997   2–22

Objective.—Whereas irreparable tear of the subscapularis is rare, its rupture is believed to be a contributing factor to continuing instability of the glenohumeral joint. The procedure, together with results of a transfer of the pectoralis muscle to treat an irreparable tear of the subscapularis

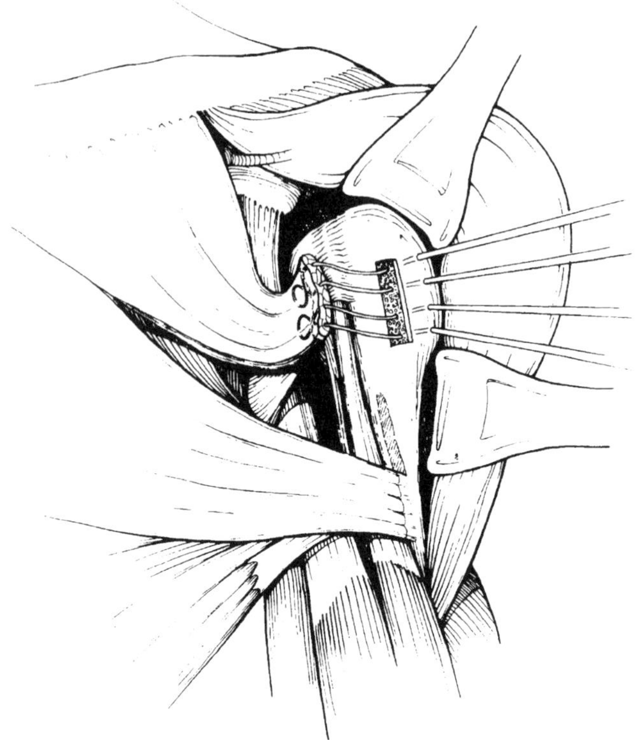

FIGURE 3.—Stay sutures, which had been placed in the pectoralis major, are passed into the bone trough and out through the cortical drill holes. (Courtesy of Wirth MA, Rockwood CA Jr: Operative treatment of irreparable rupture of the subscapularis. *J Bone Joint Surg Am* 79-A:722–731, 1997.)

muscle associated with symptomatic anterior glenohumeral subluxation or dislocation, was discussed.

Methods.—Reconstruction of the scapularis for irreparable tear was performed on 13 patients (6 women), 10 of whom had had 2 to 6 previous reconstructions.

> *Technique.*—The deltopectoral muscles are retracted and the clavipectoral fascia is divided while protecting the musculocutaneous and axillary nerves. The capsule is divided from the superior glenohumeral ligament to the inferior aspect of the capsule. The joint is cleaned and explored for abnormalities. Capsular imbrication is performed, if necessary, and capsular reconstruction is begun by double-breasting the medial aspect. The superior end of the pectoralis major tendon is released from its insertion, and its lateral edge is sutured with 3 or 4 stay sutures. A 5 × 25–mm trough is cut into the internally rotated proximal uterus. Three or 4 holes are drilled in the lateral edge of the trough, Dacron sutures are passed

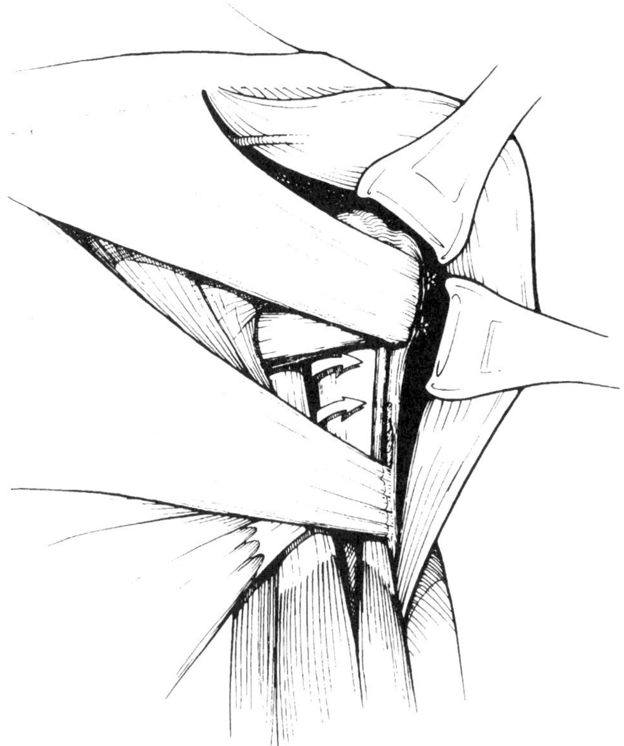

FIGURE 4.—The pectoralis major tendon is transferred lateral to the bicipital groove and is secured into the bone trough. (Courtesy of Wirth MA, Rockwood CA Jr: Operative treatment of irreparable rupture of the subscapularis. *J Bone Joint Surg Am* 79-A:722–731, 1997).

through, and the tendon is pulled into the trough (Fig 3). The tendon is secured (Fig 4).

The pectoralis minor tendon is similarly transferred across the bicipital groove and secured into a bone trough carved into the distal half of the greater tuberosity. The patient begins gentle pendulum exercises on the first postoperative day, progressing to passive flexion exercises 4–6 times a day. After 2 weeks of shoulder immobilization, the patient begins rehabilitation. At 2 weeks, the sutures and sling are removed, and the patient begins functional exercises for 6–8 weeks. After that, the patient begins a formal strengthening program.

Results.—Patients were followed for an average of 5 years. Results were satisfactory in 10 shoulders, which showed active contraction of the transferred pectoralis major muscle and decreased anterior instability, and unsatisfactory in 3.

Conclusion.—Transfer of the pectoralis major muscle is an effective procedure for reconstruction of irreparable rupture of the subscapularis and provides satisfactory functional results.

▶ In concluding that transfer of the pectoralis muscle is effective for reconstruction of the shoulder in patients with irreparable rupture of the subscapularis, the authors attribute increased glenohumeral stability to "a checkrein effect of the transferred muscle-tendon unit, similar to that found after a Magnuson-Stack procedure . . ." Here we have a major inconsistency in that, in the past. the position of the senior author has been that procedures that were not anatomical were contraindicated. It appears that we are never too old to recognize and/or learn new tricks.

J.S. Torg, M.D.

Subacromial Impingement Syndrome

Bigliani LU, Levine WN (Columbia-Presbyterian Med Ctr, New York; Univ of Maryland, Baltimore)
J Bone Joint Surg Am 79-A:1854–1868, 1997   2–23

Introduction.—For patients with shoulder pain, subacromial impingement syndrome has become an increasingly common diagnosis. Because the clinical presentation may be confusing, it is difficult to diagnose. It must be differentiated from glenohumeral instability, cervical radiculitis, calcific tendinitis, adhesive capsulitis, degenerative joint disease, isolated acromioclavicular osteoarthrosis, and nerve compression.

Etiologic Factors.—The etiologic factors can be extrinsic (extratendinous) or intrinsic (intratendinous) and may also be characterized as primary or secondary. A number of soft-tissue structures are situated between 2 rigid structures that move within the subacromial space, and interposed between 2 osseous structures are the rotator cuff tendons, the long head of the biceps tendons, the bursa, and the coracoacromial ligament. Intrinsic factors include muscle weakness, overuse of the shoulder, and degenerative tendinopathy. Extrinsic factors include glenohumeral instability, degeneration of the acromioclavicular joint, impingement by the coracoacromial ligament, coracoid impingement, os acromial, and impingement on the posterosuperior aspect of the glenoid.

Evaluation and Diagnosis.—In the anterosuperior part of the shoulder, subacromial impingement syndrome is probably overdiagnosed. An integral component is taking the history of the patient, with pain being the most common symptom with accompanying weakness and stiffness. Patients should also have a physical examination and a radiographic evaluation. Other imaging modalities may include US, MR imaging, or arthroscopy.

Treatment Options.—Often, nonoperative treatment is successful, with most patients who have impingement syndrome recovering with nonoperative intervention, including modification of activity, the use of nonsteroidal anti-inflammatory medications, subacromial injections of steroids, and physical therapy. If symptoms persist for more than 6 months, operative treatment with open or arthroscopic acromioplasty may be necessary, and both treatments have been associated with a low rate of complications and a high percentage of successful results.

▶ This article is a comprehensive presentation of the etiology, diagnosis, and nonoperative and operative management of subacromial impingement syndrome. It is a most comprehensive presentation of the subject matter and is recommended reading for those dealing with athletes with shoulder complaints.

J.S. Torg, M.D.

Non-operative Treatment of Subacromial Impingement Syndrome
Morrison DS, Frogameni AD, Woodworth P (Southern California Ctr for Sports Medicine, Long Beach)
J Bone Joint Surg Am 79-A:732–737, 1997   2–24

Objective.—A study of the outcome after nonoperative treatment of subacromial impingement syndrome also assessed the influence of sex, shoulder dominance, acromial morphology, tenderness of the acromioclavicular joint, age, and duration of symptoms.

Methods.—Subacromial impingement syndrome was diagnosed in 636 shoulders of 616 patients (230 females), aged 15–81 years, between 1985 and 1991. Patients were treated with anti-inflammatory medication and given a therapist-supervised stretching and exercise program which was to be carried out at home after discharge until at least 4 weeks after the shoulder became pain free. Patients were evaluated every 3–4 weeks.

Results.—During the first 6 weeks, 56 patients had complete symptomatic relief. Results were excellent in 186 patients and good in 227. There was no improvement in 172 patients, who subsequently underwent decompression at an average of 7 months after beginning treatment. Symptoms recurred during the follow-up in 74 of 413 patients with satisfactory results; they resolved spontaneously or after resumption of the exercise program. There were no significant differences in outcome based on sex or shoulder dominance. Satisfactory results were obtained in 91% of patients with a type I acromion, 68% of patients with a type II acromion, and 64% of patients with a type III acromion. Patients with a type I acromion had significantly better results than did patients with either a type II or type III acromion. More patients with symptoms for less than 4 weeks (78% of 86 patients) had a satisfactory result compared with patients who had symptoms for 1–6 months (63% of 228 patients) or patients who had symptoms for more than 6 months (67% of 302 patients). Patients aged 20 years or less had significantly better results that did patients aged 21–64 or patients aged over 60. Significantly more patients with acute symptoms (78%) than patients with nonacute symptoms (63%) or chronic symptoms (67%) had satisfactory results.

Conclusion.—Age and acromion type—but not shoulder dominance, sex, or concomitant tenderness of the acromioclavicular joint—significantly affected outcome after nonoperative treatment of subacromial impingement syndrome.

▶ The title of this article is somewhat misleading in that 28% of the patients eventually had arthroscopic subacromial decompression. Perhaps the judicious use of subacromial steroid injection would have reduced the surgical population even further. To be noted, the authors attributed much of the success to a physical therapy program directed at increasing the depressor effect of the rotator cuff while avoiding any increase in the elevating effect of the deltoid.

J.S. Torg, M.D.

A Taping Technique for the Treatment of Acromioclavicular Joint Sprains: A Case Study
Shamus JL, Shamus EC (HealthSouth Sports Medicine and Rehabilitation Ctr, Plantation, Fla; Lynn Univ, Boca Raton, Fla)
J Orthop Sports Phys Ther 25:390–394, 1997   2–25

Background.—Conservative treatment of grade III injuries to the acromioclavicular joint usually consists of arm immobilization in a sling for 2 to 4 weeks, followed by physical therapy. However, initial rehabilitation is compromised when sling removal exacerbates the patient's symptoms. The resultant increase in pain results in muscle guarding and spasms that then limit the extent of range of motion and strengthening exercises. This article describes a taping technique designed to decrease the patient's pain to facilitate gains in range of motion, strength, and function.

Technique.—After the sling is removed, the clinician measures and cuts hypafix tape to fit from the insertion of the middle deltoid inferiorly to 2.5 cm proximal to the acromioclavicular joint superiorly, and the coracoid process of the scapula anteriorly to the spine of the scapula posteriorly. The tape is laid gently on the skin, and leukotape is measured and cut to form 2 pieces 0.5 cm shorter than the first piece of hypafix tape, and 2 pieces 0.5 cm shorter than the second piece of hypafix tape. The first piece of leukotape is anchored at the deltoid insertion and pulled superiorly with enough force so that the arm is supported firmly. The clinician approximates the joint simultaneously with the other hand by supporting the elbow and pushing the humerus superiorly. The patient's shoulder must be relaxed during this maneuver, and wrinkles should appear in the hypafix. The upper trapezius muscle belly should not be taped, because it interferes with muscle recruitment and is very

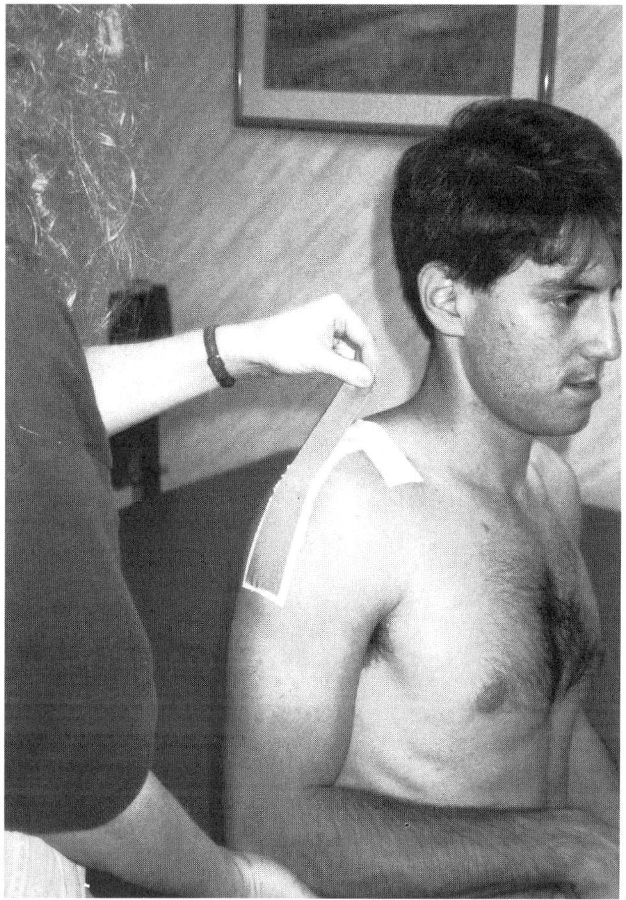

FIGURE 2.—Application of the first piece of leukotape. (Courtesy of Shamus JL, Shamus EC: A taping technique for the treatment of acromioclavicular joint sprains: A case study. *J Orthop Sports Phys Ther* 25(6):390–394, 1997.)

uncomfortable (Fig 2). The clinician applies the second piece of leukotape beginning over the coracoid process, pulling posteriorly to secure the tape near the spine of the scapula. This piece of tape should minimize superior translation of the distal end of the calvicle, serving as an anchor for the first piece of tape (Fig 3). The leukotaping is repeated to provide extra reinforcement and extend the efficacy of the tape over time.

Findings and Conclusions.—The benefits of this taping procedure appear promising in the 2 patients described. Physical therapists are urged to explore the benefits of this technique and its possible application to grades I and II sprains.

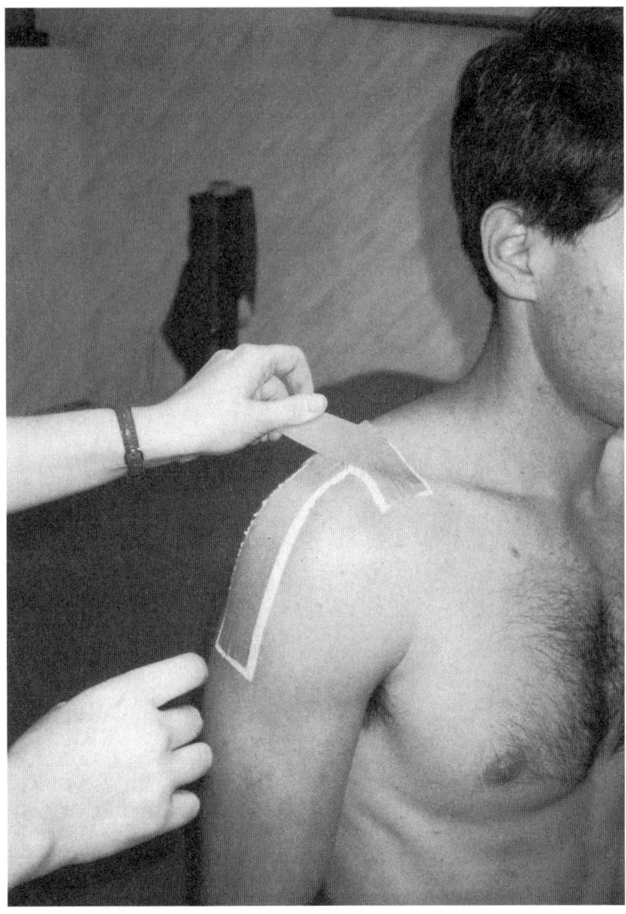

FIGURE 3.—Application of the second piece of leukotape. (Courtesy of Shamus JL, Shamus EC: A taping technique for the treatment of acromioclavicular joint sprains: A case study. *J Orthop Sports Phys Ther* 25(6):390–394, 1997.)

▶ The authors describe a method of taping grade III acromioclavicular joint sprains to relieve pain and improve mobility. The techniques they describe appear promising and deserve further investigation and trials. The authors caution us that the upper trapezius muscle belly should not be taped and, when the sling is discontinued, the involved extremity should not be used for lifting until adequate healing has occurred.

F.J. George, A.T.C., P.T.

Resection Arthroplasty of the Sternoclavicular Joint

Rockwood CA Jr, Groh GI, Wirth MA, et al (Univ of Texas, San Antonio)
J Bone Joint Surg Am 79-A:387–393, 1997   2–26

Introduction.—Surgical procedures on the sternoclavicular joint must preserve, repair, or reconstruct the costoclavicular ligament to maintain the stability of the medial portion of the clavicle in relation to the manubrium. Cephalad displacement and instability of the remaining portion of the clavicle can occur with resection of the medial portion of the clavicle if the resection included a portion of the clavicle that was lateral to the costoclavicular ligament. The results of resection of the medial portion of the clavicle were reviewed in 2 groups of patients, one group who had the ligament maintained and the other who had the ligament reconstructed.

Methods.—A retrospective review was conducted of 15 patients who had resection of the medial end of the clavicle to treat a painful sternoclavicular joint. Eight patients had a primary costoclavicular ligament that was left intact and 7 patients had revision of a failed arthroplasty of the sternoclavicular joint in which the costoclavicular ligament was reconstructed. Reconstruction involves using nonabsorbable suture passed around the remaining medial end of the clavicle and its periosteal tube (Fig 7). At an average of 7.7 years after surgery, the results of these 2 groups were compared. Routine radiographs and a CT scan were used to evaluate each patient's sternoclavicular joint and to compare it with the contralateral, normal joint.

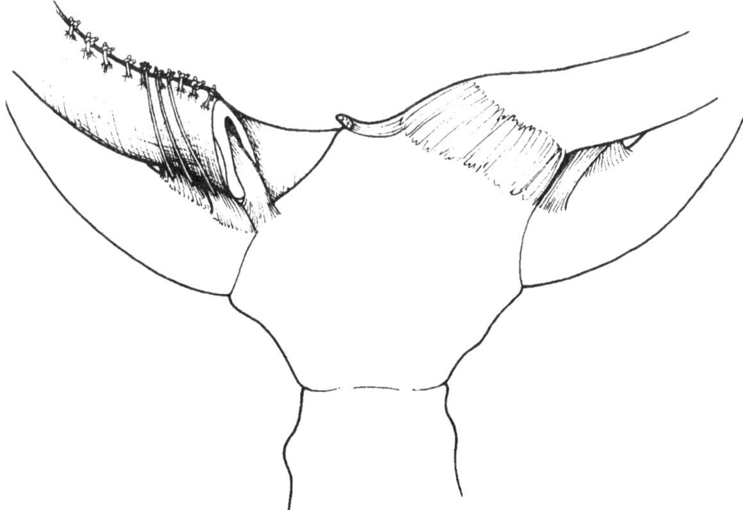

FIGURE 7.—Illustration demonstrating how closure of the periosteal tube includes sutures that pass through the stump of the old costoclavicular ligament on the first rib when the costoclavicular ligament is not intact. It may be necessary to pass sutures through drill holes or around the first rib for stability. (Courtesy of Rockwood CA Jr, Groh GI, Wirth MA, et al: Resection arthroplasty of the sternoclavicular joint. *J Bone Joint Surg Am* 79-A, 387–393, 1997.)

Results.—Excellent results were seen in all 8 patients who had their costoclavicular ligament left intact. In all but 2 patients, the pain had resolved completely, and 3 patients had slight limitation in the performance of strenuous activities or sports requiring overhead motion. In the other group, 3 patients had an excellent result, 3 had a fair result, and 1 had a poor result.

Conclusion.—To obtain a satisfactory result, preservation or reconstruction of the costoclavicular ligament is necessary at the time of resection of the medial portion of the clavicle.

▶ To be noted, spontaneous traumatic anterior dislocations and subluxations of the sternoclavicular joint are nonsurgical problems. It is further pointed out that persistent traumatic anterior displacement of the medial end of the clavicle requires surgery only in those patients who have continued severe pain and marked functional impairment. Critical to the operative procedure is stabilization of the medial portion of the clavicle to the first rib. Surgery is also indicated for chronic unreduced posterior dislocation because of the potential for compression and/or erosion of the great vessels, trachea, or esophagus by the medial end of the clavicle. Also, the potential to injure these structures, particularly the great vessels, during surgery must be recognized and injury avoided.

J.S. Torg, M.D.

The Efficacy of an Injection of Steroids for Medial Epicondylitis: A Prospective Study of Sixty Elbows

Stahl S, Kaufman T (Rambam Med Ctr, Haifa, Israel)
J Bone Joint Surg Am 79-A:1648–1652, 1997   2–27

Introduction.—The use of nonoperative measures is an accepted approach to medial epicondylitis, a clinical entity characterized by pain in the median aspect of the elbow. Some studies have reported success when patients received an injection of methylprednisolone, but the use of a local injection of steroids is controversial. A prospective, randomized, double-blind study examined the short- and long-term effects of a single injection of methylprednisolone to treat medial epicondylitis.

Methods.—All 58 patients (60 elbows) enrolled in the study had isolated epicondylitis. Physical examinations were performed and radiographs obtained in all cases. A pain-phase scale was used to assess pain before the injection and at 6 weeks, 3 months and 1 year after. Patients also evaluated intensity of pain on a 10-point scale. All patients had failed to respond to conservative therapy, and none had previously been managed with injections of steroids. Thirty elbows were treated with an injection of 40 mg of methylprednisolone with 1 mL of 1% lidocaine; 30 controls elbows received an injection of lidocaine and saline solution.

Results.—All patients were available for follow-up. The 2 groups were similar in age, gender, duration of symptoms, and number of dominant limbs involved. Six weeks after the injection, the mean pain-phase score was significantly lower for the experimental group than for the control group. Mean scores did not differ significantly, however, at 3 months or 1 year. The 2 groups were also similar in mean values for intensity of pain during follow-up. The injection of methylprednisolone did not cause local complications.

Conclusion.—Compared with controls, patients with medial epicondylitis who received an injection of methylprednisolone had a significantly better pain-phase score and a significantly faster decrease in the intensity of pain. Control and experimental groups had similar outcomes at 3 months and 1 year, suggesting that the benefits of a local steroid injection are short-term. Subsequent improvement in both groups would appear to reflect the natural history of medial epicondylitis.

▶ This well-devised study has effectively differentiated between pain resulting from normal daily activities and that elicited by more strenuous activities. It should be pointed out that the authors have failed to state whether the methylprednisolone preparation was in crystalline or suspension form. Nevertheless, their conclusion that "the local injection of a steroid has only short-term beneficial effects in the treatment of medial epicondylitis" is in keeping with my own clinical experience. I also agree that "the institution of other well known therapeutic modalities, such as rest, physical therapy, and the use of non-steroidal anti-inflammatory agents are probably the best ways to treat this clinical entity."

J.S. Torg, M.D.

Salvage Surgery for Lateral Tennis Elbow
Organ SW, Nirschl RP, Kraushaar BS, et al (Nirschl Orthopaedic Sportsmedicine Clinic, Arlington, Va)
Am J Sports Med 25:746–750, 1997   2–28

Objective.—A large number of patients fail surgical intervention for repair of lateral tennis elbow, possibly because surgeons fail to identify and resect pathologic tissue. Records of patients who had failed surgical intervention for lateral tennis elbow were analyzed retrospectively before salvage surgery.

Methods.—Salvage surgery was performed between 1979 and 1994 in 35 elbows in 34 patients (16 men), aged 28 to 70 (see Fig 1). Sixteen patients (17 elbows) were workers' compensation patients, 12 were athletes, and 6 were nonworkers' compensation patients with occupational injuries. Previous surgeries included 19 slide and release procedures, 6 slide and release procedures with partial resection of the annular ligament (Bosworth), 7 unknown procedures, 2 primary radial nerve decompressions, and 1 Nirschl procedure.

Results.—At surgery, 34 elbows showed residual tendonitis in the extensor carpi radialis brevis tendon origin, with absence of intervention

A
Lateral
epicondyle

B
Extensor carpi
radialis longus
Lateral
epicondyle
Damage to
extensor aponeurosis
due to prior surgery

C
Extensor carpi
radialis longus
Extensor carpi
radialis brevis tendon
Lateral
epicondyle
Degenerative
tendinosis
original pathology
Damage to extensor aponeurosis
due to prior surgery

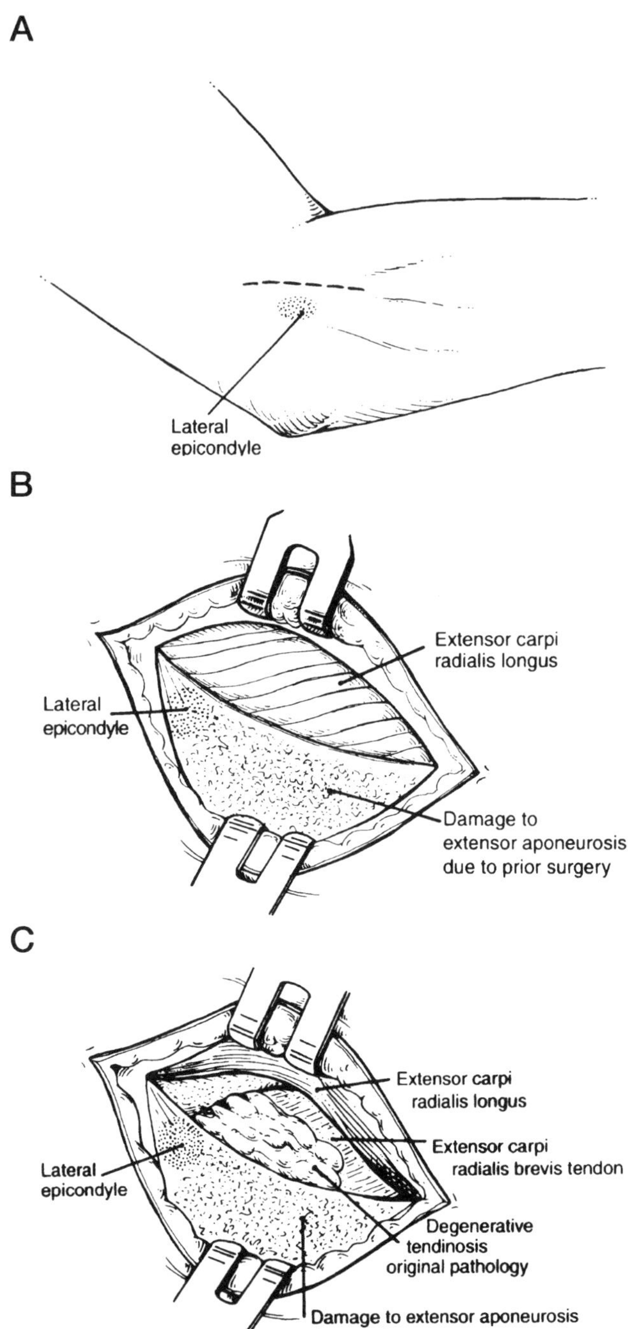

(Continued)

FIGURE 1 (cont.)

D

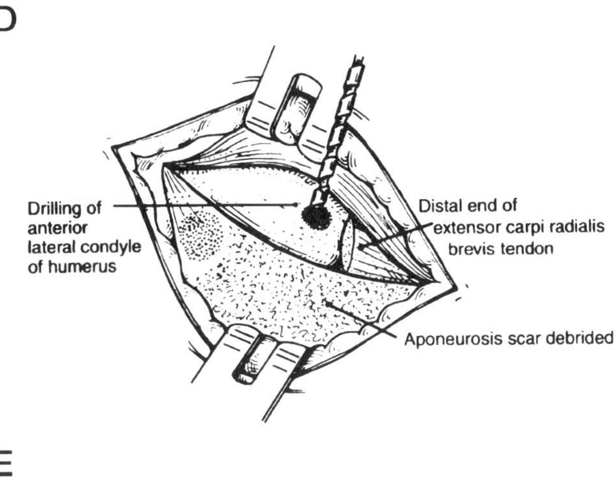

E

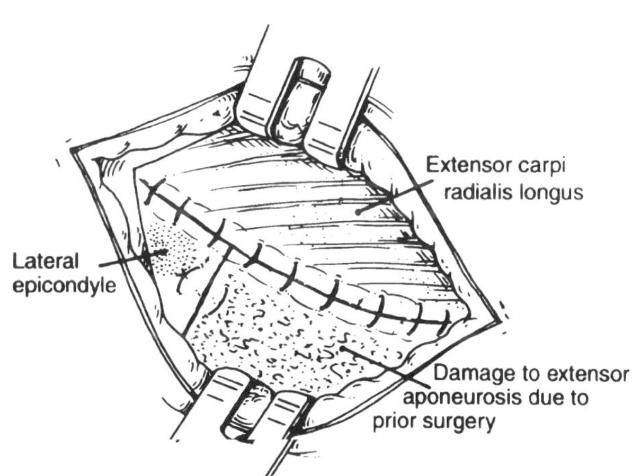

FIGURE 1.—Salvage surgical procedure for lateral tennis elbow. A, incision of damaged extensor exposure. C, deep exposure allows identification of damaged extensor carpi radialis brevis tendon. D, excision of the damaged tendon and vascular enhancement. E, closure (if aponeurosis is unstable, suture repair into bone). (Courtesy of Organ SW, Nirschl RP, Kraushaar BS, et al: Salvage surgery for lateral tennis elbow. *Am J Sports Med* 25:746–750, 1997.)

during previous surgery in 27 elbows, and incomplete intervention in 7. In these latter 7, extensor carpi radialis brevis tendon origin surgical trauma was apparent. Scarred or altered areas over the extensor aponeurosis were débrided or repaired in 34 elbows. Results of salvage surgery were excellent in 20 elbows, good in 9, fair in 5, and poor in 1, at an average of 64 months after surgery. Patients with good or excellent results were able to return to their pre-injury work or activity levels.

Conclusion.—Identification and resection of pathologic tissue, usually seen in the extensor carpi radialis brevis tendon, improves outcome after salvage surgery for lateral tennis elbow. Release operations that weaken the extensor aponeurosis should be avoided.

▶ In addition to analyzing the need and describing the preferred technique for revision of failed surgical intervention for tennis elbow, the authors make two important points. First, they emphasize that most patients with lateral tennis elbow, including those with incapacitating symptoms after prior surgery, will respond to an adequate rehabilitation program and not require surgery. Second, to avoid initial surgical failure, the authors recommend that release of the extensor aponeurosis be avoided.

J.S. Torg, M.D.

Management of an Uncomplicated Posterior Elbow Dislocation

Blackard D, Sampson J-A (Northern Michigan Univ, Marquette; Fairview Health Systems, Cleveland, Ohio)
J Athletic Train 32:63–67, 1997   2–29

Background.—Traditional management of uncomplicated posterior elbow dislocation is splint immobilization for several weeks. Recent research indicates that a shorter period of immobilization and early active motion may be more beneficial. It is known that extended immobilization can have negative effects on the human body, such as muscle atrophy, joint cartilage ulceration, osteoporosis, skin necrosis, infection, thrombophlebitis, contracture tendon collagen disorganization, and collagen fibril size reduction. Of the major joints, the elbow is the second most frequently dislocated joint, the dislocation often occurring during recreational activity or sports. The use of passive extension is one contraindication to early mobilization of posterior elbow dislocations. The case of a world-class competitive athlete with an uncomplicated posterior elbow dislocation is discussed, as well as the rehabilitation program.

> *Case Report.*—A young female athlete who participated in freestyle ski events as a member of the United States ski team sustained an uncomplicated posterior dislocation of her left elbow during competition. Reduction of the elbow was performed at the on-site first aid station, and a compression bandage and sling were applied. Rehabilitation consisted of 5 phases (Table 2). In phase 1, the main goal was to decrease inflammation then maintain strength and range of motion in the wrist, hand, and shoulder. In phase 2, treatment goals included active range of motion with gravity eliminated, proprioceptive awareness, and isometric strengthening. In phase 3, the treatment goals were to increase active range of motion with gravity, increase proprioceptive awareness, and begin isotonic strengthening exercises. In phase 4, the goals were to begin

TABLE 2.—Goals and Phases of Rehabilitation of an Uncomplicated Posterior Elbow Dislocation

Goals	Phases of Rehabilitation				
	I	II	III	IV	V
Swelling	Severe	Moderate	Moderate	Mild	Minimal
Strength	—	Isometrics	Isotonics	Isokinetics/functional activity	Return to activity
Range of Motion (Ext-Flex)	Sling	Active ROM (no gravity)	Active ROM (with gravity)	Passive ROM	Normal
	30°–125°	27°–140°	20°–140°	5°–140°	5°–140°
Proprioceptive neuromuscular facilitation	—	D1 flexion D1 extension D2 flexion D2 extension (no resistance)	D1 flexion D1 extension D2 flexion D2 extension	D1 flexion D1 extension D2 flexion D2 extension	—
			Elbow "Punch" Elbow "Pull" Elbow "Extension" Elbow "Flexion" (with resistance)	Elbow "Punch" Elbow "Pull" Elbow "Extension" Elbow "Flexion" (with resistance)	
Days	8	5	6	13	13
Total days postinjury	8	13	19	32	45

(Courtesy of Blackard D, Sampson J-A: Management of an uncomplicated posterior elbow dislocation. *J Athletic Train* 32:63–67, 1997.)

isokinetic and functional activity by using various exercise and modality techniques. The goal of phase 5 was a return to full activity with a physician's approval. Full activity included skiing, trampoline jumping, aerial stunts from ramps, skiing the bumps in moguls, and pole flips in ballet.

Discussion.—The rehabilitation of this athlete with an uncomplicated posterior dislocation of the elbow involved limited immobilization and early active motion. This athlete returned to World Championship competition 6 weeks after the injury, had no long-term complications at one year, and competed at the Winter Olympics the following year. The goal of rehabilitation in athletic training is safe and rapid return to competition. This rehabilitation program was safe and effective. The athlete's high motivation affected the success of this program.

▶ The authors have presented an aggressive management and rehabilitation program for an uncomplicated posterior elbow dislocation. The elbow was immobilized with only a sling for 11 days, and a posterior splint was never used. This treatment allowed for early range of motion and strengthening exercises and a much quicker total rehabilitation time. Passive elbow extension exercises are contradicted in the early phases of rehabilitation.

F.J. George, A.T.C., P.T.

Subacute Scaphoid Fractures: A Closer Look at Closed Treatment
Mack GR, Wilckens JH, McPherson SA (Naval Med Ctr, San Diego, Calif)
Am J Sports Med 26:56–58, 1998   2–30

Introduction.—Scaphoid fracture is a relatively common injury in the young athletic and military population. A union rate greater than 90% is reported in most studies. The best treatment for subacute scaphoid fracture is still not known. These are fractures that are recognized at least 4 weeks but not more than 6 months, after injury. The efficacy of nonoperative treatment of subacute fractures treated by cast immobilization during a 5-year period was determined retrospectively.

Methods.—A total of 23 subacute scaphoid fractures were treated in a 5-year period. Between 4 weeks and 6 months of injury, all patients sought medical attention, and their fractures were classified according to location and stability. There were 19 patients followed up until radiographic union or until closed treatment was abandoned.

Results.—In an average of 19 weeks with a range of 11–38 weeks, 9 of 10 stable, subacute middle-third scaphoid fractures healed with cast immobilization. These were compared with a randomly selected group of acute middle-third fractures that healed in an average of 10 weeks, with a range of 6–13 weeks. In an average of 20 weeks, 5 of 6 unstable, subacute middle-third fractures healed. A symptomatic humpback deformity treated by cheilectomy was found in one of these. Only 1 of 3 subacute proximal-third fractures healed after 29 weeks of closed treatment.

Conclusions.—Cast treatment is successful with stable, subacute middle-third scaphoid fractures, but may take twice as long as stable acute middle-third fractures. Closed treatment is less likely to result in satisfactory healing with unstable, subacute middle-third scaphoid fractures and subacute proximal-third fractures. An open reduction and internal fixation of the fracture may be elected by the preseason athlete with a subacute, middle-third nondisplaced scaphoid fracture, whereas cast immobilization may be the preferred treatment for a postseason athlete.

▶ This article serves to further define criteria for open vs. closed treatment of scaphoid fractures. To be noted, the authors' recommendation for closed treatment of nondisplaced subacute fractures distal to the junction of the proximal and middle thirds involved use of a long thumb-spike cast for the first 6 weeks. Also, immobilization of the wrist is performed in slight radial deviation.

J.S. Torg, M.D.

3 Injuries to the Lower Limbs

Fasciotomy of the Posterior Femoral Muscle Compartment in Athletes
Orava S, Rantanen J, Kujala UM (Hosp Meditori, Turku, Finland; Univ Hosp of
Turku, Finland; Univ of Helsinki)
Int J Sports Med 19:71–75, 1998   3–1

Background.—Acute and chronic compartment syndrome can occur in
athletes as a result of overuse and direct or indirect injuries, and usually
occurs in the lower extremities. Anterior thigh compartment syndrome is
usually associated with acute complicating fractures or severe contusion
trauma. Exercise-induced femoral compartment syndrome has been reported in the anterior and posterior compartments.

Methods.—During a period of 13 years, 46 fasciotomies were performed in 46 athletes with chronic pain in the posterior femoral muscle
compartment. In 26 patients, the etiology was exertion. Most patients in
this group competed in endurance sports, and symptoms appeared without
any sudden trauma. In 20 patients, the etiology was trauma. Patients in
this group had a history of hamstring muscle rupture or recurrent injury,
and symptoms were dull pain, stiffness, cramps, and weakness of the
posterior thigh during and after training.

Results.—Preoperatively, conservative treatment did not eliminate
symptoms during a long follow-up period. Posterior fasciotomy (minimum
length 20 cm) of the thigh was performed through 1 or 2 incisions (Fig 1).
Four patients also had simultaneous liberation, division, or suturing of the
muscle scar. Follow-up was 19 months. Results of fasciotomy were good
or excellent in 39 patients, and moderate in 6 patients. One patient had a
poor outcome because of a moderate hamstring rupture that did not
respond to fasciotomy or later plastic repair. Seven patients had complications, but these did not significantly affect final results.

Discussion.—In athletes, pain in the posterior thigh muscle compartment can become chronic and affect training. Most patients respond well
to conservative treatment. Those with recurrent, worsening, or chronic
symptoms and who are physically very active may be candidates for

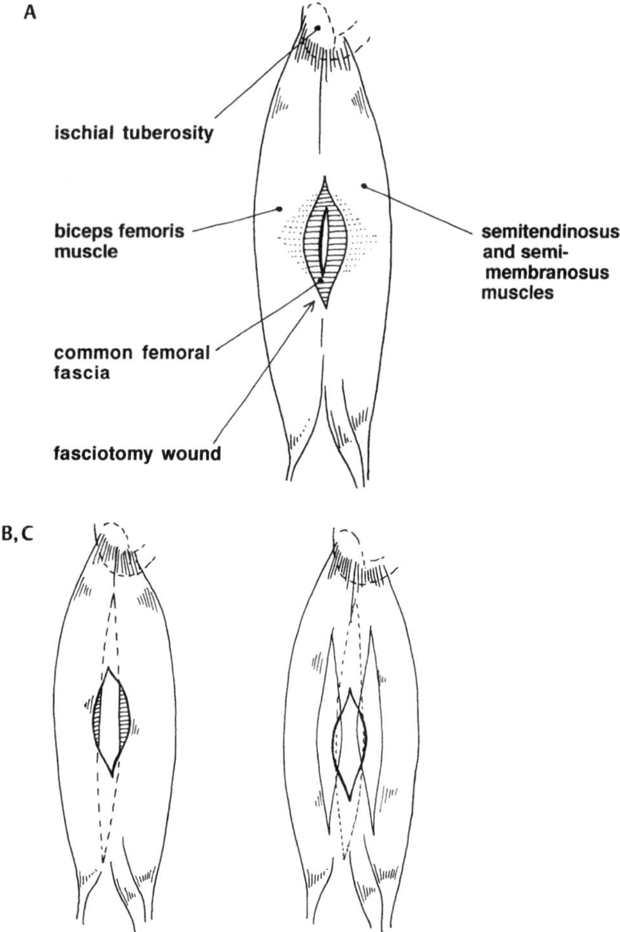

FIGURE 1.—Schematic presentation of the posterior femoral fasciotomy. **A,** division of the common fascia (see transversal fibers). **B,** length of the fascial division. **C,** fasciotomy of biceps femoris and semitendinosus-semimembranosus muscle lodges. (Courtesy of Orava S, Rantanen J, Kujala UM: Fasciotomy of the posterior femoral muscle compartment in athletes. *Int J Sports Med* 19:71–75, 1998. Georg Thieme Verlag.)

fasciotomy. This procedure can help athletes return to their preoperative level of sports activity.

▶ An interesting approach to a problem in which neither the etiology nor pathology has been identified. Described are 46 cases of "chronic exercise-induced or post-traumatic pain syndrome in athletes, located at the posterior femoral muscle compartment" treated with fasciotomy. Although the authors infer that "the dramatic effect of fasciotomy speaks about a compartment syndrome," posterior femoral compartment pressures were not performed. Somewhat disconcerting is the lack of objective indications for surgery. However, not to be denied is that 39 of the 46 athletes had good or excellent results.

J.S. Torg, M.D.

Adverse Neural Tension: A Factor in Repetitive Hamstring Strain?

Turl SE, George KP (Charing Cross Hosp, London; Manchester Metropolitan Univ, Alsager, England)
J Orthop Sports Phys Ther 27:16–21, 1998   3–2

Objective.—Hamstring injuries, common in sprinters, tend to heal slowly and to recur. Because the sciatic nerve is close to the hamstrings, any resulting adverse neural tension could be a causative factor in individual or recurring hamstring injuries. The presence of adverse neural tension was investigated in currently asymptomatic Rugby Union players with a history of repetitive, grade I hamstring strain and a matched control group with no hamstring injury history. The degree of hamstring flexibility associated with injury and/or positive slump in this cohort and the response of those with positive initial slump tests to a period of modified flexibility training were investigated.

Methods.—Fourteen male rugby players, aged 18 to 35 years, with 2 or more grade I hamstring strains in the same leg in the previous 2 years were age-, height-, weight- and playing position–matched with 14 controls with no major lower limb pathology. Active knee extension was performed 3 times on each leg while the subject was lying and a mean angle of extension was recorded for each leg. The slump test was performed by 2 different testers to assess adverse neural tension by measuring knee extension when the knee was passively extended as a tester exerted overpressure on the neck and shoulders. Data were compared between groups.

Results.—Whereas 8 patients (57%) had positive slump test results, none of the controls had positive results. There was no difference in flexibility between groups or between patients with and without a positive slump test.

Conclusion.—The positive slump test results suggest that adverse neural tension could be an underlying cause of repetitive hamstring strain. Reduced flexibility was not a finding in this group. Additional studies need to be conducted to establish a definitive relationship and to assess the value of warm-up techniques on injury incidence and the proper types, if any.

▶ An in-depth review of hamstring injuries was commented on in the 1995 YEAR BOOK.[1] Neural tension may be a factor that should be addressed when evaluating, treating, and rehabilitating hamstring injuries. The tests and exercises are easy to perform and should be included in the affected athletes' warm-up and cool down regimes.

F.J. George, A.T.C., P.T.

Reference

1. 1995 YEAR BOOK OF SPORTS MEDICINE, p 171.

Osteochondritis Dissecans of the Femoral Condyles: Long-term Results of Excision of the Fragment

Anderson AF, Pagnani MJ (Lipscomb Clinic, Nashville, Tenn)
Am J Sports Med 25:830–834, 1997   3–3

Objective.—Osteochondritis dissecans resulting from an injury to subchondral bone that leads to avascular necrosis is generally treated by excision. Results of excision of the fragment in patients with osteochondritis were reviewed.

Methods.—Nineteen patients (4 women) with 20 lesions of the knee, treated by excision of the fragment between 1973 and 1991, were studied for an average of 9 years. Sixteen fragments were grade IV and 4 were grade III. Knees were evaluated using criteria of the International Knee Documentation Committee (IKDC), and the Hughston rating scale. Clinical examinations and anteroposterior, lateral, and tunnel radiographs were performed at follow-up.

Results.—Five patients had no significant pain during strenuous activities, 11 had pain during daily activities, and 3 had pain during light activities. Subjective IKDC criteria identified 4 normal knees, 3 nearly normal, 3 abnormal, and 9 severely abnormal knees. Objective IKDC criteria rated 2 knees as normal, 6 as nearly normal, 4 as abnormal, and 8 as severely abnormal. Whereas preoperative radiographs showed normal joint space in all knees, postoperative radiographs revealed 6 normal knees, 6 knees with mild degenerative changes, and 8 with moderate degenerative changes. The Hughston scale indicated 1 excellent knee, 4 good, 4 fair, 6 poor, and 5 failed knees. Ten knees needed an additional arthroscopic procedure. Results for patients who had symptoms before attaining skeletal maturity were similar to those who had symptoms after attaining skeletal maturity.

Conclusion.—Whereas patients with osteochondritis dissecans who had fragments removed had good short-term results, their long-term results were very poor.

▶ This article certainly makes an interesting and important point. However, in view of the fact that there was no comparison group treated with either replacement of the fragment or bone grafting, the conclusion that "the long-term results are better than those after excision" is not supported by data. I certainly agree that the knee that has excision of the osteochondritic fragment eventually will have arthritic changes. However, over the long term, I do not believe that anyone has demonstrated that those with grafting or replacement of the fragment do better.

J.S. Torg, M.D.

A Comprehensive Treatment Approach for Patellofemoral Pain Syndrome in Young Women

Thomeé R (Sahlgrenska Univ, Göteberg, Sweden)
Phys Ther 77:1690–1703, 1997

3–4

Introduction.—Patellofemoral pain syndrome consists of anterior knee pain without intra-articular pathology, peripatellar tendinitis, or bursitis. It is one of the most common knee problems among physically active adolescents and young adults. Exercise is the most frequently recommended treatment, but the effects of exercise programs on this syndrome are not well documented. In a group of patients with patellofemoral pain syndrome, the effects of a comprehensive treatment approach consisting of an educational and training component were evaluated by analyzing physical activity level, pain, and muscle function. A treatment program of predominantly isometric contractions was compared with a treatment program consisting of predominantly eccentric contractions.

Methods.—There were 40 female patients, aged 15–28 years, who had patellofemoral pain syndrome. They were assigned to a group using isometric muscle contractions or a group using eccentric muscle contractions (Fig 1). They participated in a 12-week program that included education and training. They were evaluated for physical activity pain and muscle function at 3 and 12 months.

Results.—Between the 2 groups, no differences were found, except in one of the torque measurements. In both groups after treatment, there was a reduction in pain and improvements in torque, vertical jumping ability, and physical activity level. Eighty-five percent of patients were able to participate in sports without having pain at the 12-month follow-up, with 37 patients rating their overall knee function as good or excellent.

Conclusions.—Spontaneous recovery over time, education given to the participants, the pain monitoring system, the adjusted physical activity, and the gradually progressive training program may have resulted in the improvements seen in the study patients. Monitoring of pain and gradual progression of load and repetitions of lower-extremity exercises seem to be warranted in training programs for patients with patellofemoral pain syndrome.

▶ Patellofemoral pain syndrome is more common in women than in men. There are several factors related to the syndrome. Common causes include patellar malalignment, quadriceps flexibility, and quadriceps strength deficits. This study compared 2 types of strength training programs, isometric and eccentric, on self-reported knee function, pain, sports participation, and strength. The author found both types of strength training programs to be equally effective in reducing pain, and increasing strength and physical activity level after 12 weeks of treatment and after the 12-month follow up. However, no control group was recruited for comparison purposes, so the improvements may have resulted from expected recovery over time. Also, several other types of treatment were included in the training program,

EXERCISES USED IN THE TRAINING PROGRAM FOR PATELLOFEMORAL PAIN SYNDROME

Exercises used only by the group doing isometric contractions

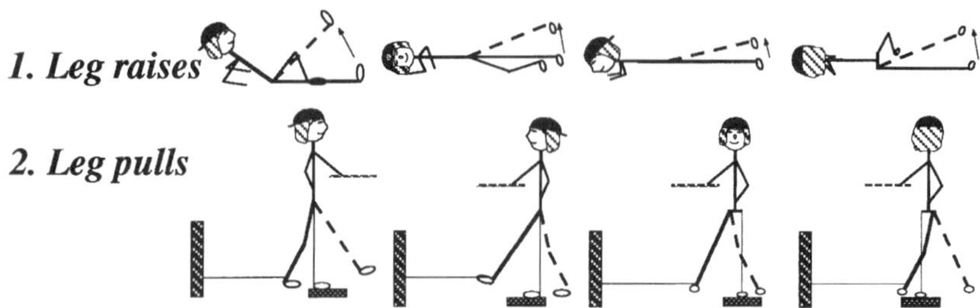

Exercises used only by the group doing eccentric contractions

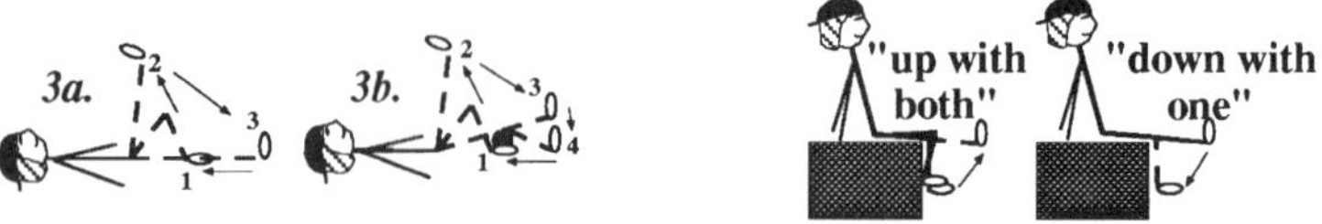

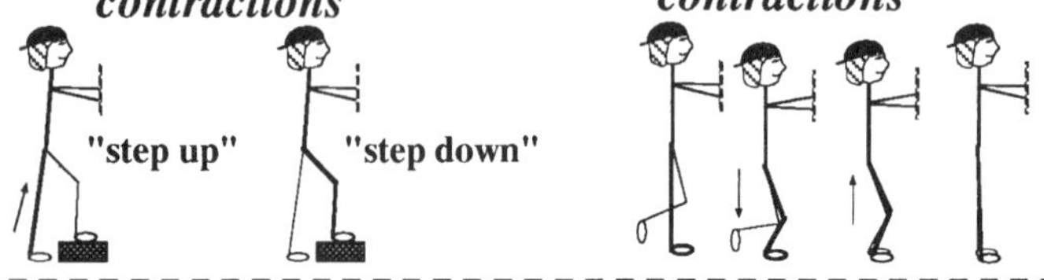

Exercises used by both groups

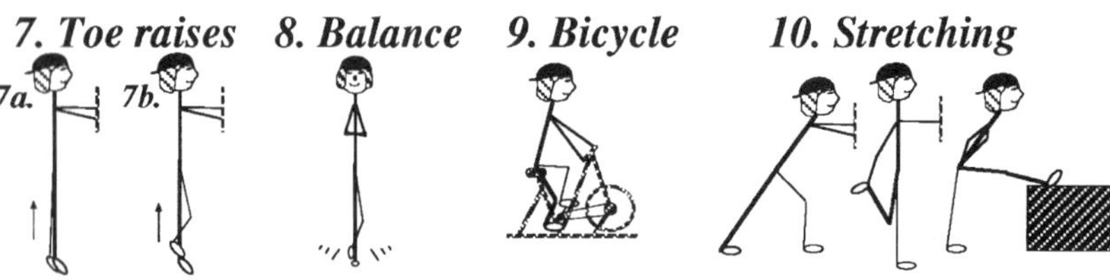

FIGURE 1.—Exercises followed by the isometric and eccentric contraction groups. (Courtesy of Thomeé R: A comprehensive treatment approach for patellofemoral pain syndrome in young women. *Phys Ther* 77:1690–1703, 1997. Reprinted from *Physical Therapy* with the kind permission of the American Physical Therapy Association.)

including education, activity modification, and pain monitoring, all of which may have led to improvements. In a multifactorial study such as this, it is difficult to determine whether the strength training exercises, the recovery time, or the patient counseling produced the greatest improvements in patellofemoral function.

M.J.L. Alexander, Ph.D.

On the Mechanical Effects of Knee Bandages in the Therapy of Patellar Chondropathy

Farkas R, Glitsch U, Paris M (German Sport Univ, Cologne, Germany)
Clin Biomech 12:116–121, 1997

3–5

Introduction.—Use of the infrapatellar bandage (IPB) has been reported to give substantial relief of perceived pain and instability during walking, running, and stepping down stairs. Underlying physiologic mechanisms that can be attributed to this therapeutic effect have not been defined. Some reports indicate that there is a significant decrease in electromyographic (EMG) activity of the knee after applying an IPB. The influence of the IPB on kinetic and EMG activity was evaluated in 10 patients with patellar chondropathy.

Methods.—Six male and 4 female patients, with a mean age of 27.6 years, underwent measurement of EMG, kinematic, and dynamic param-

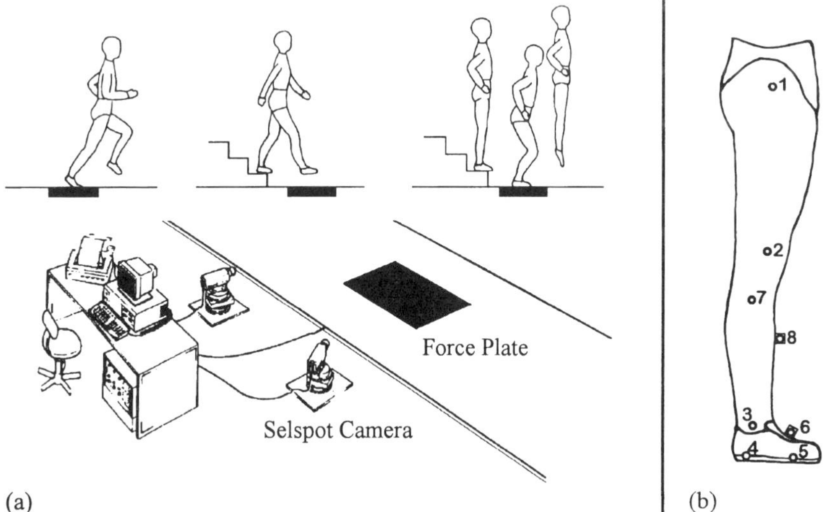

FIGURE 2.—**A**, Laboratory setup for the 3-D motion analysis of the selected movements (running, walking downstairs, drop jump). **B**, Disposition of the active SELSPOT markers (LEDs) at the lower extremity of interest. (Reprinted from Farkas R, Glitsch U, Paris M: On the mechanical effects of knee bandages in the therapy of patellar chondropathy. *Clin Biomech* 12:116–121, copyright 1997 with kind permission from Elsevier Science Ltd, The Boulevard, Langford Lane, Kidlington OX5 1GB UK.)

eters, with and without IPB, during the following 3 different movement activities: (1) running, (2) drop jump, and (3) walking down stairs (Fig 2).

Results.—There was a significant decrease in the neuromuscular activity of selected muscles during the drop jumping while wearing the IPB compared with performing drop jumping without the IPB. The load in the knee joint was not significantly reduced while wearing the IPB during walking down stairs or running.

Conclusion.—The effect of wearing the IPB is probably not the result of decreased joint load because of a general movement adaptation. It probably is because of a neural influence on the nociception.

Clinical Significance.—The therapeutic success of IPB does not coincide with a general decrease in the knee load. The still unknown neurologic effects that allow improvements in perceived pain and function have no influence on the kinetic factors causing the joint disorder in patients with patellar chondropathy. For therapeutic effect, the IPB is better compared with an analgesic medicine than with an orthotic device.

▶ This study examines the mechanical effects of an infrapatellar bandage on the movements of patients with patellofemoral dysfunction. Ten patients were filmed while running, walking downstairs, and performing a drop jump onto a force plate. EMG data also were collected during these activities. There was found to be a decrease in the activity in the hamstring and quadriceps muscle groups during these activities following the application of the knee bandage. The dynamic loads on the knee joint were not found to be significantly altered with the wearing of the bandage during any of these activities. It was suggested that the bandage altered the neurologic activity around the knee joint, and so acted like an analgesic in decreasing pain and discomfort in the joint. The bandage has no influence on the kinetic factors causing the patellofemoral problems, but it does improve knee function and alleviates pain in many of the patients who use it.

M.J.L. Alexander, Ph.D.

Patella Position and Biomechanical Properties of the Patellar Tendon 1 Year After Removal of its Central Third

Hanselmann K-F, Dürselen L, Augat P, et al (Universität Ulm, Germany)
Clin Biomech 12:267–271, 1997
3–6

Background.—Reconstruction of the anterior cruciate ligament is frequently performed using a patellar tendon graft. Although the usefulness of the tendon as a ligament replacement has been studied, the consequences for the function of the remaining tendon have not been well characterized. The effect of removal of a patellar tendon graft on the mechanical properties of the remaining patellar tendon and the position of the patella at the knee joint were investigated in a sheep model of cruciate ligament reconstruction.

Methods.—Ten adult male merino sheep underwent anterior cruciate ligament reconstruction using the middle third of the patellar tendon. After 1 year, the animals were sacrificed, and the length of the patella and patellar tendon, the patella position, cartilage damage and consistency, cross-sectional area, tensile strength, tendon length, stiffness and elasticity were assessed. These results were compared with the contralateral nonoperated control tendons.

Results.—The patella position did not change in the operated joints, compared with the nonoperated contralateral control joints. The cross-sectional area of the operated tendon was significantly increased by scar tissue formation at the site of operation. The inferior mechanical properties of the scar tissue reduced the tendon modulus of elasticity, but the increased cross-sectional area permitted structural stiffness similar to that of the control tendons.

Conclusions.—The effect of patellar tendon grafting on the remaining tendon was investigated in a sheep model. Although the removal of the central portion of the patellar tendon had no effect on patellar position within the joint, it was associated with the formation of scar tissue with reduced elasticity. The increased cross-sectional area of the scar tissue region permitted continued tendon function.

▶ One of the most common grafts for a torn anterior cruciate ligament (ACL) is the use of the central third of the patellar tendon attached to a piece of the patella and the tibial tuberosity, the bone-ligament-bone preparation. The technique has met with limited support in the past few years because of the resulting losses in strength and flexibility of the remaining patellar tendon following this surgery and because of success using other muscles such as semimembranous and gracilis.

In this study, the central third of the tendon was removed from 10 sheep, and, after 1 year of healing, the tendon and patella were compared to nonoperated controls. It was reported that the tendon regained stiffness and load to failure characteristics, but the scar tissue has a lower stiffness and is not replaced by normal tendon tissue after 1 year. Therefore, function may be compromised. This study further supports caution and prudence in the use of the patellar tendon graft in repair of the torn ACL in active individuals.

M.J.L. Alexander, Ph.D.

Soft Tissue Restraints to Lateral Patellar Translation in the Human Knee
Desio SM, Burks RT, Bachus KN (Fallon Med Ctr, Worcester, Mass; Univ of Utah, Salt Lake City)
Am J Sports Med 26:59–65, 1998   3–7

Objective.—Little is known about the soft tissue restraints to lateral patellar dislocation. This is a difficult condition with a high recurrence rate after conservative or operative treatment. Selective cutting studies have offered useful insights into the restraining forces about the tibiofemoral joint, though with some limitations. This cadaver study examined the restraints to lateral patellar translation under conditions of free patellar rotation, leaving the lateral structures intact initially and maintaining the relationship between the lateral femoral condyle and patella.

Methods.—Nine cadaver knees underwent biomechanical testing on a universal testing device to study restraints to lateral patellar translation at 20 degrees of knee flexion. The tissues were first preconditioned, then the patella of each specimen was translated laterally until a force of 200 N was reached. The distance required to achieve this force was used in patellar translation of the remaining structures to be sectioned. The restraints were then sectioned in a predetermined order; the difference between the restraining force before and after sectioning was used to define that structure's contribution to the total restraining force.

Results.—The main restraint to lateral patellar translocation was the medial patellofemoral ligament, which provided 60% of total restraining force. Less important were the medial patellomeniscal ligament and the lateral retinaculum, which provided 13% and 10% of total force, respectively. No important restraining force was provided by the medial patellotibial ligament or the superficial fibers of the medial retinaculum.

Conclusions.—The major soft tissue restraint to lateral patellar translation at 20 degrees of knee flexion is the medial patellofemoral ligament, followed by the medial patellomeniscal ligament and the lateral retinaculum. The involvement of the lateral retinaculum questions the use of isolated lateral release for patellar instability. This could explain the high clinical failure rate noted in several studies of this procedure.

▶ The authors introduce a concept certainly worth considering; that is, they demonstrate that the lateral retinaculum represents 10% of the total restraining force on the patella, and proposed that its sectioning will adversely affect the purpose of the lateral release procedure, which is to reduce propensity for a lateral patella translation. The authors point out several limitations of their experimental design. Most important appears to be the fact that patella subluxation/dislocation occurs in younger individuals, and their determinations were made on cadaver specimens with presumed decreases in the viscoelastic properties of the soft tissues. Ideally, from a clinical standpoint, it would be advantageous if the surgeon could predict which knees will and will not benefit from lateral retinacular release procedures, in view of these reported observations by Desio et al.

J.S. Torg, M.D.

Patellar Dislocation: The Long-term Results of Nonoperative Management in 100 Patients
Mäenpää H, Lehto MUK (Tampere Univ, Finland)
Am J Sports Med 25:213–217, 1997   3–8

Background.—There is no standard treatment for acute or recurrent dislocation of the patella. Although more than 100 operative techniques have been described since 1888, no single treatment method has been universally adopted. There have been reports of results of 1 or 2 surgical procedures, but there is little information on different nonsurgical treatments of patellar dislocation.

Methods.—One hundred men and women were treated nonoperatively for primary acute patellar dislocation. The mean patient age was 23 years. A plaster cast was used in 60 patients, a posterior splint was used in 17 patients, and a patellar bandage or brace was used in 23 patients. The average follow-up was 13 years. Clinical examination included evaluation of restriction of knee joint movement, retropatellar crepitation, and an apprehension test.

Results.—There were 0.17 redislocations per follow-up year overall. The number of redislocations for each patient group was 0.29 for patients who had a patellar bandage or brace, 0.12 for those who had a plaster cast, and 0.08 for those treated with a posterior splint. Patients who were treated with a posterior splint had fewer recurrences and a lower rate of patellofemoral pain and subluxation than the other 2 groups. Patients treated with a plaster cast had the most significant restriction of knee joint movement. Subjective evaluation of treatment was similar for all groups. Treatment of redislocations and management of later problems were also evaluated. Patients who were treated operatively for a redislocation had a better outcome than those treated nonoperatively. Surgery did not relieve the symptoms of patients with later problems.

Discussion.—These long-term results indicate that patients treated nonoperatively for patellar dislocation manage reasonably well compared with patients in similar studies, but the results depend on the type of treatment. More than 50% of these 100 patients had symptoms after 13 years. Attention should be paid to immobilization time, knee joint restriction, retropatellar crepitation, and other problems, such as patellofemoral pain and subluxation. Recommended treatment includes posterior splint for primary dislocation, operation for redislocation, and nonoperative management of further problems. More research is needed in this area.

▶ The important conclusion to be drawn from this study is that those patients treated operatively for redislocations had better outcomes than those treated nonoperatively. The conclusion that "careful prospective studies are needed to define the types of patients who require operative interventions" appears superfluous. That is, the authors have answered that question. Those who fail with conservative management and have a redislocation should have an operative realignment.

J.S. Torg, M.D.

Results of Isolated Patellar Debridement for Patellofemoral Pain in Patients With Normal Patellar Alignment
Federico DJ, Reider B (Univ of Chicago)
Am J Sports Med 25:663–669, 1997   3–9

Introduction.—Most patients with patellofemoral pain will benefit from nonoperative treatment, but arthroscopic surgery may be indicated if conservative measures fail to provide relief after 4 to 6 months. Patients found to have significant chondromalacia patellae at surgery commonly undergo debridement of loose or damaged cartilage. The long-term results of this procedure were examined in a review of 36 cases.

Methods.—The patients underwent arthroscopic patellar debridement for isolated chondromalacia patellae between 1985 and 1990. Excluded were those with a history of patellar instability or dislocation and those who had other surgery, an abnormally tight lateral retinaculum, or patellar malalingment. Patients were 23 women and 13 men with an average age of 31 years. Nineteen were classified as having traumatic and 17 as having atraumatic chondromalacia patellae. Patients were evaluated at an average of 59 months postoperatively. The surgical goal was to remove all loose or damaged cartilage, leaving a smooth and stable chondral surface.

Results.—Grade 3 lesions were the most common finding in this series (61% of all patients; 73% of traumatic and 47% of atraumatic patients). Most lesions involved an area of at least 1.5×1.5 cm. A subjective rating system found 32 patients better at the time of follow-up, 2 unchanged, and 2 worse. All improved to at least some extent with surgery as determined by the Fulkerson-Shea Patellofemoral Joint Evaluation score. Overall, there was significant improvement from the preoperative level to the maximal postoperative level and from the preoperative level to the final postoperative level. Surgery yielded good or excellent results in 57.9% of traumatic cases and in 41.1% of atraumatic cases.

Conclusion.—Patellar debridement may benefit patients whose patellofemoral pain does not respond to nonoperative care. Improvement can be obtained even when chondral damage is considerable, and most postoperative improvement is sustained at 5 years postoperatively.

▶ Despite its widespread prevalence, management of patients with chondromalacia patellae can be difficult at times. From this article, 3 important points can be discerned regarding this problem. First, as the authors point out, most patients with patellofemoral pain can be treated nonoperatively. The surgical procedure proposed by the authors simply consists of arthroscopic debridement, by shaving or curet, to remove all loose and involved patellar articular cartilage, leaving a smooth and stable chondral surface.

Second, patient selection is crucial. Excluded were those with tight lateral structures, malalignment, and tracking abnormalities. Also to be noted, those patients with patellofemoral pain of traumatic origin appear to do better. Lastly, improvement can be obtained regardless of the degree of chondral damage.

J.S. Torg, M.D.

Recalcitrant Patellar Tendinitis: Magnetic Resonance Imaging, Histologic Evaluation, and Surgical Treatment
Popp JE, Yu JS, Kaeding CC (Ohio State Univ, Columbus)
Am J Sports Med 25:218–222, 1997   3–10

Introduction.—Patellar tendinitis is a particular risk in basketball, football, and volleyball players. Some athletes with patellar tendinitis do not respond to conservative treatments, and continue to play with pain. This can lead to chronic and recalcitrant pain, affecting both their training and performance. Various surgical procedures have been used in the treatment of chronic patellar tendinitis. An experience with surgical management of recalcitrant patellar tendinitis is reported, including the MRI findings, surgical results, and pathologic findings.

Methods.—Surgery was performed in 11 knees of 9 athletes with recalcitrant patellar tendinitis. There were 8 men and 1 woman, mean age 20. Four were volleyball players, 3 were football players, and 2 were basketball players. Symptoms of patellar tendinitis had been present for more than 2 years in every case, including pain and tenderness at the inferior pole of the patella. All patients showed no response to traditional nonoperative treatment, and demonstrated thickening of the proximal patellar tendon on MRI scanning. The scans showed abnormal signal intensity in the proximal portion of the patellar tendon.

All patients were treated by surgical exploration and debridement. One surgeon performed all operations, including multiple longitudinal tenotomies, debridement of abnormal tissue, and scarification of the inferior patellar pole. Debridement focused on the areas of greatest pathologic change on MRI and clinical examination. All patients were followed up for at least 1 yr.

Results.—The results were considered excellent in 7 knees, good in 3, and poor in 1. The only failure was in a football player who returned to competition prematurely. Pathologic examination of the debrided tissue revealed "angiofibroblastic tendinosis," corresponding to the abnormal MRI findings in the proximal third of the infrapatellar tendon.

Discussion.—For properly selected patients with recalcitrant patellar tendinitis, surgical treatment can produce excellent results. Criteria include Blazina stage III jumper's knee with symptoms lasting longer than 1 yr, no response to at least 3 months of nonoperative therapy, abnormal MRI findings corresponding to the physical findings, and a desire to return to competitive sport. This study demonstrates correlation between the histologic and MRI findings of recalcitrant patellar tendinitis.

▶ I certainly agree that recalcitrant patella tendinitis should be managed surgically. The 91% good and excellent results reported by Popp et al., compared with the varied results in the literature, is explained on their ability to identify and debride the area of "angiofibroblastic tendinosis." This appears to have been accomplished by correlating MRI findings with their surgical technique, which involves making 3 longitudinal tenotomies in the patella tendon, dividing it into 4 equal segments, then exploring and debriding the area with greatest pathologic changes seen on the MRI. Although not employed in this series, it is noted that exploration and debridement can be performed under local anesthetic, thus aiding the surgeon in identifying the most tender area. This is my own approach to the problem.

J.S. Torg, M.D.

A Cross Sectional Study of 100 Athletes With Jumper's Knee Managed Conservatively and Surgically
Cook JL, for the Victorian Institute of Sport Tendon Study Group (Univ of Melbourne, Australia)
Br J Sports Med 31:332–336, 1997   3–11

Introduction.—Jumper's knee is responsible for considerable morbidity in athletes, especially those participating in basketball, volleyball, and soccer. Treatment starts with conservative therapy, with surgery reserved for patients whose symptoms do not respond. However, there is no scientific evidence in support of either approach, and the treatment outcome remains unpredictable. The clinical course of jumper's knee in a large patient cohort was described.

Methods.—A total of 100 patients with jumper's knee treated at a sports medicine clinic during a 9-year period were retrospectively studied. There were 80 men and 20 women with a mean age of 27 years. The patients responded to a questionnaire seeking data on their sports participation, symptoms, and time away from their sport. Radiologic reports of the ultrasound findings were analyzed. The histopathologic findings in 12 patients who underwent open patellar tenotomy were reviewed as well.

Results.—In nearly half of patients, the first symptoms of jumper's knee developed before 20 years old. Time away from sports exceeded 6 months in 33 patients, 18 of whom could not participate for longer than 1 year. About half of the patients had 2 or more episodes of jumper's knee symptoms. The characteristic ultrasound findings included a hypoechoic region at the junction of the inferior patellar pole and the deep surface of the patellar tendon. Polarized light microscopy of the surgical specimens demonstrated separation and disruption of the collagen fibers. The specimens also showed increased mucoid ground substance, suggesting the presence of tendon collagen damage without inflammation. It generally took 7–12 months to resume sports participation after surgery.

Conclusions.—Jumper's knee can cause long-term symptoms in young athletes, more than one third of whom may eventually require surgery. Pathologically, the lesion consists of tendon degeneration or microtears, rather than inflammation. Jumper's knee in athletes cannot be classified as a benign, self-limiting condition. Its course is consistent with the pathologic diagnosis of tendinosis, rather than tendinitis.

▶ I certainly agree with the authors' conclusion that jumper's knee can cause long-term symptoms in the athlete and that the problem is "not that of a self-limiting benign condition." However, it has not been our experience that if the lesion is debrided surgically, that a protracted postoperative course necessarily follows. Precise localization of the lesion can be facilitated if the procedure is performed under local anesthesia; that is, infiltration of the skin with a 2% xylocaine and 1:100,000 epinephrine solution, with subsequent localization of the lesion in an awake, alert patient.

J.S. Torg, M.D.

The Effect of Patellar Taping on the Onset of Vastus Medialis Obliquus and Vastus Lateralis Muscle Activity in Persons With Patellofemoral Pain

Gilleard W, McConnell J, Parsons D (Univ of Sydney, New South Wales, Australia)
Phys Ther 78:25–32, 1998   3–12

Introduction.—Taping of the patellofemoral joint in patients with patellofemoral pain syndrome (PFPS) may affect timing of the vastus medialis oblique (VMO) and vastus lateralis (VL) muscles and thus alter the way the patella tracks in the trochlea of the femur. Changes in pain level could also alter timing of muscle activity. The confounding effects of pain on the kinematics of a task need to be evaluated to determine the effects of tape on the onset of muscle activity. Taping of the patellofemoral joint was assessed in patients with PFPS to determine its effects on the timing of activity of the VMO and VL muscles during walking up and down stairs.

Methods.—Mean age of 14 women with untreated PFPS was 22.7 years. Research subjects walked up and down stairs without patellar taping and with the patellofemoral joint of the painful lower extremity taped to reduce pain by at least 50% on a pain provocation test. Surface EMG data were collected during both procedures.

Results.—There was no significant difference in the onset of activity between the VMO and VL during step-up and step-down tasks without taping. With taping, the onset of VMO activity occurred earlier, and there was no change in the onset of VL activity during the step-up task. During the step-down task with the knee taped, the onset of VMO activity occurred earlier and the onset of VL activity was delayed. During both step-down and step-up tasks, onset of VMO activity occurred earlier than onset of VL activity.

Conclusion.—Timing of VMO and VL was altered with taping of the patellofemoral joint in patients with PFPS during step-up and step-down tasks. The earlier activation of the VMO may change the movement of the patella. Further investigation should evaluate whether this occurs and whether it is helpful.

▶ The authors do state that a controversy exists regarding EMG activity of the VMO relative to the VL in individuals with and without PFPS. This study indicates that during the step-down activity the onset of VMO activity occurred earlier and the onset of VL activity was delayed. This delaying of VL activity would somewhat support the study done by Witvrouw et al.[1] and my comments in the 1997 YEAR BOOK OF SPORTS MEDICINE, page 137, The authors of the study recommend that a rehabilitation program for PFPS should retard the firing of the VL rather than accelerate the VMO reflex response. Their reasoning was that both reflex responses of VL and VMO are already significantly shorter in the individual with PFPS.

F.J. George, A.T.C., P.T.

Reference

1. Witvrouw E, Sneyers C, Lysens R, et al: Reflex response times of vastus medialis obliquus and vastus lateralis in normal subjects and in subjects with patellofemoral pain syndrome. *J Orthop Sports Phys Ther* 24:160–165, 1996.

Patella Fractures Associated With Accelerated ACL Rehabilitation in Patients With Autogenous Patella Tendon Reconstructions
Brownstein B, Bronner S (SOAR Research, New York)
J Orthop Sports Phys Ther 26:168–172, 1997   3–13

Background.—Anterior cruciate ligament (ACL) reconstruction with an autogenous patella tendon graft can be complicated by patella fracture, typically resulting from a fall. The incidence of this injury is about 0.5%. Patella fractures can also occur when "accelerated" rehabilitation protocols are used without consideration of the healing tissue, the patient's preoperative condition, neuromuscular status, and appropriate individual goals.

Discussion.—In many rehabilitation programs, knee function recovery is pursued in the order of range of motion, strength, and functional movement. The authors suggest that functional movement be pursued before strength, redirecting the rehabilitative emphasis to neuromuscular factors that improve reaction time, promote proximal stability and control of distal components, and restructure the movement patterns that guide function. Excessive joint forces may instigate negative feedback from local receptors that may inhibit rather than promote muscle function. Assessment of the mechanism of nontraumatic fractures of the patella implicates sudden, forceful quadriceps contractions as a contributing factor, which may be mitigated through neuromuscular training to improve the patient's ability to control and modulate lower extremity muscle activity. Such training should include feedback and feedforward control activities to integrate sensorimotor defects resulting from the rupture of the ACL, graft removal, associated effusion, and loss of quadriceps control. Rehabilitation methods that generate large joint forces along with large muscle forces require careful patient assessment before initiation.

Conclusions.—Patella fracture resulting from rehabilitation efforts should be an avoidable complication of ACL reconstruction. Accelerated programs focusing on early return to sports activities and incorporating early high-stress exercises need to consider the previous activity level of the patient. The patella should be considered at risk during the first 8–12 weeks of rehabilitation.

▶ The reasons for patella fractures with ACL repairs are described by the authors. They recommend a change in rehabilitation philosophy, namely that functional movement be pursued before a strengthening program. Their emphasis is on neuromuscular factors that improve reaction time, promote proximal stability, and restructure movement patterns. They warn us that the patella is at risk for 8–12 weeks after surgery.

F.J. George, A.T.C., P.T.

Knee Dislocation: Initial Assessment and Implications for Treatment
Wascher DC, Dvirnak PC, DeCoster TA (Univ of New Mexico, Albuquerque)
J Orthop Trauma 11:525–529, 1997   3–14

Introduction.—Narrowly defined, knee dislocation is the radiographically confirmed complete loss of the tibiofemoral articulation. This traditional definition has been expanded to include bicruciate knee injuries, even when the knee is reduced on initial presentation. A retrospective review of knee dislocations was conducted to determine whether this injury was more common when the broader definition was applied and whether this had implications regarding vascular injuries.

Methods.—During an 8-year period, 50 knee dislocations were treated in 47 patients at the study institution. Included were both patients with radiographically proven or clinically documented knee dislocations and those with bicruciate ligament injuries. Injuries were classified by 2 methods: (1) the direction of the dislocation, based on clinical and radiologic findings and (2) the knee ligament injury pattern, together with the presence or absence of a major periarticular fracture. The patients' charts and radiographs were reviewed for these findings and for mechanism of injury, presence of vascular and nerve injuries, and location of associated trauma.

Results.—Patients were 36 men and 11 women with a mean age of 28 years. All 10 dislocations that occurred during recreational athletic activities were isolated, low-energy injuries. The remaining 40 injuries resulted from high-energy trauma; there were 8 open dislocations and 3 bilateral dislocations in this group. Most patients with high-energy dislocations had coexisting major trauma; 2 died from abdominal trauma sepsis during the first week post injury. Twenty-two knees had classic knee dislocations and 28 were "reduced" bicruciate ligament injuries. All complete popliteal artery disruptions were secondary to high-energy trauma, and more than half occurred in spontaneously reduced bicruciate knee injuries. Vascular injury was as common in bicruciate ligament injuries as in knee dislocations. Neither the ligament injury pattern nor the presence of arterial injury could be predicted by the direction of knee dislocation.

Conclusion.—All bicruciate knee injuries should be considered knee dislocations. Even if reduced, the residual functional disability and coexisting injuries are the same as those of obvious dislocations and have an equivalent risk of major popliteal artery injury.

▶ I fully concur with the authors' conclusion that "Bicruciate ligament injuries are reduced knee dislocations and are at equivalent risk of major popliteal artery injury." This is explained on the basis of spontaneous reduction of the dislocation. The authors express a particular interest in determining what the implications regarding vascular injuries were in this situation. Their answer to this question is not really well defined. They state that their data support selective arteriography based on serial physical examination of patients with bicruciate ligament injuries.

J.S. Torg, M.D.

A Prospective Outcome Study of Rehabilitation Programs and Anterior Cruciate Ligament Reconstruction
Schenck RC Jr, Blaschak MJ, Lance ED, et al (Univ of Texas, San Antonio; Northern Illinois Univ, Dekalb; Univ of Central Arkansas, Conway)
Arthroscopy 13:285–290, 1997   3–15

Introduction.—Early weight-bearing and functional rehabilitation programs have contributed significantly to the restoration of function in the reconstructed anterior cruciate ligament(ACL)-deficient knee. The outcomes of 2 programs, one home-based rehabilitation (HR) and the other clinic based rehabilitation (CB), were compared in a study of 37 patients who had undergone midpatellar autograft reconstruction of the ACL.

Methods.—Fifteen patients were randomized to CB and 22 to HR. With HR, patients took part in an exercise-based functional program monitored by a physical therapist (Table 1). They were also provided with a therapist-directed preoperative education session approximately 30 to 45 minutes in length. Both CB and HR groups received preoperative education by the therapist and physician. Those in CB were prescribed 3 visits a week for 6 weeks. Brace-free rehabilitation was used for both groups for 6 weeks after surgery, and return to cutting/jumping sports was planned for 4 to 6 months after surgery. Patients completed the Sickness Impact Profile.

TABLE 1.—Home-Based Rehabilitation Model

Time	Instructions/Exercises	Goals	Warning Signs
Preoperative (surgeon/ therapist)	Explain diagnosis and proposed surgery Explain time line of postoperative function and specific exercises Discuss postoperative function, including early ambulation activities Quadriceps retraining, co-contractions, single-leg raise, partial squats (wall slides) are explained Discuss use of physical agents (ice) Teaching period: 45 minutes	Full motion, particularly terminal extension	Loss of motion, specifically flexion and extension Abnormal pain response Abnormal gait
Day of surgery or postoperative day 1 (usually surgeon only)	Quadriceps co-contractions Emphasize passive motion, active flexion/ assisted extension in sitting or prone position Discuss ice after activity and for patient to "let swelling after activity be the guide" to dosing of activity Begin gait training with crutches; weight bearing as tolerated	Maintain terminal extension Perform adequate co-contractions Leg control (able to flex hip and lift the leg of involved extremity against gravity without assistance)	Loss of terminal extension Loss of leg control Abnormal swelling
Postoperative day 3 (surgeon/therapist)	Focus on gait training and other ambulation activities Terminal extension exercises Passive flexion Continue quadriceps activity, introduce partial squat* (with progression from bilateral to unilateral, placing increased body weight on involved extremity—no more than 45° of flexion)	Maintain terminal extension Progression toward 90° of flexion Ambulation: weight bearing as tolerated with normal heel-toe gait on involved extremity	Signs of infection at site of incision Poor leg control Abnormal pain response More than minimal swelling Loss of terminal extension Not progressing in abulation

(Continued)

TABLE 1 (cont.)

Time	Instructions/Exercises	Goals	Warning Signs
Postoperative day 10 (surgeon, therapist)	Progress from partial squat to wall slide-squat* or stepper/stationary bike as tolerated Continue to emphasize terminal extension, progressive flexion, and ice after activity	Terminal extension 90° flexion 3-minute squats with good form Full weight bearing with normal heel-toe gait *If patient has not achieved these goals, frequency of therapy should be increased*	Inability to passively extend knee fully Has not achieved 90° of flexion Has not achieved full weight bearing with normal or near-normal gait
3 Weeks after operation (surgeon, therapist as needed)	Stepper Stationary bike Loaded squats Swimming	Normal ambulation	More than minimal swelling after activity
6 Weeks after operation (surgeon, therapist)	Release to light jogging, bicycling Patient will begin slow return to function	Performing weight-bearing loaded activities such as stepper with only minimal swelling	More than minimal swelling after activity
12 Weeks and beyond (surgeon, therapist as needed)	Gradual return to activities	Activity performance with minimal swelling	Let swelling after activity be the guide

Note: The patients were started with mini-squats against the wall to aid balance. When they were able to do 3 minutes of squats against the wall, they were started on squats without wall support. They returned to wall support for unilateral squats and progressed to unsupported unilateral squats.

(Courtesy of Schenck RC Jr, Blaschak MJ, Lance ED, et al: A prospective outcome study of rehabilitation programs and anterior cruciate ligament reconstruction. *Arthroscopy* 13:285–290, 1997.)

Results.—Patients were 28 men and 9 women with a mean age of 24.1 years. Thirty-six patients, including all 15 in the HR group, reported satisfaction with knee function at 3 months and 1 year after ACL reconstruction. Neither group exhibited evidence of arthrofibrosis or fixed flexion contractures. Postoperative Sickness Impact Profile scores did not differ significantly between treatment groups. Visual analogue scale pain scores averaged 5.1 preoperatively for both groups and 0.89 at 1 year. The average number of visits in the HR group was 5.1, vs. 14.2 in the CB group; average costs were $225 and $930, respectively.

Conclusion.—All patients in the study reported a high level of satisfaction with ACL reconstruction and rehabilitation, a decrease in pain, and improved quality of life. Functional and subjective outcomes were similar in the HR and CB groups, but there was significant cost savings with the HR program.

▶ The concept of an exercise-based HR program after ACL reconstruction is sound. The stated goal of such a program was to "obtain full range of motion and normal gait as soon as reasonably possible." Unfortunately, this rehabilitation protocol does not deal with the important subject of muscle strength rehabilitation. Our approach to this aspect of the problem, after a trainer/therapist-directed home exercise range of motion program, is to have our patients continue with a closed chain program at their local health club. Again, the patients are given written instructions with explanations and demonstrations by our trainer/therapist. This approach is not only cost effective, it omits the application of needless modalities that many physical therapists seem prone to use.

J.S. Torg, M.D.

Early Season Anterior Cruciate Ligament Tears: A Treatment Dilemma
Shelton WR, Barrett GR, Dukes A (Mississippi Sports Medicine & Orthopaedic Ctr, Jackson)
Am J Sports Med 25:656–658, 1997   3–16

Introduction.—Athletes with anterior cruciate ligament (ACL) tears are typically treated by surgical reconstruction or a nonoperative regimen of exercise, bracing, or life-style modification. An ACL tear in the preseason or early season in competitive athletes is a treatment predicament for physicians. The choices are immediate surgery, which ends the playing season, or rehabilitative exercises and bracing to quickly return the athlete to competition. Forty-three athletes (44 tears) who elected to rapidly return to their sport by treatment with exercise and bracing were followed prospectively to determine the criteria for return to play and whether an early return is safe.

Methods.—All athletes had an acute injury in a previously normal knee, a positive Lachman test, and KT-1000 arthrotomy demonstrating ligament abnormalities. All patients had ACL tear and no meniscus tear on MRI.

The athletes were followed for episodes of knee buckling in the brace after their return to play.

Results.—Thirty patients with 31 tears treated with rehabilitation/bracing returned to play at an average of 5.7 weeks after injury. Seventy percent (30 of 43 patients, 31 of 44 knees) completed their season wearing knee braces. Only 12 patients were able to return to their sport without recurrent buckling of the injured knees. Eighteen patients (19 knees) experienced recurrent buckling during play. Thirteen patients were not able to return to play after rehabilitation. Patients were followed until they had ACL reconstruction (29 patients, 29 tears), discontinued their sport because of instability but did not elect surgery (3 patients), or returned to play in a brace and refused surgery (11 patients, 12 tears). All patients who underwent reconstruction had recurrent knee buckling. There were 23 meniscal tears (17 knees) in 29 patients who underwent reconstruction. The meniscal tears were not observed on MRI before patients returned to play.

Conclusion.—Nineteen of 30 athletes who returned to play after rehabilitation/bracing experienced knee buckling in the brace. All athletes with recurrent buckling reported that instability hampered their ability to return to 100% of preinjury performance levels. Fifty-nine percent of knees that underwent ACL reconstruction had torn menisci from return to play.

▶ This article deals with 1 of the major dilemmas of the sports medicine practitioner: Should an individual return to athletic activities after acute disruption of his or her ACL? Unfortunately, the subjects were not segregated into cutting and noncutting activity groups. Certainly, the success, or lack thereof, after returning to such activities as basketball and football should not be grouped with that of a swimmer or a distance runner. It is important to note that 59% of those who returned to their activity, and ultimately had an ACL reconstruction, had torn menisci. My own approach to this problem is to advise youngsters participating in cutting sports to have the ACL reconstruction before returning to their activity. Clearly, the goal of patient management should be to pursue a course that insures the best chances for a healthy knee over ones lifetime.

J.S. Torg, M.D.

The Effect of Anterior Cruciate Ligament Reconstruction on Symptoms of Pain and Instability in Patients Who Have Previously Undergone Meniscectomy: A Prereconstruction and Postreconstruction Comparison
Barrett GR, Ruff CG (Mississippi Sports Medicine and Orthopaedic Ctr, Jackson)
Arthroscopy 13:704–709, 1997   3–17

Introduction.—Functions of the meniscus include distribution of stress across the knee, shock absorption, nutrition, joint lubrication, and joint stability. The absence of meniscal tissue and the presence of anterior cruciate ligament (ACL) deficiency can cause arthritic changes in the knee. It is possible that the symptoms and complaints of patients who have undergone earlier meniscectomy can be improved with ACL reconstruction. The effects of ACL reconstruction on 21 symptomatic patients with coexisting knee problems from an earlier meniscectomy and chronic ACL insufficiency were retrospectively evaluated.

Methods.—The average patient age was 31 years. The average time from meniscectomy to ACL reconstruction was 6.6 years. Arthroscopic examination revealed that all patients were ACL deficient. Five and 1 patients, respectively, had a new medial or lateral meniscus tear. Patients underwent arthroscopically assisted intra-articular ACL reconstruction using a middle, one-third patella-tendon autograft. Preoperative and postoperative comparisons were made for range of motion, stability, and subjective evaluations.

Results.—The average follow-up was 37.4 months (range, 24–67 months). Five patients needed further surgery. These included 3 diagnostic arthroscopies, 1 debridement with manipulation, 1 metal removal, manipulation and lysis of adhesions, shaving of scar tissue and removal of an osteophyte, and debridement of the articular cartilage and removal of an osteophyte. Three patients had pathologic, ligament laxity. A 2+ Lachman, a 2+ pivot shift, and a greater than 5-mm difference on KT-1000 maximum manual testing was detected in 1 patient; 2 patients had a 1+ Lachman and a 1+ pivot shift. Preoperative and postoperative range of motion were similar. All preoperative measurements on a panel of 15 visual analogue scales were improved, and intensity of pain and instability were significantly improved.

Conclusion.—Successful ACL reconstruction in an already arthritic knee can protect the knee from further damage. Patients in this series experienced a decrease in pain and instability and were able to continue a satisfactory activity level and life-style.

Anterior Cruciate Ligament Reconstruction With Autogenous Patellar Tendon Graft in Patients With Articular Cartilage Damage

Noyes FR, Barber-Westin SD (Cincinnati Sportsmedicine and Orthopaedic Ctr, Cincinnati, Ohio; Deaconess Hosp, Cincinnati, Ohio)
Am J Sports Med 25:626–634, 1997   3–18

Introduction.—Few investigations in the English literature have reported results of anterior cruciate ligament (ACL) reconstruction in patients with chronic ruptures and advanced articular cartilage damage observed by direct arthroscopic visualization. Fifty-three patients with arthroscopically documented advanced cartilage damage were evaluated to determine whether ACL reconstruction with autogenous patellar tendon could relieve symptoms and functional limitations and increase activity levels.

Methods.—The mean time between original injury and reconstruction was 7.5 years. Ninety prior surgeries had been performed in 53 patients. Preoperative and postoperative knee displacement testing was performed with a KT-2000 arthrometer and knees were assessed with the Cincinnati Knee Rating System.

Results.—After surgery, all patients achieved immediate motion and early functional rehabilitation. At a mean follow-up of 27 months, patients had significant improvements in pain, swelling, giving way, functional limitations in daily and sports activities, and the overall rating score. Seventy-nine percent of patients (42) returned to some type of athletic activity. Six percent of patients (3) had failed results. Fifty-one patients rated overall knee condition as follows: 8 (16%), normal; 28 (55%), very good; 7 (14%), good; 5 (10%), fair; and 3 (6%), poor.

Conclusion.—Most patients with advanced articular cartilage damage benefited from arthroscopically assisted ACL reconstruction. The operation decreased discomfort and giving way and allowed increased activity without aggravating the pre-existing arthrosis.

▶ Barrett and Ruff observe that the symptoms of pain and instability in patients with chronic ACL deficiency who have previously undergone meniscectomy can be improved by ACL reconstruction if objective stability is obtained. This is in keeping with my own experience. However, it should be pointed out that the authors' suggestion that a successful ACL reconstruction will protect an arthritic knee from further deterioration is not supported by the data. To be noted is the observation of Noyes et al. that patients with severe articular cartilage damage with bone exposure on 2 opposing articular surfaces, those with secondary degenerative changes that provide stability, and those whose symptoms are related to the arthrosis rather than instability are not candidates for ACL reconstruction.

J.S. Torg, M.D.

An Analysis of Anterior Cruciate Ligament Reconstruction in Middle-aged Patients

Heier KA, Mack DR, Moseley JB, et al (Baylor College of Medicine, Houston)
Am J Sports Med 25:527–532, 1997   3–19

Objective.—Whether surgical or nonsurgical treatment is best for rupture of the anterior cruciate ligament (ACL) is controversial. Moreover, outcome after treatment of ACL ruptures in older patients has not been specifically studied. This article studies complications and outcomes for patients older than 40 years who had arthroscopically assisted reconstruction of their ACLs.

Methods.—Interviews, physical examinations, radiographs, Biodex dynamometer testing, and KT-1000 arthrometer testing were performed on 45 patients (17 men), aged 40–62 years at the time of surgery, at an average of 37 months after ACL reconstruction.

Results.—Twenty patients had early reconstruction, 14 had delayed reconstruction, and 11 had late reconstruction. Baseline Lysholm and Gillquist scores averaged 91. All but 1 patient was satisfied with the results. Scores from the International Knee Documentation Committee were normal in 4 patients, nearly normal in 25, abnormal in 14, and severely abnormal in 2. After surgery, KT-1000 arthrometer testing results showed a significant decrease in laxity between sides at 30 pounds: 3 mm or less in 31 patients, 3–5 mm in 10 patients, and more than 5 mm in 12 patients. At follow-up, 34 patients had returned to their preoperative levels of activity. There were 5 complications, 2 patients with ruptures and 3 who required a second arthroscopic procedure.

Conclusion.—Outcome after ACL reconstruction in older patients is similar to that in younger patients.

▶ It should be noted that there were no absolute criteria for exclusion in this study, except that patients with severe osteoarthritis were discouraged from having the procedure, which consisted of the standard arthroscopic ACL reconstruction using a two-incision approach with autogenous patellar tendon graft. The authors point out that "a potential weakness of this study is the lack of a non-surgically treated control group." However, Ciccotti et al[1] demonstrate 83% satisfactory outcome for 30 middle-aged patients ages 40–60 treated conservatively. The authors point out that the surgical treatment for ACL ruptures in older patients is not necessarily the treatment of choice. However, their results should alleviate reluctance to operate on "selected, motivated patients."

J.S. Torg, M.D.

Reference

1. Ciccotti MG, Lombardo SS, Norweiler B, et al: Non-operative treatment of ruptures of the anterior cruciate ligament in middle-aged patients. Results after long-term follow-up. *J Bone and Joint Surg* 76-A:1315–1321, 1994.

The Science of Reconstruction of the Anterior Cruciate Ligament
Frank CB, Jackson DW (Univ of Calgary, Alta; Southern California Ctr for Sports Medicine, Long Beach)
J Bone Joint Surg (Am) 79-A:1556–1576, 1997   3–20

Introduction.—There is no consensus regarding when or how to optimally perform reconstruction of the anterior cruciate ligament (ACL). A review of the current scientific understanding of reconstruction of the ACL was presented.

Current Concepts in Anterior Cruciate Ligament Reconstruction.— Carefully performed reconstruction of the ACL usually improves short-term function of the knees. It is not easy to decide which are the best methods of reconstruction. All methods seem to be improving. Increasing attention is being given to details of structure, function, and biology of the normal ACL; patient selection; operative techniques; and rehabilitation protocols. Current techniques are unable to return more than a few reconstructed knees to normal. A normal ACL has yet to be recreated. The duration of follow-up has not been sufficient and assessments of outcomes are too varied to adequately determine whether or how reconstruction affects the long-term natural history of an injured ACL. A combined clinical and basic-research effort could dramatically advance the science of reconstruction over the next decade. The goal of operative treatment should always be the safe and effective restoration of all knees with an injury of the ACL to their pre-injury state.

Conclusion.—Current operative techniques of ACL reconstruction are superior to earlier approaches, but none are able to recreate normal ACL function. The goal of treatment must always be the safe and effective restoration of all knees with ACL injury to their pre-injury condition.

▶ This article appeared as a Current Concepts Review in *The Journal of Bone and Joint Surgery*. It presents much of what you need to know regarding ACL function, criteria for patient selection, reconstruction timing, and operative techniques, through postoperative care and rehabilitation. Importantly, the article points out that ". . . few reconstructed knees are returned to normal with use of current techniques, and a normal anterior cruciate ligament has not yet been recreated." Most impressive is the fact that the article is based on 316 reference citations.

J.S. Torg, M.D.

Reconstruction of the Anterior Cruciate Ligament in Patients Who Are At Least Forty Years Old: A Long-term Follow-up and Outcome Study
Plancher KD, Steadman JR, Briggs KK, et al (Steadman Hawkins Clinic, Vail, Colo)
J Bone Joint Surg Am 80-A:184–197, 1998   3–21

Background.—The best treatment of a torn anterior cruciate ligament in patients older than 40 years has not been determined. Most patients are treated nonoperatively because of concern that operative reconstruction of the anterior cruciate ligament in this population is associated with a higher rate of arthrofibrosis and decreased arc of motion. Studies suggest that patients who are managed nonoperatively have a high rate of reinjury after they return to preinjury activity levels, and that use of a brace does not lower reinjury rates.

Methods.—The long-term results of 72 patients who had a bone-patellar ligament-bone intra-articular reconstruction of the anterior cruciate ligament in 75 knees were reviewed. The mean patient age was 45 years. A questionnaire, functional results, and objective clinical data were analyzed. The clinical examination included range-of-motion evaluation, Lachman and pivot-shift tests, and measurements with a KT-1000 arthrometer. The Lyshom and Gillquist scale, The Hospital for Special Surgery scale modified by Insall et al., and the International Knee Ligament Standard Evaluation Form were used.

Results.—The main causes of injury were skiing, tennis, and soccer. Follow-up was 26–117 months. At the last follow-up examination, 3 patients had pain or swelling. There were no reports of giving-way or symptoms related to the patellofemoral joint. The mean range of extension was −8–42 degrees preoperatively, and −12–6 degrees at the last postoperative examination. The mean range of flexion was 52–154 degrees preoperatively, and 112–150 degrees postoperatively. In 1 patient, flexion was limited to 112 degrees, but this was 5 degrees greater than in the unaffected knee. The pivot-shift test was negative in 80% of knees, and 13% of knees had a grade of 1+. Testing with the KT-1000 arthrometer at maximum manual pressure showed that the mean difference between the injured and uninjured knees improved by 5.1 mm. On the International Knee Ligament Standard Evaluation Form, 96% of knees had a grade of C or D preoperatively, and 93% of knees had a grade of A or B postoperatively. Mean scores on the Hospital for Special Surgery scale were 69 points preoperatively and 92 points postoperatively. Mean scores on the Lyshom and Gillquist scale were 63 points preoperatively and 94 points postoperatively. All patients were pleased with their results. Bicycling was resumed at a mean of 4 months, jogging was resumed at a mean of 9 months, skiing was resumed at a mean of 10 months, and tennis was resumed at a mean of 12 months.

Discussion.—These patients older than 40 years had a satisfactory outcome after reconstruction of the anterior cruciate ligament. The range of active and passive motion was excellent. There was no arthrofibrosis, and reinjury rates were lower than those reported in studies of younger patients treated nonoperatively. A satisfactory outcome after operative treatment is very likely when strict patient selection criteria are followed.

▶ To be noted, the operative technique used in this study was an arthroscopically assisted 2-incision technique using a bone-patella ligament bone autograft from the ipsilateral limb. Seventy-six percent of the patients were able to return to their preinjury level of sports activity, 20% modified their level of activity, and 4% no longer participated in athletic activity. Seven percent of the knees in the study sustained a reinjury after return to activities. However, the authors point out that this is in contrast with that of 37% of the group of middle-aged patients who were managed nonoperatively (reported by Ciccotti, see citation after comment on Abstract 3–19).

J.S. Torg, M.D.

Ablation Rates of Human Meniscal Tissue With the Ho:YAG Laser: The Effects of Varying Fluences

Vangsness CT Jr, Ghaderi B, Brustein M, et al (Univ of California, Los Angeles)
Arthroscopy 13:148–150, 1997

3–22

Introduction.—In arthroscopic knee surgery, lasers are used as an adjunctive tool because surgeons have easier access in tight joints with small laser handpieces. The laser has the ability to resect and coagulate with good contouring abilities. Partial meniscectomy has been the most promising clinical use for lasers within the knee joint. Meniscal tissue is ablated, a small thermal damage zone is produced with the laser, which must also have fiberoptic capability and be able to irradiate tissue in a saline environment. For arthroscopy, the holmium:yttrium aluminum garnet (Ho:YAG) laser at a wavelength of 2.1 µm offers many desirable characteristics. Using the Ho:YAG, the effect of different fluence levels (energy per unit area) on laser ablation rates and depth of thermal injury of meniscal tissue was evaluated.

Methods.—An in vitro experiment was established to measure ablation rates and the concomitant thermal injury to define the operating parameters for the Holmium laser meniscectomy. Energy levels were varied between 167 and 927 J/cm² per pulse to measure meniscal ablation rates using an experimental setup with a laser fiber penetrating through meniscal tissue slices Hematoxylin and eosin and trichrome staining were used to evaluate the adjacent thermal effects after each experiment.

Results.—At 927 J/cm² per pulse, the fastest ablation rate was found. The increases in energy levels were directly proportional to the increase in ablation rates. The average lateral thermal change was 400–500 µm, according to histologic examination, with no demonstrated relation to the pulse level of energy. The higher levels of energy per pulse showed better ablation of human meniscal tissue without increasing thermal effects in adjacent tissue at these laser parameters.

Conclusions.—For more efficient arthroscopic meniscectomy with the Holmium laser, higher energy levels and fluences appeared desirable. Human meniscal tissue can be quickly and precisely ablated with the Holmium laser. During arthroscopic meniscectomy, the properties provided by the Holmium wavelength give it a strong potential for use.

▶ This somewhat technical article indicates that higher energy level fluences result in more effective arthroscopic meniscectomy with the Holmium (Ho:YAG) laser. The recent literature indicates that there appears to be a problem with femoral necrosis of bone with both the Nd:YAG and the Ho:YAG laser systems. Unfortunately, this study did not determine the effect of laser repetition rates on tissue cooling as it related to the phenomenon of thermal superposition and thermal damage to tissue. As the authors point out, "the pulse width and repetition rate must be kept low enough during clinical laser energy delivery to minimize any cumulative thermal injury imparted to adjacent tissue." The advantages of making these determinations in vitro are obvious.

J.S. Torg, M.D.

Failure Strength of a New Meniscus Arrow Repair Technique: Biomechanical Comparison With Horizontal Suture
Albrecht-Olsen P, Lind T, Kristensen G, et al (Gentofte Univ, Denmark; Aalborg Univ, Denmark)
Arthroscopy 13:183–187, 1997   3–23

Introduction.—Even partial resection of the meniscus can result in cartilage degeneration and future arthrosis. Described was a new method of arthroscopic all-inside repair of vertical meniscus lesions using a meniscus arrow, a biodegradable fixation device. The failure strength of this meniscus repair technique was compared with that of the horizontal suturing technique.

Methods.—The arrow is made of self-reinforced biodegradable polylactic acid and consists of a T-handle and a stem with a diameter of 1.1 mm. Twenty-four fresh frozen bovine medial menisci were defrozen and separated into 3 groups. An artificial vertical lesion was created 3 mm from the peripheral rim and repairs were performed with 1 of the following: a single horizontal Maxon-0 suture using an Acufex double-barrel cannula with a knot tied on the capsular side (group I); a 13-mm Biofix Meniscus arrow (Fig 4) (group II); or repair as in group II, but with the menisci incubated in isotonic saline at 21°C for 24 hours before testing (group III). After the repair procedures, the vertical cut was completed through the meniscus horn so that only the repair site would be tested. Pull-out tests to failure were completed in a computer-based Nene M5 testing machine with a load cell of 5 kN connected to a computer.

Results.—There were no between-group differences in failure loads.

Conclusion.—Repair with 1 meniscus arrow had about the same failure strength as a horizontal suture loop.

▶ The conclusion of this in vitro biomechanical study confirms our clinical observation that the meniscal arrow repair technique effectively stabilizes peripheral tears of both medial and lateral menisci. Of course, long-term clinical follow-up will be necessary to substantiate the effectiveness of the technique in vivo.

J.S. Torg, M.D.

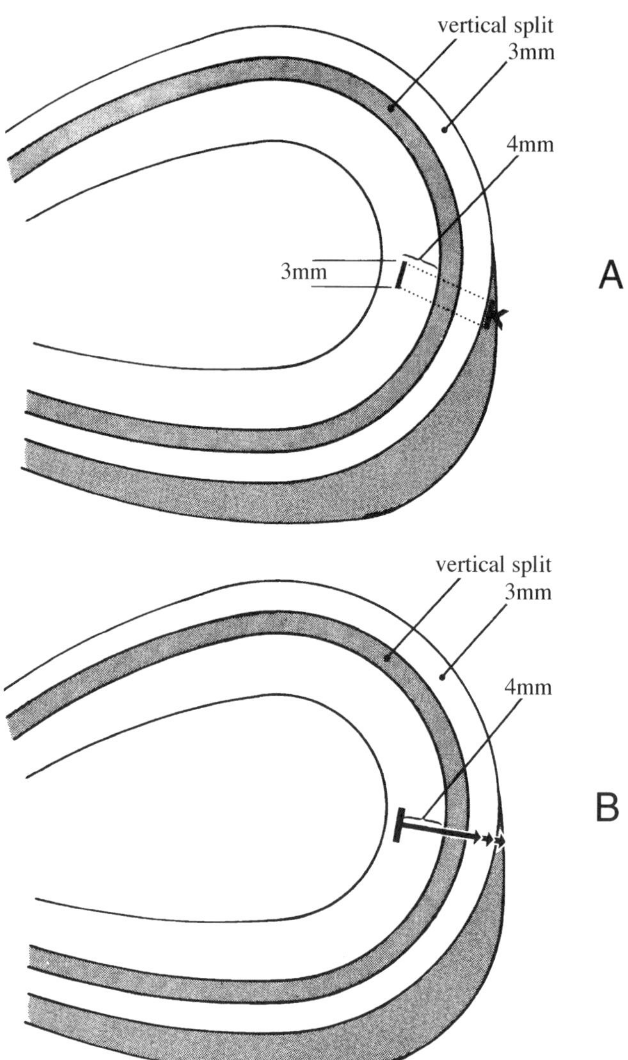

FIGURE 4.—**A,** horizontal suture. **B,** meniscus arrow repair. (Courtesy of Albrecht-Olsen P, Lind T, Kristensen G, et al: Failure strength of a new meniscus arrow repair technique: Biomechanical comparison with horizontal suture. *Arthroscopy* 13:183–187, 1997.)

The Outcome of Operatively Treated Anterior Cruciate Ligament Disruptions in the Skeletally Immature Child
Lo IKY, Kirkley A, Fowler PJ, et al (Univ of Western Ontario, London, Canada; The Toronto Hosp)
Arthroscopy 13:627–634, 1997   3–24

Background.—There are 4 main options for treating anterior cruciate ligament (ACL) disruption: (1) conservative therapy (2) ACL reconstruction with transphyseal drill holes, (3) ACL reconstruction without drill holes, and (4) extra-articular procedures. It has been thought by many that growth plate disturbance would result in skeletally immature children who underwent ACL reconstruction. The outcome of transphyseal ligament reconstruction for children with ACL disruption was evaluated.

Methods.—Physicians performed intra-articular reconstruction of the ACL on 5 patients between the ages of 8 and 12 years (mean 12.9 years) with open growth plate who were projected to grow more than 5 additional centimeters. Two of the reconstructions utilized the quadriceps patellar tendon and 3, the hamstring tendons. All surgeons drilled through an open physis using a tibial drill hole smaller than 6 mm. Grafts were placed "over the top" of the femur.

Results.—An average of 7.4 years after surgery, all patients had negative pivot shift, Lachman, and anterior drawer tests. No more than 3 mm of anteroposterior displacement (mean ±SD =1.0 ±1.6 mm) was found using the KT-100 arthrometer test. The height of patients increased a mean of 17.7 cm. Orthoroentgenograms showed that patients' legs did not vary significantly in length (−0.8 mm ± 3.4 mm). In all patients, MR imaging revealed symmetric fusing of 4 tibial physes with 1 remaining open.

Conclusion.—The International Knee Documentation Committee (IKDC) method for evaluation revealed 4 patients to have grade A and 1, grade C. The patient with grade C had suffered additional knee injuries (patellar dislocation with osteochondral fracture). Hence, normal future growth does not appear to be inhibited by this procedure.

▶ Management of ACL injuries in the skeletally immature child is controversial. The concern that drill holes across an open epiphyseal plate will result in growth disturbances has resulted in many surgeons treating this problem in the skeletally immature child either nonoperatively or with extra-articular procedures. The literature clearly indicates that conservative treatment not only incapacitates the youngsters with regard to return to sports because of symptoms of instability, but, most important, results in subsequent injury to the menisci and joint surfaces. There's no question in my mind that complete tears of the ACL should be treated surgically with a graft passed through both tibial and femoral bone tunnels. Fear of growth plate disturbance is based on animal models, and to my knowledge, this problem has not been demonstrated in humans. The observations of the authors are in keeping with my own experience.

J.S. Torg, M.D.

A Biomechanical Study of Replacement of the Posterior Cruciate Ligament With a Graft: Part I: Isometry, Pre-tension of the Graft, and Anterior-Posterior Laxity

Markolf KL, Slauterbeck JR, Armstrong KL, et al (Univ of California, Los Angeles)

J Bone Joint Surg Am 79-A:375–380, 1997

3–25

Introduction.—A growing number of reports suggest that many patients experience excessive posterior laxity after reconstruction of the posterior cruciate ligament. Possible explanations for increased laxity are gradual stretching of the graft, improper placement of the graft, and failure to pre-tension the graft correctly. A cadaver study was conducted to examine the biomechanics of posterior cruciate reconstructions.

Methods.—An apparatus was designed for testing the 12 fresh-frozen, normal stable knees obtained from cadavera of individuals aged 49–79 at the time of death. Specimens were subjected to anterior-posterior laxity testing with 200 newtons of force applied to the tibia. After removal of the posterior cruciate ligament, the proximal end of a thin trial isometer model was attached to 1 of 4 points designated on the femur. Displacement of the distal end of the wire relative to the tibia was measured over a 120-degree range of motion.

Results.—Attaching the wire to the proximal part of the femur resulted in the least amount of change in the relative displacement of the trial wire over the 120-degree range of flexion. The greatest change in relative displacement was associated with the anterior point. The mean relative displacements of the trial wire when attached to a point at the center of the femoral origin of the ligament were not significantly different from the corresponding mean displacements of the distal end of the graft when the proximal end of the graft was centered at this point. As recorded by a load cell, the laxity-matched pre-tension of the graft at 90 degrees of flexion ranged from 6–100 newtons.

Discussion.—It is important to avoid anteriorly placed femoral tunnels, for isometer readings indicated increased tension, with flexion of the knee, in a graft placed in this region. The femoral end of the graft should be tensioned, and the pre-tension should be greater than 53 newtons in all cases so that normal laxity can be restored.

A Biomechanical Study of Replacement of the Posterior Cruciate Ligament With a Graft: Part II. Forces in the Graft Compared With Forces in the Intact Ligament

Markolf KL, Slauterbeck JR, Armstrong KL, et al (Univ of California, Los Angeles)

J Bone Joint Surg Am 79-A:381–386, 1997

3–26

Objective.—Patients undergoing reconstruction of the posterior cruciate ligament (PCL) may be left with increased posterior laxity, the result of incorrect graft pretensioning or graft stretching over time. Recommendations regarding bracing, rehabilitation, and postoperative activities require knowledge of the forces developing in the PCL graft. A cadaver study was performed to analyze the biomechanics of PCL replacement grafts.

Methods.—Tibial-loading tests were performed in 12 fresh-frozen cadaver knees. Measurements of force at the femoral origin of the PCL were obtained using a femoral load cell installed in the knee. After removal of the PCL, a bone-patellar ligament-bone graft, measuring 10 mm in width, was placed. With the knee in 90 degrees of flexion, graft pretensioning was performed to achieve the same anterior-posterior laxity as recorded after the load cell was installed. The loading tests were then repeated. The study sought to measure the effects of tibial prerotation on the forces generated in the intact PCL in response to a posterior tibial force; to compare the forces in the intact PCL vs. the pretensioned grafts; and to compare tibial rotation before and after PCL replacement, in the presence and absence of tibial torque.

Results.—The mean force in the intact PCL—with a 200–newton posterior force applied to the tibia, which was locked in neutral rotation—ranged from 220 newtons in 90 degrees of flexion to 36 newtons in full extension. This force was reduced with the tibia locked in external rotation during the posterior drawer test and the knee flexed 10 to 70 degrees. With the tibia locked in internal rotation, the mean force was reduced at 30 and 45 degrees of flexion only. Compared with the intact PCL, mean forces in the graft were not significantly different in response to a straight posterior tibial force, a 15 newton meter flexion or extension moment, a 10 newton meter varus or valgus moment, or a 10 newton meter internal or external tibial torque. The intact PCL and graft were similar in terms of mean tibial rotations at any angle of flexion, whether or not tibial torque was applied.

Conclusion.—With some exceptions, the forces measured in grafts used to replace the PCL are similar to those measured in the intact PCL. The findings suggest that, after healing of graft fixation, low-level rehabilitation activities need not be restricted. In both the graft and intact ligaments, high forces may be generated during hyperextension and hypertension. Thus, patients undergoing PCL reconstruction should be braced during the early postoperative period to prevent these motions.

▶ One of the major unsolved problems of ligamentous reconstructive knee surgery is the technical management of PCL reconstruction. These 2 articles (Abstracts 3–25 and 3–26) attempt to deal in vitro with the technical aspects of tunnel placement, isometry, graft tensioning, as well as the determination of forces generated in the ligament. Presumably, the latter information will have relevance with regard to rehabilitation activities and the advisability of bracing. Of course, the value of this information will be determined by clinical results.

J.S. Torg, M.D.

Injuries to the Posterolateral Aspect of the Knee: Association of Anatomic Injury Patterns With Clinical Instability

LaPrade RF, Terry GC (Hughston Clinic, PC, Columbus, Ga)
Am J Sports Med 25:433–438, 1997   3–27

Objective.—Whereas injuries to the posterolateral aspect of the knee at surgery have been described, no association of the injuries with abnormal clinical limits-of-motion testing has been provided. The association between clinical examination tests demonstrating abnormal limits of joint motion and specific anatomical injury patterns was prospectively investigated in a group of patients with injuries to the posterolateral structures of their knees.

Methods.—Clinical examinations, performed in 71 patients (22 females) treated for posterolateral knee injuries, included the anterior drawer test with the knee at 90 degrees of flexion, the posterolateral external-rotation test with the knee at 90 degrees of flexion, adduction and abduction with the knee at 30 degrees of flexion, the posterolateral external-rotation test with the knee at 30 degrees of flexion, the pivot shift test, the reverse pivot shift test, and the external rotation-recurvatum test (Fig 5). Patterns of injury to the anatomical component of the posterolateral aspect of the knee, to the anterior cruciate ligament, the posterior cruciate ligament, the menisci, the mid-third medial capsular ligament, chondral and osseous surfaces, and other structures were recorded at surgery . The ability of clinical examination to predict specific anatomical injuries was evaluated using multiple logistic regression.

Results.—Numerous tears were found at surgery (Table 1). Reverse pivot shift was associated with damage to the fibular collateral ligament, popliteal components, or mid-third lateral capsular ligament. Posterolateral external rotation at 30 degrees of flexion was associated with damage to the fibular collateral ligament and lateral gastrocnemius tendon. Adduction at 30 degrees of flexion was associated with damage to the posterior arcuate ligament. Because the fibular collateral ligament was injured in only 23% of knees, clinicians who suspect an injury to the posterolateral aspect of the knee should look further.

Conclusion.—There is an association between injured anatomical structures and abnormal clinical stability tests.

▶ The importance of understanding and recognizing the effects of injuries to the posterior lateral aspect of the knee deserves emphasis. Failure of the clinician to recognize an injury resulting in posterolateral instability can create a situation that is difficult, if not impossible, to reconstruct surgically. Although the material presented here is certainly not new, its value is in reiterating important concepts regarding posterolateral instability.

J.S. Torg, M.D.

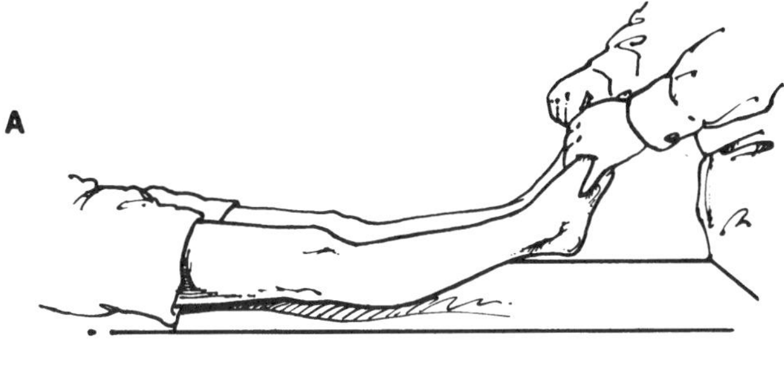

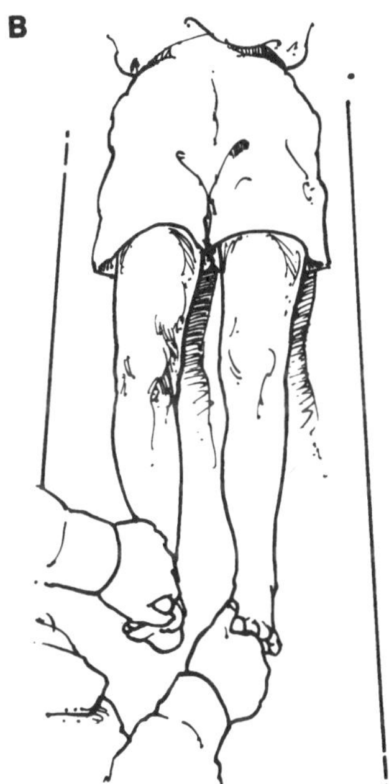

FIGURE 5.—External rotation-recurvatum test. **A**, patient is supine with both legs extended. The examiner grasps the great toes of both feet and simultaneously lifts both legs. **B**, a positive test is indicated by increased recurvatum, varus, and apparent internal rotation of the tibia on the injured leg caused by posterolateral opening of the joint. (Courtesy of LaPrade RF, Terry GC: Injuries to the posterolateral aspect of the knee: Association of anatomic injury patterns with clinical instability. *Am J Sports Med* 25:433–438, 1997).

TABLE 1.—Tears Found in Posterolateral Knee Anatomical Structures
During Surgical Exploration

Anatomic structure	No. of tears	Percentage of patients
Capsuloosseous layer of ITT	53	75
Deep layer of ITT	51	72
Components of posterior arcuate ligament	47	66
Components of short head of biceps femoris muscle*	45	63
Lateral aponeurotic components of biceps femoris muscle	41	58
Midthird lateral capsular ligament	37	52
Fabellofibular ligament	28	39
Popliteal components	25	35
Fibular collateral ligament	16	23
Components of long head of biceps femoris muscle*	9	13
Superficial layer of ITT	4	6
Lateral gastrocnemius tendon	3	4
Arciform layer of ITT	2	3

*Excluding lateral aponeurotic components.
Abbreviation: ITT, iliotibial tract.
(Courtesy of LaPrade RF, Terry GC: Injuries to the posterolateral aspect of the knee: Association of anatomical injury patterns with clinical instability. *Am J Sports Med* 25:433–438, 1997.)

Arthroscopic Meniscal Repair Using Fibrin Glue: Part I. Experimental Study

Ishimura M, Ohgushi H, Habata T, et al (Nara Med Univ, Kashihara, Japan; Nara Shin-oomiya Seikeigeka Clinic, Japan)
Arthroscopy 13:551–557, 1997

3–28

Introduction.—It is hard to achieve good outcomes when suturing tears in the avascular area of menisci. A purified fibrin glue has been used with some success in repairing this tissue. The healing-promoting properties of fibrin glue were assessed in an experimental trial of rabbit menisci.

Methods.—The fibrin glue was made from rabbit blood. A 1.5-mm–diameter defect was created in the left knee of 60 rabbits. Twenty rabbits each were placed in 1 of 3 groups: in C group, the defect was left empty; in F group, the defect was filled with fibrin glue; and in M group, the defect was filled with fibrin glue–containing marrow cells. Five animals from each group were sacrificed at 1, 3, 6, and 12 weeks postoperatively. The removed menisci were photographed and the vacant areas remaining in the punched-out defect were quantified using a color image processor. Samples of each menisci underwent histologic examination.

Results.—At each time point, the remaining defect was significantly smaller in the F group and the M group, compared with the C group. Histologic evaluation revealed earlier mature healing of the defects in the M group than the F group. There were no adverse reactions.

Conclusion.—Defects filled with fibrin glue–containing marrow cells had earlier histologic maturation and more rapid healing, compared with defects filled with acellular fibrin glue. Fibrin glue–containing marrow cells may be more effective in enhancing meniscal healing than fibrin glue by itself.

Arthroscopic Meniscal Repair Using Fibrin Glue: Part II. Clinical Applications

Ishimura M, Ohgushi H, Habata T, et al (Nara Med Univ, Kashihara, Japan; Nara Shin-oomiya Seikeigeka Clinic, Japan)
Arthroscopy 13:558–563, 1997   3–29

Introduction.—A recurrence rate of 11% to 30% has been reported in patients with isolated meniscal tears who undergo suture repair. Posterior segment tears are difficult to suture without arthrotomy. The long-term follow-up of patients who underwent arthroscopic repair of meniscal tears using a purified fibrin-based glue was reported.

Methods.—Forty patients underwent 61 meniscal repairs beginning in 1984. The average patient follow-up was 8 years. The average patient age was 20 years (range, 12–45 years). Ten knees had isolated meniscal tears (isolation group) and 30 knees also had anterior cruciate ligament (ACL) lesions (combined group).

Operative Technique.—There are 2 solutions in the fibrin adhesive system. Solution A is composed of purified dense fibrinogen, aprotinin, and factor. Thrombin and calcium chloride make up solution B. When the tear was in the medial meniscus, the inner margin of the torn meniscus was held with a grasping forceps and the position at reduction was confirmed. The glue was injected with a 20-gauge, 90-mm needle around the anterior border of the medial collateral ligament. For tears in the lateral meniscus, the needle was inserted around the anterior border of the lateral collateral ligament (Fig 2). When there was an associated ACL lesion, the meniscus repair was done immediately after ligament reconstruction. Meniscal sutures were used when the torn meniscus was degenerated. Recreational sports activities were allowed at 3 and 6 months, respectively, in the isolation and combined groups.

Results.—In 35 repairs in 27 patients with early repair, 77% of results were good, 11.5% were fair, and 11.5% were poor. Six patients (6 repairs) complained of meniscal symptoms (2 locking, 4 catching) at an average of 2.8 years after initial repair, and they underwent partial meniscectomy. Factors most significantly correlated with recurrent symptoms were insufficiency of the associated ACL, repairs of fresh tears, and repairs requiring supplementary meniscal sutures.

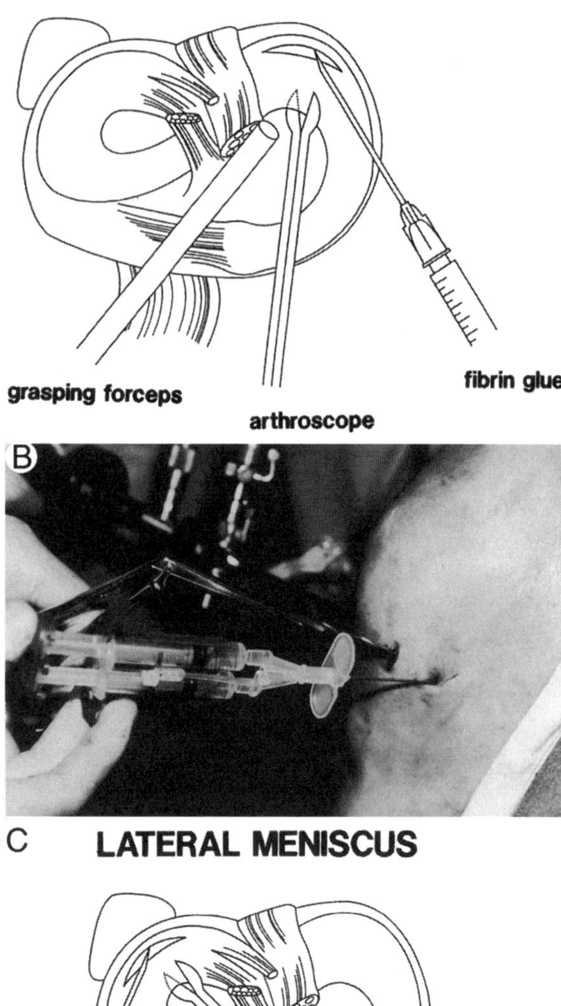

FIGURE 2.—Operative procedures. **A,** schematic drawing of meniscal repair using fibrin glue for a tear of the medial meniscus in the right knee. **B,** corresponding intraoperative photograph. **C,** schematic drawing of meniscal repair using fibrin glue for a tear of the lateral meniscus in the right knee. (Courtesy of Ishimura M, Ohgushi H, Habata T, et al: Arthroscopic meniscal repair using fibrin glue: Part II. Clinical applications. *Arthroscopy* 13:558–563, 1997.)

Conclusion.—The recurrence rate in patients undergoing arthroscopic meniscal repair using fibrin glue was 10%. This method is easier to perform than other methods because it minimizes the need for suturing. It may be used concomitantly with ACL reconstruction.

▶ Both the importance and the difficulty of meniscal repair are well recognized. The literature indicates an 11% to 30% recurrence rate for isolated meniscal repairs treated with suturing techniques. The recurrence rate reported in this clinical study using fibrin glue is most impressive. Also, this failure rate can be explained on the basis of associated ACL instability, meniscal degenerative changes, unstable tears, and tears in the white zone. One problem with the study by Ishimura et al is that there was no evaluation with regard to the level of functional activities post operation. An interesting approach to dealing with meniscal tears might be combining the fibrin glue with the currently available biodegradable meniscal arrows.

J.S. Torg, M.D.

Preliminary Results of the T-fix Endoscopic Meniscus Repair Technique in an Anterior Cruciate Ligament Reconstruction Population
Barrett GR, Treacy SH, Ruff CG, et al (Mississippi Sports Medicine and Orthopaedic Ctr, Jackson)
Arthroscopy 13:218–223, 1997   3–30

Background.—The menisci have a basic role in shock absorption, load transmission, and joint stability in the knee. It is important to preserve meniscal tissue; studies of total and partial meniscectomies show an increasing rate of degenerative changes over time. The most effective technique of maintaining maximum functional meniscal tissue in cases of a peripheral vascularized tear is controversial. A recently introduced technique uses the T-fix suture anchor for repair of meniscal tears. Potential advantages are avoidance of a posterior incision, ease of placement, and fewer complications, such as neurovascular injury. There have been no reports on the results of studies of this device.

Methods.—The T-fix suture anchor was used in 21 meniscus repairs in 20 patients. There were 11 medial tears and 10 lateral tears. Fourteen tears were in the peripheral third of the meniscus (zones 0–1) and 7 tears were in the central third (zone 2). All patients had anterior cruciate ligament reconstruction. Follow-up was 12 to 28 months.

Results.—At follow-up, 4 patients were symptomatic, and 3 of these had complex tears in zone 2. Radiographs showed that 3 patients had a mild progression Fairbank's change. All sutures were removed in 1 patient because of infection. In 4 patients, second-look arthroscopy showed that 3 patients had healed and 1 had not.

Discussion.—Good clinical results were seen after arthroscopic meniscus repair with the T-fix suture anchor device at short-term follow-up. These results indicate that meniscus healing can occur after repair using the T-fix endoscopic technique if principles of meniscus repair are followed, such as blood supply, synovial rasping, and stable fixation. There was a high failure rate in cases of complex meniscal tears or tears in circumferential zone 2. Long-term follow-up data and more extensive second-look data are needed.

▶ In view of the fact that all of the patients in this study had their anterior cruciate ligament reconstructed in addition to T-fix endoscopic meniscus repair and were released to full activity at 6 months, renders the minimum follow-up of 1 year most inadequate. Therefore, other than the observation that this technique does not work well in complex meniscal tears for tears located in the red/white zone, no other conclusion can be drawn regarding the efficacy of the T-fix device.

J.S. Torg, M.D.

Tissue Engineered Meniscus: A Potential New Alternative to Allogeneic Meniscus Transplantation
Ibarra C, Jannetta C, Vacanti CA, et al (Harvard Med School, Boston; Univ of Massachusetts, Worcester)
Transplant Proc 29:986–988, 1997   3–31

Introduction.—Attempts to replace a massively torn or absent meniscus have not yielded encouraging results. An ideal alternative for the patients who had to undergo a total meniscectomy would be a new meniscus, created from the patient's own cells and with the shape and size to fit the knee exactly. "Tissue-engineered" meniscal tissue was created for this purpose.

Methods.—Bovine fibrochondrocytes were isolated by collagenase digestion of both menisci harvested from newborn calf knees. Prepared cells were seeded onto polyglycolic acid (PGA) scaffolds or suspended in a 1% calcium alginate gel at a concentration of 2.5×10^7 cells/mL. The cell-polymer constructs were planted subcutaneously in 24 nude mice for 4, 8, and 16 weeks (8 mice at each time point). In a control condition, 6 PGA scaffolds without cells were similarly implanted. Harvested tissue specimens were analyzed and compared with normal meniscus samples.

Results.—Histologic sections of 4-week specimens exhibited matrix architecture similar to meniscal repair tissue, and by 16 weeks the tissue formed had the gross appearance of meniscal tissue, had maintained the size and shape of the original polymer scaffolds, and had a pattern of fiber orientation similar to that of normal meniscus (Fig 2).

Discussion.—Fibrochondrocytes can be isolated from menisci, expanded in culture, and loaded onto synthetic biodegradable polymer scaffolds and injectable gels. Some areas of meniscal tissue had matrix architecture almost identical to normal meniscal tissue, suggesting that the cells have an intrinsic ability to form specific tissue structures. Meniscal tissue

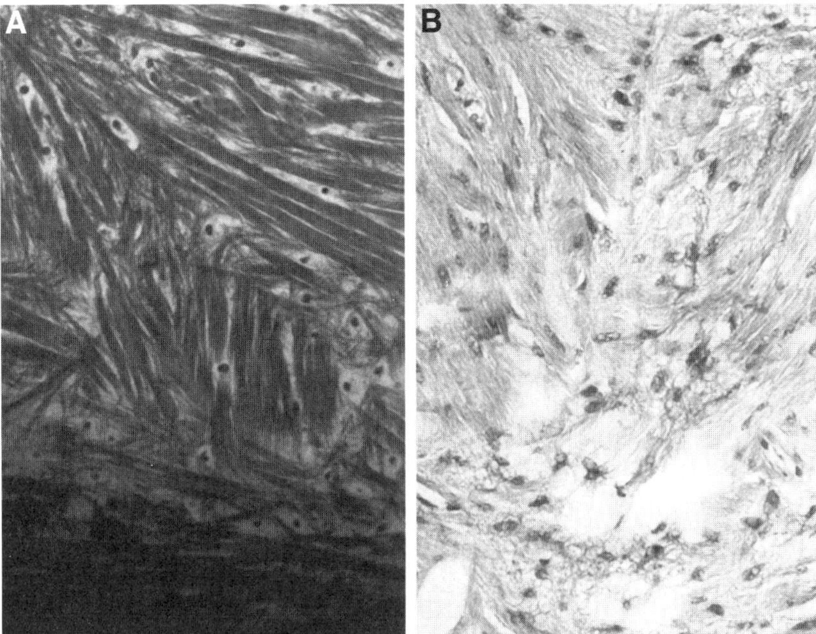

FIGURE 2.—**A,** histologic section stained with Masson's trichrome of a specimen of normal bovine meniscus (20×). Notice the orientation pattern of the collagen fibers. **B,** histologic section stained with hematoxylin and eosin of tissue engineered meniscus after 16 weeks of implantation (20×). Notice the similarity in fiber orientation pattern to normal meniscus. (Courtesy of Ibarra C, Jannetta C, Vacanti CA, et al: Tissue engineered meniscus: A potential new alternative to allogeneic meniscus transplantation. *Transplant Proc* 29:986–988. Copyright 1997, reprinted by permission of Appleton & Lange, Inc.)

engineered from autologous cells could substitute for allografts in meniscus transplantation.

Regeneration of Meniscal Cartilage With Use of a Collagen Scaffold: Analysis of Preliminary Data

Stone KR, Steadman JR, Rodkey WG, et al (Stone Clinic, San Francisco; Steadman-Hawkins, Vail, Colo; ReGen Biologics, Redwood City, Calif)
J Bone Joint Surg Am 79-A:1770–1777, 1997   3–32

Introduction.—Most methods used to replace damaged or removed meniscal cartilage have yielded poor results. Seeking an alternative to artificial materials and autogenous or allograft tissue, researchers have successfully used collagen scaffolds as templates for regeneration of meniscal cartilage in dogs. This article reports the first clinical trial of such a collagen implant in humans.

Methods.—Six criteria were required for collagen implant materials: they had to be biocompatible, have a physical shape similar to that of the normal meniscus, have a pore structure that would facilitate cellular

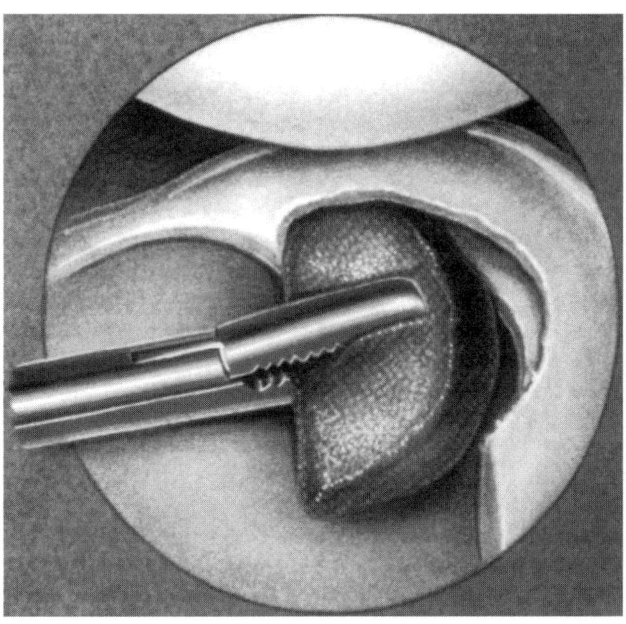

FIGURE 3.—Drawing showing insertion and suturing of the collagen meniscal implant. (Courtesy of Stone KR, Steadman JR, Rodkey WG, et al: Regeneration of meniscal cartilage with use of a collagen scaffold: Analysis of preliminary data. *J Bone Joint Surg Am* 79-A:1770–1777, 1997.)

ingrowth, have an initial mechanical strength suitable for operative implantation, be permeable to macromolecules for nutrient supply, and have an initial in vivo stability. The material developed consisted of purified collagen fibers from bovine Achilles tendon. After independent laboratories tested the collagen meniscal implant for safety, 10 patients with an irreparable tear or major loss of meniscal cartilage were enrolled in a phase-1 trial of the implant. The implant was inserted (Fig 3) via an anterior medial miniarthrotomy incision of approximately 2 cm. Sutures placed through arthroscopic cannulae were tied directly over the posterior part of the medial aspect of the capsule (Fig 4). Patients were followed for effects of the implant on the immune system and examined with MRI for regeneration of tissue.

Results.—Nine patients remained in the study for 36 months. The collagen scaffold was found to be safe and to support regeneration of tissue in meniscal defects of various sizes. Sequential serological testing revealed no adverse immunological reactions. Second-look arthroscopy, performed 3 or 6 months after implantation, confirmed that newly formed

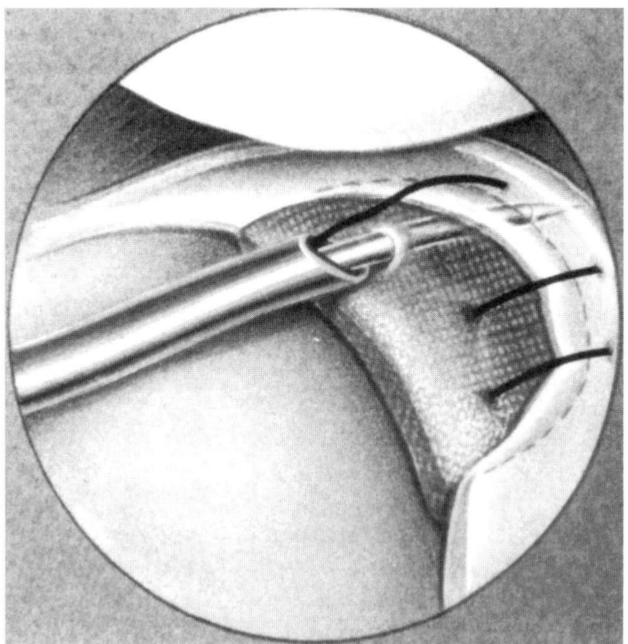

FIGURE 4.—Drawing showing insertion and suturing of the collagen meniscal implant. (Courtesy of Stone KR, Steadman JR, Rodkey WG, et al: Regeneration of meniscal cartilage with use of a collagen scaffold: Analysis of preliminary data. *J Bone Joint Surg Am* 79-A:1770–1777, 1997.)

tissue was replacing the implant as it was resorbed. At 6 months, the gross appearance of the regenerated tissue was similar to that of the fibrous tissue of meniscal cartilage Three years after receiving the implant (Fig 7), patients reported a decrease in symptoms and an increase in their ability to perform strenuous activities.

Conclusion.—Regeneration of meniscal cartilage can be accomplished in humans by means of an implanted collagen scaffold. With 3 years of follow-up, the implant was found to be safe and effective.

▶ These 2 articles make several noteworthy points. First, the "use of a new meniscus created from the patient's own cells, with the exact shape and size to fit the patient's knee, would be an ideal alternative for the patient that had to undergo a total meniscectomy." Second, "these studies suggest that regeneration of meniscal cartilage through a collagen scaffold is possible." Third, "additional studies are needed to determine long-term efficacy."

J.S. Torg, M.D.

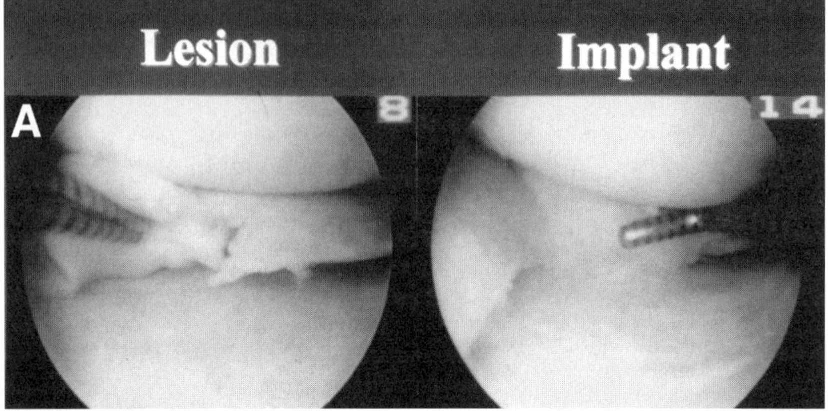

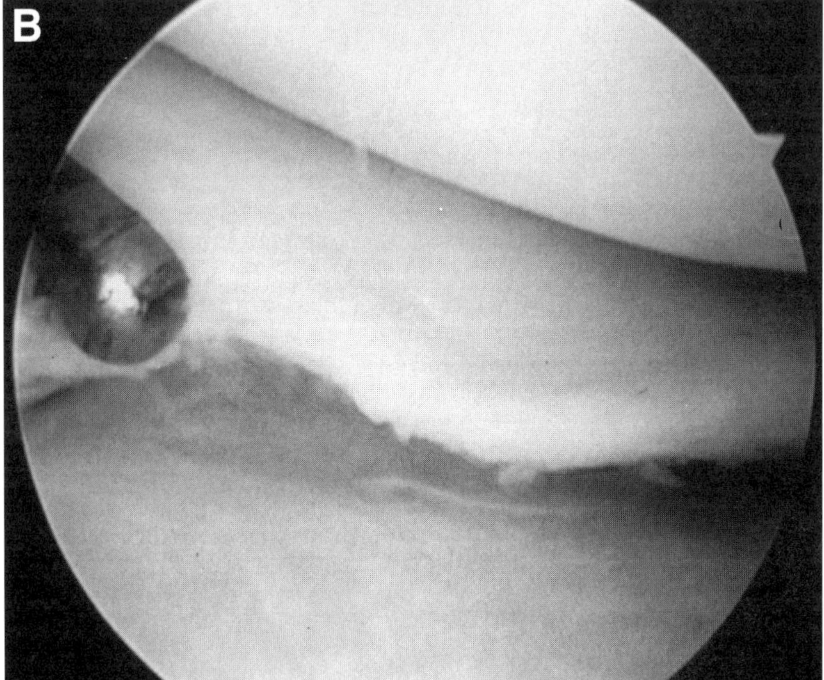

FIGURE 7.—**A,** intraoperative photograph of a meniscal lesion before and after placement of the collagen meniscal implant. **B,** photograph of a meniscal lesion, made at second-look arthroscopy, 6 months after placement of the collagen meniscal implant. (Courtesy of Stone KR, Steadman JR, Rodkey WG, et al: Regeneration of meniscal cartilage with use of a collagen scaffold: Analysis of preliminary data. *J Bone Joint Surg Am* 79-A:1770–1777, 1997.)

Total Knee Replacement in Young, Active Patients: Long-term Follow-up and Functional Outcome

Diduch DR, Insall JN, Scott WN, et al (Beth Israel North Med Ctr, New York)
J Bone Joint Surg Am 79-A:575–582, 1997   3–33

Objective.—For the young patient with a painful, osteoarthrotic knee, the choice is between conservative therapy, which provides little lasting benefit; surgery, which interferes with activity; and knee replacement, which carries the risk of later prosthetic complications. Knee replacement is generally reserved for patients older than 60 years, yet there is no evidence showing the outcomes of knee replacement in younger patients. An experience with total knee arthroplasty in patients aged 55 years or younger was reviewed.

Methods.—A total of 114 knee replacements were performed in 88 patients with severe osteoarthrosis. Their average age was 51 years. The surgeons used a cemented technique and a posterior stabilized, posterior cruciate–substituting prosthesis in nearly every case. Survivorship analysis included 108 knees of 48 patients. Clinical evaluation, including the Hospital for Special Surgery and the Knee Society scores, was performed in 103 unrevised knees at an average follow-up of 8 years. Follow-up of longer than 10 years was available for 36 knees. Patient activity was assessed using the activity score of Tegner and Lysholm. Radiographic evidence of component loosening was retrospectively sought.

Results.—The average Hospital for Special Surgery score increased from 55 points before knee replacement to 92 afterward. The average Knee Society score was 94 points and the average functional score was 89 points at the most recent follow-up examination. On both scoring systems, all knees had a good or excellent result. The average activity score improved from 1.3 points before surgery to 3.5 points at last follow-up. The activity score improved after knee replacement in all patients but 2. Nearly one fifth of patients had an increase in their activity score of 5 points or greater. They were able to take part in such recreational activities as tennis, skiing, and bicycling, as well as in farm or construction labor.

Nonprogressive tibial radiolucent lines were observed in 9% of knees. Late infections developed in 2 patients, requiring revision. Another patient had polyethylene wear requiring replacement of a tibial component, which was well fixed at the time. Loosening required revision of the patellar component in 3 patients, and instability led to spacer exchange in another. Overall 18-year survival was 94% when failure was defined as revision of the femoral or tibial component, and 90% when failure was expanded to include patellar revisions.

Conclusions.—Good results are reported in younger patients undergoing arthroplasty with a cemented posterior stabilized total knee prosthesis. Knee replacement should be considered in younger patients when less invasive treatments have failed. Despite their high activity level during 8 years' follow-up, these patients have few problems with polyethylene wear, osteolysis, or prosthetic loosening. However, the outcomes could change with longer follow-up. The decision to perform arthroplasty in a younger patient should always be considered carefully, and the patient advised to avoid activities involving impact.

▶ A most creditable report on the results of total knee replacement in young active patients with an average age of 51 years. Unfortunately, however, the long-term evaluation was based on 2 knee scoring systems and was not activity specific for each of the 108 knees reported. With regard to specific activities, it appears that postoperatively 24% regularly participated in such activities as tennis, skiing, bicycling, or strenuous farm or construction work. Importantly, loosening that necessitated revision was not a notable problem in this group. The authors do conclude that "until additional information is available, total knee arthroplasty in younger patients should continue to be considered with caution and activities that involve impact should be avoided. For some younger patients, deferment of definitive operative treatment may be the best option."

J.S. Torg, M.D.

Technique for Arthroscopic Suture Fixation of Displaced Tibial Intercondylar Eminence Fractures
Kogan MG, Marks P, Amendola A (Lake in the Hills, Ill; Orthopaedic and Arthritic Hosp, Toronto; Univ of Western Ontario, London, Canada)
Arthroscopy 13:301–306, 1997   3–34

Background.—Open reduction and immobilization have been recommended for type II fractures of the tibial intercondylar eminence—those with complete separation of the fracture fragment. Although operative techniques and fixation methods have varied, this recommendation has held over the years. Recent reports have described arthroscopic suture fixation of these fractures. A technique of arthroscopic reduction and suture fixation of displaced avulsion fractures of the tibial intercondylar eminence, including comminuted fractures, was reported.

Technique.—After routine diagnostic arthroscopy, full radius resection is performed to removes hematoma and loose fragments from the fracture site. The fracture fragment is approximated to the tibial fracture bed. A 2-cm longitudinal incision is made and a commercial anterior cruciate ligament (ACL) tibial drill guide is introduced. A guide pin is drilled through the fracture bed into the avulsed fragment to hold it in place. Another guide pin is placed into the anteromedial edge of the fracture bed or through the reduced fragment, then removed for a Hewson suture passer. A Caspari punch is passed through the loop of the suture passer to place a No. 0 or 1 PDS suture into the medial base of the ACL. After this step is repeated, the suture passer is retracted through the tibia, bringing the 2 sutures through the drill hole. Another guide pin is placed into the anterolateral aspect of the fracture, and sutures are placed as before. Through tension on the sutures and use of a probe, the fracture is reduced, and normal ACL position and tension are restored.

The knee is observed through the arthroscope as it is put through a full range of motion. An additional drill hole can be placed anterior to the avulsed fragment, if necessary, to prevent anterior lifting of the fragment with the knee in extension. The knee is kept immobilized in full extension for 2–3 weeks, followed by range-of-motion exercises. After protected weight-bearing on crutches for 6 weeks, strengthening exercises are started.

Experience.—This technique has been used in 6 adult patients with displaced fractures of the tibial intercondylar eminence. Four patients achieved full range of motion by 6 weeks. The other 2 patients reached −2 degrees of extension by 8 weeks. The patients were followed up for an average of 22 months. All were satisfied with their results and were able to return to their previous level of activity. None of the patients had any problems with instability or required additional surgery.

Conclusions.—A modified technique for arthroscopic reduction and suture fixation of displaced tibial intercondylar eminence fractures is technically simple, can be used even in comminuted fractures, and leaves no hardware behind in the knee. Good results have been achieved using this arthroscopic technique, combined with a relatively aggressive rehabilitation program.

▶ On the basis of this article and my own experience in the arthroscopic management of this problem, I would agree that reduction and suture fixation can restore the necessary tension on the ACL in a reproducible and simplified manner without the need for metal hardware.

J.S. Torg, M.D.

The Effect of a Pneumatic Leg Brace on Return to Play in Athletes With Tibial Stress Fractures

Swenson EJ Jr, DeHaven KE, Sebastianelli WJ, et al (Univ of Rochester, NY; Penn State Univ, Univ Park, Pa; Orthopaedic Inst of Pennsylvania, Camp Hill)
Am J Sports Med 25:322–328, 1997   3–35

Objective.—Approximately half of the stress fractures that occur are tibial stress fractures, and most occur from running. Although some stress fractures have been treated with pneumatic leg braces, allowing immediate return to sports without disabling symptoms, there have been no prospective reviews or controlled studies conducted of the outcome. Results of a prospective, randomized study evaluating the effect of the pneumatic leg brace on return to play in recreational and competitive athletes with tibial stress fractures were reported.

The progression is designed for a 1/4 mile track (i.e., 220 yards, half lap; 440 yards, 1/4 mile, one lap; 880 yards, 1/2 mile, two laps; 3/4 mile, three laps; 1 mile, four laps). If a 1/4 mile track is not available, estimate distances as closely as possible.

Stage I
1. Walk 1 mile
2. Walk 330 yards (three-quarter lap), jog 110 yards (one-quarter lap), walk 330 yards, jog 110 yards, walk 330 yards, jog 110 yards, walk 330 yards, jog 110 yards, walk 110 yards.
3. Walk 220 yards, jog 220 yards, walk 220 yards, jog 220 yards, walk 220 yards, jog 220 yards, walk 440 yards.
4. Walk 440 yards, jog 440 yards, walk 440 yards, jog 440 yards, walk 100 yards.
5. Walk 440 yards, jog 880 yards, walk 440 yards.
6. Walk 220 yards. jog 3/4 mile, walk 220 yards.
7. Walk 100 yards, jog 1 mile, walk 100 yards.

Stage II
8. Jog 330 yards, run 110 yards, jog 330 yards, run 110 yards, jog 330 yards, run 110 yards, jog 330 yards, run 110 yards, jog 110 yards.
9. Jog 220 yards, run 220 yards, jog 220 yards, run 220 yards, jog 220 yards, run 220 yards, jog 440 yards.
10. Jog 440 yards, run 440 yards, jog 440 yards, run 440 yards, jog 110 yards.
11. Jog 440 yards, run 880 yards, jog 440 yards.
12. Jog 440 yards, run 3/4 mile, jog 220 yards.
13. Jog 440 yards, run 1 mile, jog 220 yards.

Stage III—Progression to Sprint Running Step 13 may be used as warmup for "sprint running" to include stretching. Walk for 440 yards and then complete the sprint running as indicated in Step 14. Complete a cool-down jog for 440 yards. Rest between intervals is completed by walking. Code: 220 (distance) × 2 (repeats) with 3 minutes (rest).
14. Run 50 yards at 50% speed then at 75% for two repetitions and finally at 100% speed for two repetitions taking as much time as needed to rest between intervals.
15. 100 × 2 with 5 minutes.
16. 100 × 4 with 5 minutes.
17. 40 × 6 with 3 minutes.
18. 40 × 10 with 2 minutes.

Stage IV—Agility Drills
Agility activities are used for the sports that involve jumping and cutting. Complete a warmup of 1 mile and then initiate agility exercise A. Complete one cycle of each exercise at 50% of full speed and then progress to one cycle at 75% and then one cycle of 100%. If disabling pain occurs stop and proceed as directed in the introduction. Certain people may find that they can complete the agility activities within one session. Distance and sprint running are then completed.
   A. *Figure-of-8 Running:* Run a figure-of-8 pattern with two 10-foot diameter circles and then with two 5-foot diameter circles. Complete 3 repetitions of each figure-of-8 at 50%, 75%, and 100% effort.
   B. *Carioca:* Run sideways crossing legs in front of and then behind the lead leg for 20 yards, rest 5 seconds, and return in other direction. Repeat 4 times for each cycle.
   C. *Backward Running:* Run for 20 yards, rest 5 seconds, and repeat 4 times for each cycle.
   D. *Box Running:* Select an area and mark out a 5 yard square box for the run. Initiate the run by running the box 5 times clockwise and then 5 times counterclockwise.
   E. *Vertical Jumping:* Jump with 50% effort and mark a spot on a wall. Repeat jumping to that mark 10 times. Change the mark to 75% and jump 10 times. Change the mark to 100% and jump 10 times.

Stage V—Progression to Practice and Games
Practice sessions are not initiated until functional rehabilitation is successfully completed. All practice sessions are initiated with a warmup that includes 1) light running and stretching, 2) gradual increase in speed to full speed running, 3) completion of agility activities with gradual increase in intensity, and 4) gradual increase in speed and intensity of movements specific to sport. After practice complete a cooldown of running and stretching.

(Courtesy of Swenson EJ, DeHaven KE, Sebastianelli WJ, et al: The effect of a pneumatic leg brace on return to play in athletes with tibial stress fractures. *Am J Sports Med* 25:322–328, 1997.)

Methods.—Eighteen athletes, aged 15 to 44 years, with a tibial stress fracture were randomly assigned to treatment with a pneumatic leg brace (10 patients) and gradual return-to-activity guidelines or the traditional non–weight-bearing treatment (8 patients) of 3 days of rest and gradual return to activities (Appendix). Radiographs were taken at baseline and at 6 and 12 weeks after treatment. Pain and tenderness were evaluated at each visit.

Results.—The median time from initiation of treatment to the beginning of light activity was 7 days for the brace group and 21 days for the traditional group. Resolution of swelling, tenderness to palpation, percussion, and vibratory pain were similar between groups. The median time to disappearance of pain was 14 days for the brace group and 45 days for the traditional group. The median time from beginning of treatment to completion of functional progression was 21 days for the brace group and 77 days for the traditional group.

Conclusion.—When the pneumatic leg brace was used for treating athletes with tibial stress fractures, athletes returned to light activity, experienced disappearance of pain, and completed functional progression significantly faster than athletes treated in the traditional way.

▶ The pneumatic leg brace used in this study was the long (15.5 inches) Air-Stirrup (Aircast Corporation, Newark, New Jersey) leg brace.[1] The results indicate that the athletes wearing this brace returned to activity in significantly less time than those who did not. This brace may also be used to alleviate symptoms in those athletes with suspected stress fractures.

F.J. George, A.T.C., P.T.

Acute Atraumatic Compartment Syndrome in an Athlete: A Case Report

Stollsteimer GT, Shelton WR (Mississippi Sports Medicine & Orthopaedic Ctr, Jackson)
J Athletic Train 32:248–250, 1997   3–36

Introduction.—An uncommon complication of participation in athletics is acute, atraumatic, exercise-induced compartment syndrome of the leg. Delay in diagnosis can lead to disastrous consequences. Complications can be prevented by understanding the pathogenesis, diagnosis, and treatment of this disease. A case report is presented.

> *Case Report.*—Male football player 18, complained of severe anterolateral left leg pain on his second day of training and was diagnosed with shin splints. On the fourth day, the patient told the physician the pain worsened with ambulation, and he had a tense, swollen, anterolateral compartment of the left leg. Palpation over the anterolateral compartment caused excruciating pain.

Results.—After receiving a diagnosis of atraumatic compartment syndrome, he was transferred to the hospital for emergency surgery. An anterolateral compartment fasciotomy was performed. Debridement of the dead muscle was performed and a free-flap latissimus dorsi graft was used to cover the wound At 6 weeks post injury, the patient had a persistent foot drop and a persistent sensory loss in the distributions of the superficial peroneal nerve and the deep peroneal nerve.

Conclusion.—Acute compartment syndrome is potentially more devastating than the more frequent causes of leg pain, such as chronic exertional compartment syndrome, stress fracture, or medial tibial syndrome, but it is much less common. The soft tissue can become ischemic and cells can die when the increased intracompartment pressure within a closed tissue space exceeds capillary perfusion pressure and tissue perfusion is decreased. Pain with passive stretching of the compartment and pain out of proportion to the results of the physical examination are the most important clinical diagnostic signs of compartment syndrome.

▶ The authors emphasize that the 5 "P's" commonly used to diagnose acute compartment syndrome are not a reliable diagnostic tool. They stress that the most important diagnostic sign is pain with passive stretching of the compartment and pain greater than one would normally expect. This particular case occurred with no documented contact; however, maximal exertion in an unconditioned athlete was reported.

F.J. George, A.F.C., P.T.

Functional Bracing for Rupture of the Achilles Tendon: Clinical Results and Analysis of Ground-reaction Forces and Temporal Data
McComis GP, Nawoczenski DA, DeHaven KE, et al (Univ of Rochester, NY)
J Bone Joint Surg Am 79-A:1799–1808, 1997   3–37

Introduction.—Classic treatment for rupture of the Achilles tendon is surgery or immobilization in a plaster cast. Surgery is associated with a lower rate of repeat rupture and also with increased risk of morbidity related to an open procedure and higher cost. The functional brace is a nonoperative approach that allows immediate weight-bearing, active plantar flexion of the ankle, and limited dorsiflexion. Clinical and functional performance was compared in 15 patients managed with a functional bracing protocol for treatment of ruptured Achilles tendon and 15 age- and gender-matched normal controls.

Methods.—Patients were studied for a mean of 31 months. Participants were given numeric scores (100–point scoring system) based on subjective responses to a questionnaire, clinical measurements of the range of motion of the ankle and the circumference of the calf, and results of the Thompson squeeze test and a single-limb heel-rise test. Ground-reaction forces and temporal data were evaluated during functional dynamic activities, including walking, a single-limb power hop, and a 30-second single-limb heel-rise endurance test.

Results.—Results of functional testing were: 3 excellent, 9 good, 2 fair, and 1 poor. The only significant difference between the treatment group and normal controls was an increase in passive dorsiflexion of the treated ankle. The increase in dorsiflexion was associated with vertical force output between the mid-stance and terminal-stance phases of gait. There were no significant between-group differences in kinetic or temporal variables measured during functional dynamic activities. Patients who had less peak vertical force and vertical height during the single-limb power hop test were likely to have poorer clinical scores.

Conclusion.—Nonoperative functional bracing may be a viable alternative to surgery or plaster casting for treatment of acute rupture of the Achilles tendon. This approach may reduce the time needed for rehabilitation, facilitate an early return to work and preinjury activities, and offer a feasible alternative for patients not able to undergo surgical intervention.

▶ The authors report an innovative approach to the management of acute Achilles tendon ruptures. A major defect in the study, in addition to the small number of participants studied, was failure of the authors to include an operatively-treated cohort for comparison. Thus, their conclusion that "additional investigations involving the larger population of patients, as well as comparison with a cohort of operatively treated patients, would strengthen decisions regarding the treatment of acute ruptures of the Achilles tendon" is appropriate. It should be noted that in the group of 15 patients who did return for follow-up, 1 sustained a rerupture and 5 were unable to return to their previous activity level. It is my opinion that in physically active individuals, operative intervention with an accelerated postoperative rehabilitation program is actually the more conservative approach to management of this problem.

J.S. Torg, M.D.

Chronic Pain Following Ankle Sprains in Athletes: The Role of Arthroscopic Surgery

Ogilvie-Harris DJ, Gilbart MK, Chorney K (Toronto Hosp; Univ of Toronto)
Arthroscopy 13:564–574, 1997   3–38

Purpose.—Ankle sprains are very common injuries that can lead to significant morbidity and cost. For patients with persistent symptoms 6 months after ankle sprain, arthroscopy is an option for further treatment. Arthroscopy may reveal such chronic problems as instability, impingement, or articular lesions. The indications for and findings of arthroscopy for patients with chronic ankle pain after sprains of the ankle were studied.

Methods.—A total of 100 patients with persistent symptoms 6 months after a major acute ankle sprain were studied. All underwent arthroscopy after lack of response to the usual conservative treatment modalities. At arthroscopy, the pathologic findings were classified as instabilities, lateral and syndesmotic; impingements, anterior and anterolateral; or articular lesions, chondral and osteochondral. Arthroscopic diagnosis was followed by specific surgical interventions. The patients were then followed up in terms of pain, swelling, stiffness, limping, activity, and instability. In addition to the main outcomes of pain and activity, the patients' level of satisfaction and return to sports were assessed.

Results.—The arthroscopic pathologic findings were lateral instability in 27 patients, syndesmotic instability in 9, anterior impingement in 11, anterolateral impingement in 17, chondral fractures or loose bodies in 21, and osteochondral fractures in 7. Five patients had nonspecific findings, i.e., osteoarthritis and/or synovitis. The patients with syndesmotic instability and those with anterior or anterolateral impingement showed significant improvement after arthroscopic surgery. Seventy-five percent of patients with chondral fracture in a stable ankle had good results, compared with 33% of those with unstable ankles. For patients with osteochondritis dissecans, excision of the lesion with abrasion of the base constituted effective treatment. Chronic lateral instability required open surgical repair; in this group, arthroscopy was useful for diagnostic purposes only. Arthroscopy offered little improvement for patients with nonspecific diagnoses.

Conclusions.—The findings help to clarify the diagnostic and therapeutic uses of ankle arthroscopy in patients with chronic pain after ankle sprains. Unless the diagnosis is in question, arthroscopy is of little benefit to patients with lateral instability. For patients with other pathologic conditions, arthroscopy offers definitive treatment. All patients with ankle sprains should receive at least 6 months of conservative therapy, which will be sufficient treatment in many cases.

▶ It is important to point out that the role of arthroscopic surgery in the posttraumatic ankle resulting in lateral and syndesmotic instability is limited to a diagnostic one. Specifically, in the group of 27 patients with lateral instability, a reconstruction was carried out after arthroscopy in 21 patients. Although the authors conclude that ankle arthroscopy was a valuable aide to diagnosis in all cases, it was definitive in the treatment of those having other than lateral instability.

J.S. Torg, M.D.

Persistent Pain After Ankle Sprain: Targeting the Causes
Bassewitz HL, Shapiro MS (Univ of California, Los Angeles)
Physician Sportsmed 12:58–68, 1997   3–39

Background.—Ankle sprains are the most commonly seen injury in athletes; conservative treatment usually achieves good results. However, some patients have continued pain after an apparently routine sprain. The

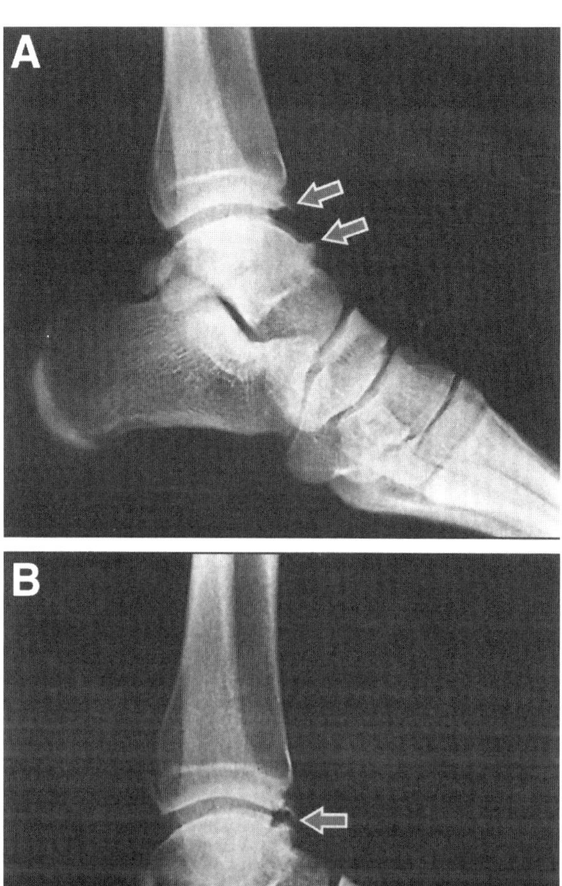

FIGURE 2.—Lateral radiographs of the ankle of a 20-year-old football player who had impingement syndrome. A view in slight plantar flexion (**A**) shows prominent anterior tibial and talar spurs (*arrows*). With the ankle in forced dorsiflexion (**B**), the "kissing osteophytes" (*arrow*) show bony impingement. Soft-tissue impingement may occur in association with bony impingement or alone. Radiographic results may be normal in the latter situation. (Courtesy of Bassewitz HL, Shapiro MS: Persistent pain after ankle sprain: Targeting the cause. *Physician Sportsmed* 12:58–68, copyright 1997. Reproduced with permission of McGraw-Hill, Inc.)

causes and management of persistent pain after ankle sprain were reviewed.

Causes of Persistent Ankle Pain.—The key to managing chronic pain after ankle sprain is to understand the relationship between ankle anatomy, mechanisms of injury, and range of ankle injuries. Inadequate rehabilitation is the most frequent cause of persistent ankle pain. Symptoms and signs may include stiffness, weakness, loss of proprioception, and recurrent instability. Pain, capsular contracture, or intra articular adhesions may lead to limitation of motion and activities. To restore full function, these patients need a formal, rigorous rehabilitation program, including physical therapy and a home exercise program. If the problem is not resolved by 6 weeks, a more thorough workup is needed. Impingement syndromes may be caused by fibrous connective tissue forming in the anterolateral or anteromedial ankle. Chronic anterolateral pain can result from abnormal soft-tissue and/or bone spurs causing pinching in the anterior tibiotalar joint on dorsiflexion (Fig 2). The diagnosis of impingement is suggested by a side-to-side difference of 5 degrees or greater on a standing impingement test. Arthroscopic surgery is the recommended treatment for refractory ankle impingement syndrome.

Osteochondritis dissecans, subchondral cysts, or talar osteochondral lesions can occur after ankle sprain. These lesions are usually found on the posteromedial or anterolateral part of the talus and appear on plain radiographs. Once osteochondral injury is recognized, arthroscopic surgery is the treatment of choice. To avoid late degenerative changes, the injury should be recognized and treated as soon as possible. A history of dorsiflexion injury with a painful snapping sensation should prompt examination for a tear of the peroneal retinaculum. The diagnosis of peroneal tendon injury is confirmed by MRI. Surgery is indicated for patients with overt snapping. Injury to the syndesmosis complex can occur with external rotation injuries, which may occur in patients with inversion sprain. In addition to the usual findings of ankle sprain, these patients will have supramalleolar edema and pain on passive dorsiflexion and external rotation. Most syndesmosis injuries resolve spontaneously within 8 to 12 weeks, although surgery may be needed for complete ruptures with lateral talar subluxation. Lateral instability can cause swelling, lateral pain and tenderness, and recurrent giving-way. The diagnosis requires radiographic stress views, especially the inversion-varus stress view. Patients with instability during daily activities may need surgical repair or reconstruction.

Discussion.—Most ankle sprains can be successfully treated by conservative means; many injuries of greater severity can be identified and treated at presentation. For patients with continued pain 6 or more weeks after ankle sprain, further investigation is needed. With thorough clinical and radiographic examination, the physician can usually diagnose and treat the specific cause of chronic pain.

▶ This is a good review of ankle injuries and the initial management of ankle sprains. The authors include suggestions for post–ankle sprain pain which is not resolved within 6 weeks. Inadequate postinjury rehabilitation is the most common cause of persistent pain, according to the authors. The symtoms of stiffness, weakness, and loss of proprioception should be evaluated. The authors recommend a formal program of physical therapy to address these issues and a home program to insure full recovery of function.

F.J. George, A.T.C., P.T.

The Effects of Spatting and Ankle Taping on Inversion Before and After Exercise

Pederson TS, Ricard MD, Merrill G, et al (Brigham Young Univ, Provo, Utah)
J Athletic Train 32:29–33, 1997   3–40

Introduction.—The support provided by taping the ankle decreases by about 21% after a short period of exercise. Spatting the ankle is a taping technique that involves taping over the shoe and sock of the athlete to minimize the reduction in tape support during exercise. The effects of spatting, a combination of spatting and taping, conventional ankle taping, and not taping on the amount and rate of inversion of the ankle before and after exercise were evaluated.

Methods.—Fifteen male rugby players with no history of lower leg injury within the previous 6 months that limited activity for more than 2 days underwent ankle inversion range of motion and rate of inversion under 4 conditions: untaped, taped, taped and spatted, and spatted ankles. After 30 minutes of exercise, athletes were filmed at 60 Hz during testing on a platform that produced a sudden inversion of the right ankle to 35 degrees.

Results.—The most effective method for decreasing inversion rate and range of motion before and after exercise was the combination of spatting and taping.

▶ Athletic trainers, in general, have been resistant to the practice of spatting ankles. A number of different reasons have been given for this: The effectiveness of spatting has never been addressed in a study of this type. Taping alone should provide adequate support for the ankle. It takes too much time and is not worth the extra expense of the tape. It doesn't look good. If the ankle or leg should be injured, it is difficult to remove the spatting to examine the leg . . . and on and on.

This study indicates that taping and spatting are more effective than taping alone. The authors explain that the reason for this may be that more tape is applied to the ankle and/or the perpendicular distance of the tape to the subtalar joint is increased.

F.J. George, A.T.C., P.T.

Arthroscopic Treatment of Soft-Tissue Impingement of the Ankle in Athletes
DeBeradino TM, Arciero RA, Taylor DC (United States Military Academy, West Point, NY)
Arthroscopy 13:492–498, 1997   3–41

Introduction.—A number of conditions can account for anterolateral ankle pain after an inversion injury, and determining the cause of pain can be difficult. When all nonoperative approaches have failed, ankle arthroscopy is a useful diagnostic and therapeutic procedure. Findings were reported for 60 ankle arthroscopies performed on patients with chronic soft-tissue impingement of the ankle after an ankle sprain.

Methods.—The study group was drawn from patient records, operative summaries, and an ankle injury database at the United States Military Academy. From January 1989 to January 1994, nearly 5,000 ankle sprains were evaluated. Sixty of 163 patients who underwent ankle arthroscopy satisfied inclusion criteria: injury to the ankle, chronic anterolateral ankle pain and swelling with exertion, and a stable ankle with a normal preoperative radiograph. Follow-up consisted of physical examination and determination of an ankle score based upon subjective, objective, radiographic, and functional criteria.

Results.—The patients, 53 men and 7 women, failed to respond to at least 4 months of conservative therapy. Arthroscopy was performed at an average of 23 months after injury. Fifty-two patients reported loss of motion. Preoperative bone scans, performed in 34 cases, revealed increased uptake at the ankle joint. Impingement of soft tissues, confirmed in all 60 patients, was characterized as adhesions with thick fibrous bands and hypertrophic synovial tissue. The location of the impinging tissue correlated with the clinical area of maximum point tenderness. At an average follow-up of 27 months, the 31 patients available for review had an ankle score of 96.6, indicating an excellent result. Subjective pain relief was excellent in 70% of cases, good in 13.3%, fair in 15%, and poor in 1.6%. All patients were satisfied with their outcome, and none required further surgery.

Conclusion.—Most inversion injuries of the ankle resolve uneventfully, but a few require arthroscopy when chronic soft-tissue impingement develops. Synovial hyperplasia was a universal finding in this series of patients. Neither bone scans nor MRI yielded a specific diagnosis. The diagnosis of soft-tissue impingement should be suspected in the setting of inversion injury, localized tenderness, and a stable ankle examination. Resection of the tissue provided good subjective, objective, and functional results.

▶ This interesting article substantiates the success in alleviating pain caused by hypertrophic synovium, synovitis, or fibrous adhesions by arthroscopic resection of the impinging hypertrophic synovium or fibrous bands. To be noted is the fact that during the period covered by this study, 60 of nearly

5,000 ankle sprains (1.2%) seen in the United States Military Academy population had soft-tissue impingement that required ankle arthroscopy. My own approach to dealing with posttraumatic synovitis of the ankle is an intra-articular injection of a corticosteroid. I have found this to be most effective in alleviating ankle pain caused by soft-tissue impingement.

J.S. Torg, M.D.

A Prospective Study of Prognostic Factors Concerning the Outcome of Arthroscopic Surgery for Anterior Ankle Impingement
van Dijk CN, Tol JL, Verheyen CCPM (Academic Med Ctr, Amsterdam)
Am J Sports Med 25:737–745, 1997   3–42

Introduction.—The causes of anterior ankle pain are soft tissue and bony obstruction. Bony obstruction may be caused by osteoarthritic changes or spurs from repetitive minor trauma, which are commonly seen in athletes. Painful anterior ankle bone spurs may be classified according to their size and location. Sixty-two consecutive patients with painful, limited dorsiflexion of the ankle, refractory to nonoperative treatment, were evaluated to define prognostic factors for outcome of arthroscopic surgery for anterior ankle impingement.

Methods.—Forty-two males and 20 females (average age 31 years) with anterior ankle impingement underwent arthroscopic surgery. Preoperative radiographs were scored using osteoarthritic and impingement classification systems. Patients were evaluated at baseline and 4 months and at 1 and 2 years after surgery.

Results.—The degree of osteoarthritic changes was a better prognostic factor for arthroscopic surgical outcome than were size and location of spurs. At 2 year follow-up, 73% of patients had excellent or good results. Fifty percent and 90%, respectively, of patients with and without joint-space narrowing had significantly better scores 2 years postoperatively in pain, swelling, ability to work, and engagement in sports. Patients with less than 2 years of ankle pain before surgery and with spurs located antero-medially were more pleased with their surgical results than patients with longer periods of preoperative pain and with spurs located anterolaterally.

Conclusion.—The degree of osteoarthritic changes is a good prognostic factor for outcome of arthroscopic surgery for anterior ankle impinge-ment. Outcome was less desirable in patients with joint-space narrowing, a 2-year or longer history of ankle pain, and/or anteromedial versus anterolateral impingement.

▶ In addition to demonstrating the osteoarthritic classification to be more discriminative than the impingement classification for predicting outcome of arthroscopic surgery for anterior ankle impingement, this article makes several other important points. It is interesting to note that the authors believe that distraction of the joint hinders identification of structures in the anterior compartment. With regard to determining the size of spurs on x-ray examination, the details of positioning the joint are important. When taking lateral roentgenographs, "both malleoli are positioned perpendicular to the surface of the film and therefore the foot has to be placed in a sagittal angle that can be well over 45 degrees. Small variations of this angle can cause considerable variations in the radiographic appearance of the spurs." Also, "osteophytes on the anterior border of the medial malleolus are undetected on standard AP and lateral roentgenographs because of the superimposition or overprojection or both."

J.S. Torg, M.D.

A Randomized Controlled Trial of Piroxicam in the Management of Acute Ankle Sprain in Australian Regular Army Recruits: The Kapooka Ankle Sprain Study

Slatyer MA, Hensley MJ, Lopert R (1st Recruit Training Battalion, Kapooka, Australia; Univ of Newcastle, New South Wales, Australia)
Am J Sports Med 25:544–553, 1997   3–43

Background.—Ankle sprains represent a substantial burden of injury in active populations. The efficacy of the nonsteroidal anti-inflammatory drug piroxicam in the management of acute ankle sprain was investigated in Australian Regular Army recruits.

Methods and Findings.—Three hundred sixty-four recruits with acute ankle sprains sustained during training were assigned randomly to receive piroxicam or placebo. Compared with placebo recipients, piroxicam recipients had less pain, were able to resume training more rapidly, were treated at lower cost, and had increased exercise endurance on resumption of activity. Nausea was the only adverse effect reported significantly more often in the treatment than in the placebo group, with incidences of 6.8% and 0.3%, respectively. Patients given piroxicam showed some evidence of local abnormalities, such as instability and decreased range of motion.

Conclusions.—Piroxicam use resulted in better recovery at a lower cost for these army recruits with acute ankle sprain. Piroxicam treatment reduced pain, shortened time lost from training, and increased exercise endurance. Although piroxicam recipients also had more instability, less range of motion, and increased swelling, overall the use of the nonsteroidal anti-inflammatory drug was beneficial.

▶ It is difficult to understand why the piroxicam group had less difficulty performing physical activity than the placebo group, since this group had greater instability, less range of motion, and increased swelling. Despite this, there was a statistically significant difference between the 2 groups' abilities to undertake physical activity, with those in the piroxicam group performing at a higher level. Also, cost-effectiveness favors the piroxicam group.

J.S. Torg, M.D.

The Three-dimensional Passive Support Characteristics of Ankle Braces
Siegler S, Liu W, Sennett B, et al (Drexel Univ, Philadelphia; Hahnemann Univ, Philadelphia)
J Orthop Sports Phys Ther 26:299–309, 1997   3–44

Introduction.—The most common injuries in sports and recreational activities are ankle injuries. Athletic tape and ankle braces have been created to minimize the occurrence of such injuries. Ankle braces were shown to restrict range of motion in inversion as effectively as tape, but they do not lose their effectiveness during exercise, as tape does. An objective assessment of dorsiflexion/plantar flexion, inversion/eversion, and internal rotation/external rotation of ankle braces has not been conducted. A technique to measure the support provided by ankle braces in all rotational directions was developed, and 4 common braces were used to compare this technique.

Methods.—The 4 braces used were: Ascend, Swede-O, Aircast, and Active Ankle (Fig 1). The flexibility of the ankle complex was measured in 10 healthy participants, using a 6 degrees-of-freedom linkage (Fig 2). No brace support and each of the 4 braces were used on each of the participants. On 2 different occasions, testing was repeated on each participant. The 4 segmental flexibility values obtained from the loading portion of the moment-angular displacement data and the angular displacement at specified moment values were used. Significant differences among the braces and differences between each brace and the no-brace conditions were analyzed statistically.

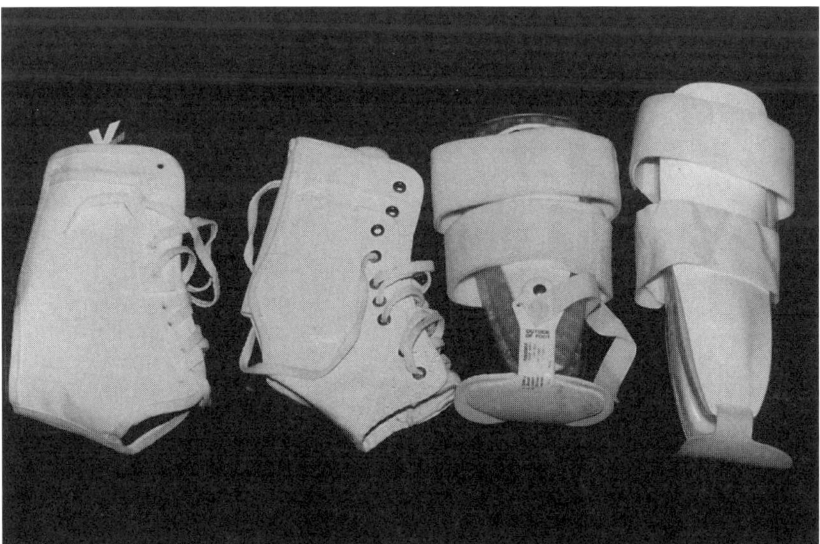

FIGURE 1.—View of the 4 different braces tested in this study: (**left to right**) Ascend; Swede-O; Active Ankle; and Aircast. (Courtesy of Siegler S, Liu W, Sennett B, et al: The three-dimensional passive support characteristics of ankle Braces. *J Orthop Sports Phys Ther* 26: 299–309, 1997.)

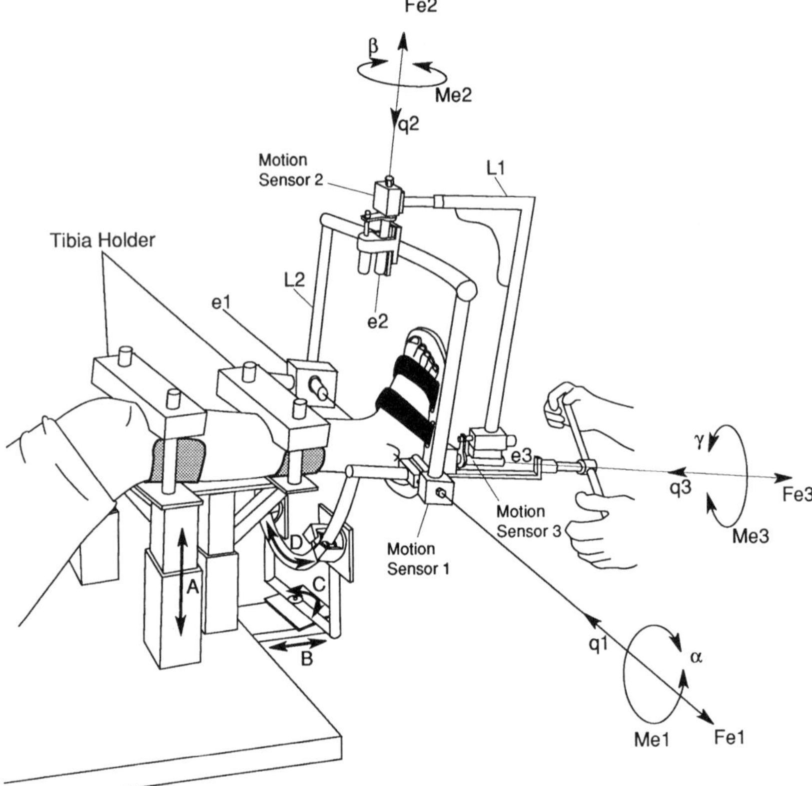

FIGURE 2.—The Ankle Flexibility Tester used to measure the passive moment-angular displacement characteristics of the ankle-brace system. A, B, C, and D are adjustments used to align the device to the subject's ankle. α, β , γ . q1, q2, q3 are the 3 rotational and 3 translational degrees-of-freedom measured by the device. (From Siegler S, Liu W, Sennett B, et al: The three-dimensional passive support characteristics of ankle braces. *J Orthop Sports Phys Ther* 26:299–309, 1997. Courtesy of Siegler S, Lapointe S, Nobilini R, et al:)

Results.—In inversion, eversion, and internal rotation, each of the 4 braces provided significant support. Among the braces, the amount of support varied significantly. Only the stirrup braces provided significant support in external rotation. In the amount of interference with dorsiflexion and plantar flexion, the braces varied significantly. In inversion/eversion and internal rotation, all 4 braces provided significant support. The Active Ankle brace was found to provide the least interference with performance while maintaining the highest lateral support in inversion.

Conclusion.—When prescribing braces to their patients, clinicians may be assisted by objective data on the amount and nature of passive support.

► This is an excellent study that employs a cutting edge and technically sophisticated assay device to determine passive support function of commercially available ankle braces. Recognizing the fact that the observations derived from the data do not necessarily correlate with protection from injury in an active exposure situation, I agree with the conclusion that "the technique presented can provide a useful tool to the brace manufacturing industry to assist in developing improved, effective ankle braces." Also, it can provide objective data to assist clinicians and trainers in selecting ankle braces with specific support properties to meet specific needs of the athlete.

J.S. Torg, M.D.

Laxity and Flexibility of the Ankle Following Reconstruction With the Chrisman-Snook Procedure

Tohyama H, Beynnon BD, Pope MH, et al (Univ of Vermont, Burlington; Univ of Iowa, Iowa City; Hokkaido Univ, Sapporo, Japan)
J Orthop Res 15:707–711, 1997   3–45

Introduction.—An inversion sprain of the ankle is the most common injury in athletics and recreational events, and patients with recurrent instability are candidates for surgical reconstruction if conservative treatment has failed. The Chrisman-Snook procedure is one of the more common techniques used and is a nonanatomical tenodesis performed with the peroneus brevis tendon. Designed to reconstruct the anterior talofibular and calcaneofibular ligaments of the ankle, the procedure has had variable results. During the anterior drawer test, the effect of reconstruction of the anterior talofibular ligament with the Chrisman-Snook procedure on neutral zone laxity (anterior-posterior displacement at low loads) and flexibility (a measure of the nonlinear load-displacement response) of the ankle was investigated in vitro.

Methods.—The magnitude of anterior-posterior displacement of the ankle joint at ±2.5 N of applied load was the definition of neutral zone laxity. The slope of a line between the natural logarithm of the anterior load applied to the ankle and the resulting displacement was the definition of the flexibility parameter.

Results.—At 0 degrees of plantar flexion, the values for neutral zone laxity of the ankle were significantly less than normal after reconstruction with the Chrisman-Snook procedure, whereas the flexibility values were significantly greater than normal. A significant effect on flexibility was seen with the procedure, whereas the plantar flexion angle and the interaction between this angle and the reconstruction procedure had no significant effect.

Conclusion.—Even if the values for neutral zone laxity are reduced to less than normal, values for ankle flexibility are not restored to normal after the Chrisman-Snook procedure. Normal kinematics of the ankle joint are not reproduced by this nonanatomical reconstruction procedure. Some of the adverse clinical reports associated with the Chrisman-Snook reconstruction procedure may be explained by these results. Future studies should investigate whether anatomical reconstruction of the lateral ligaments can restore neutral zone laxity and flexibility to within normal limits for all angles of plantar flexion of the ankle.

Biomechanics of Ankle Ligament Reconstruction: An In Vitro Comparison of the Broström Repair, Watson-Jones Reconstruction, and a New Anatomic Reconstruction Technique
Bahr R, Pena F, Shine J, et al (Univ of Minnesota, Minneapolis; Norwegian Univ, Oslo, Norway; Ullevaal Hosp, Oslo, Norway)
Am J Sports Med 25:424–432, 1997   3–46

Introduction.—To treat recurrent lateral ankle instability, many surgical procedures have been devised. The Broström repair (Fig 3), the Watson-Jones reconstruction, and a new anatomic reconstruction method were compared in a cadaveric model using biomechanical testing. The new technique approximates normal ligament position and uses an autograft with mechanical properties similar to the normal ligament's. The goal was to determine which procedure most closely approximates normal ligament function and motion patterns.

Methods.—A specially designed testing apparatus, in which the ankle position (dorsiflexion-plantar flexion and supination-pronation) could be varied in a controlled manner, was used on 8 specimens. Intact ligaments

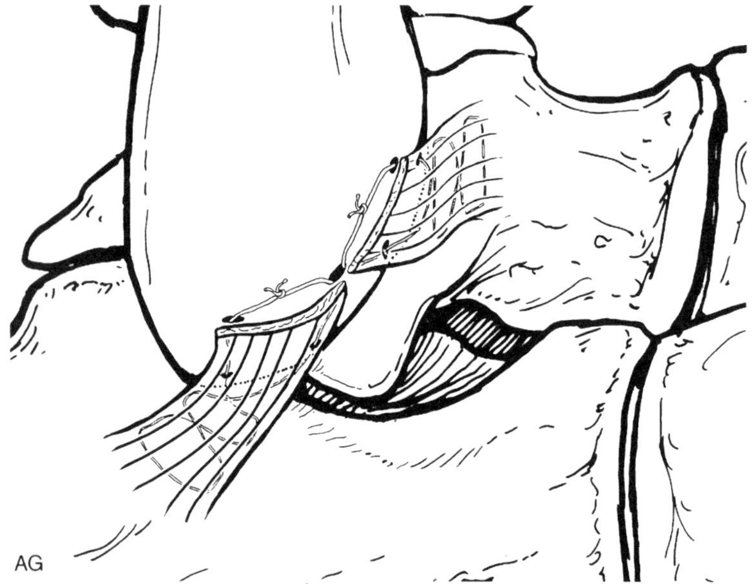

FIGURE 3.—Illustration of the Broström repair. Buckle transducers were installed on the anterior talofibular ligament and calcaneofibular ligament but are not shown. (Courtesy of Bahr R, Pena F, Shine J, et al: Biomechanics of ankle ligament reconstruction: An in vitro comparison of the Broström repair, Watson-Jones reconstruction, and a new anatomic reconstruction technique. *Am J Sports Med* 25:424–432, 1997.)

were used for testing. After sectioning of the anterior talofibular ligament and the calcaneofibular ligament, and after a Broström repair, a Watson-Jones reconstruction, and a new anatomic reconstruction, testing was repeated. Using an anterior translating force of 10–50 newtons, an anterior drawer test was performed. Using a supination torque of 1.1–3.4 newton-meters, a talar tilt test was performed. Buckle transducers were used to measure the forces in the anterior talofibular ligament and calcaneofibular ligament. An instrumented spatial linkage was used to measure tibiotalar motion and total ankle joint motion.

Results.—The 3 reconstructive techniques significantly reduced the increase in ankle joint laxity observed after sectioning of both the anterior talofibular and calcaneofibular ligaments, but not always to the level of the intact ankle. Compared with the intact ankle, joint motion was restricted after the Watson-Jones procedure. The ligament or graft force patterns seen during loading after the new anatomic technique and the Broström repair were similar to those in the intact ankle, and this was not observed with the Watson-Jones procedure.

Conclusion.—To determine whether the new anatomic technique offers any advantages over the currently used nonanatomic methods, larger clinical studies and additional biomechanical analyses are necessary. A more detailed analysis of ligament and joint function is possible with this new technique.

Functional Evaluation of the 10-Year Outcome After Modified Evans Repair for Chronic Ankle Instability

Rosenbaum D, Becker H-P, Sterk J, et al (Univ of Ulm, Germany; Military Hosp, Ulm, Germany)
Foot Ankle Int 18:765–771, 1997   3–47

Introduction.—More than 80 operative treatments for ligament repair in patients with chronic lateral ankle instability have been described, including nonanatomical reconstruction techniques using peroneal tendons and anatomical methods with direct repair of the ligaments or with replacement by endogenous or allograft material There is little documentation of the assessment of functional outcome using objective, observer-independent tests. The Evans tenodesis method is a common method used to stabilize the ankle, and is a nonanatomical procedure that does not reconstruct the anterior talofibular or calcaneofibular ligament directly. There is a hypothesis that Evans reconstruction for the treatment of ankle joint instability will demonstrate an impairment in foot function as a result of the changes induced by the procedure. Whether a modified Evans procedure led to a satisfactory clinical and functional outcome was evaluated.

Methods.—At 10-year follow-up, 19 patients were available for a clinical examination, which included a detailed questionnaire and stress radiographs. During walking, plantar pressure distributions measurements were taken to evaluate foot function. On a rapidly tilting platform, peroneal reaction time measurements were taken and recorded with surface electromyography.

Results.—A high rate of residual instability, pain, and swelling was contrasted with high subjective patient satisfaction. An increased number of exostoses was seen on radiographs. Under the lateral heel, reduced peak pressures were seen on the gait analysis. Under the longitudinal arch, increased values were found. On the operated side, the reaction times of the peroneal muscles were shorter.

Conclusion.—Foot function may be permanently altered by the disturbed ankle joint kinematics after an Evans procedure as seen by the persistent clinical problems and the functional changes. Arthrosis may develop. Only if anatomical reconstruction of the lateral ankle ligaments is not feasible, should the Evans procedure be applied.

▶ From these 3 articles (Abstracts 3–45–3–47) several important observations can be discerned. Tohyama, et al. observe that the subjective satisfaction of patients following the Evans procedure did not correlate with the objective findings of pain, swelling, and residual instability. Neither the Evans repair, Christman-Snook procedure, or Watson-Jones reconstruction was able to restore normal biomechanical function of the ankle joint. Tohyama's conclusion that "future investigations should be designed to determine if anatomic reconstruction of the lateral ligaments can restore neutral zone laxity and flexibility within normal limits for all angles of plantar flexion of the ankle" is interesting. It is my impression that Broström did this 30 years ago. Clearly, what goes around, comes around and in the interim a series of procedures have been described which are both technically difficult and unsound from a biomechanical standpoint. With regard to both acute repair and chronic reconstruction of the ankle, these articles reinforce my opinion that less is more.

J.S. Torg, M.D.

Long-term Functional Outcome After Primary Repair of the Lateral Ligaments of the Ankle
Kaikkonen A, Hyppänen E, Kannus P, et al (Univ of Tampere, Finland; Urho Kaleva Kekkonen Inst, Tampere, Finland)
Am J Sports Med 25:150–155, 1997   3–48

Objective.—Whatever treatment is given—surgical or nonsurgical—the short-term prognosis of acute lateral ankle ligament rupture is similar. However, previous outcome studies have not followed standardized protocols and have had short follow-up times: generally less than 2 years. The long-term outcomes of patients undergoing primary surgical repair of a ruptured ankle ligament were studied using a standardized performance test protocol and scoring scale for the evaluation of ankle injuries.

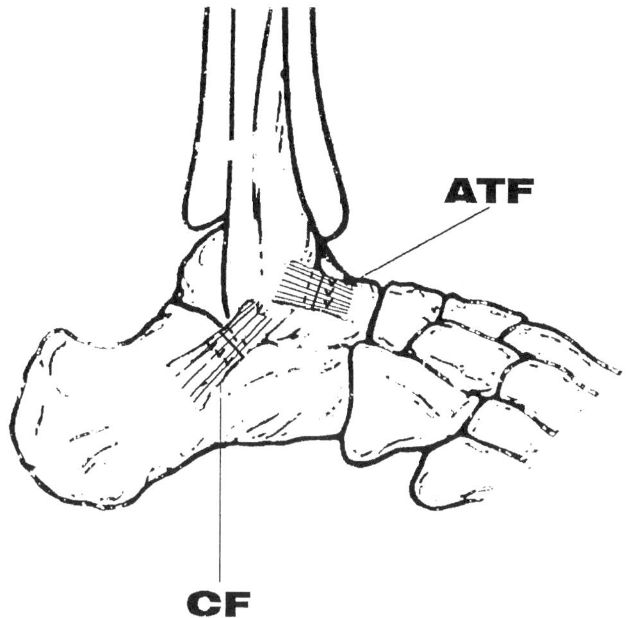

FIGURE 1.—Primary repair of the lateral ligaments of the ankle. *Abbreviations: ATF,* anterior talofibular ligament; *CF,* calcaneofibular ligament. (Courtesy of Kaikkonen A, Hyppänen E, Kannus P, et al: Long-term functional outcome after primary repair of the lateral ligaments of the ankle. *Am J Sports Med* 25:150–155, 1997.)

Methods.—A total of 193 patients who had primary repair of an acute, grade III lateral ligament injury of the ankle were retrospectively studied. Fifty-nine percent of the injuries were sports injuries, and nearly two thirds of those were volleyball injuries. All patients were operated on within 48 hours; two thirds of patients had a rupture of the anterior talofibular ligament combined with a rupture of the calcaneofibular ligament, and one third had an isolated rupture of the anterior talofibular ligament. All ruptured ligaments were primarily repaired using an end-to-end technique (Fig 1). A follow-up questionnaire was sent to 122 patients, 100 of whom underwent clinical and functional reexamination. The standardized evaluation protocol combined subjective and functional assessment of the ankle in walking and running, measurement of joint laxity and range of motion, and standardized functional testing. Mean follow-up was 7 years.

Findings.—The subjective results were rated as excellent or good in 74 of the 100 patients. Anterior drawer sign testing revealed no sign of instability in the operated ankle for 75 patients. On performance testing, the results were graded as excellent or good in 65 patients, fair in 27, and poor in 8. Forty-five patients returned to sports at their preinjury level of competition.

Conclusions.—For most patients, primary surgical repair of ruptured lateral ankle ligaments gives acceptable long-term results. However, about one fourth of patients are less than completely satisfied. Mechanical stability may not be the critical factor affecting the functional outcome of ankle injuries. Prospective, randomized trials are needed to determine whether nonoperative therapy, such as early controlled mobilization, could achieve comparable long-term results.

▶ This is an interesting report on long-term follow-up of primary repair of lateral ankle ligament disruption. However, there is no long-term nonoperative control group for comparison. Also, it is pointed out that 25% of the patients had abnormal joint laxity after surgery, leading the authors to observe that "mechanical stability is not a critical factor in determining the functional outcome." They further observe that "in some sports activities general laxity of the joints is not a disadvantage, and therefore some patients may end up with an excellent subjective assessment despite residual mechanical instability." Other noteworthy observations were that 17 patients had notable swelling of the ankle at follow-up of 7 years. Importantly, excellent recovery in this group was dependent on well-restored ankle dorsiflexion.

J.S. Torg, M.D.

Plantar Fasciitis
Singh D, Angel J, Bentley G, et al (Royal Natl Orthopaedic Hosp, Stanmore, Middlesex, England; Baylor College of Medicine, Houston)
BMJ 315:172–175, 1997   3–49

Introduction.—The most common cause of inferior heel pain is plantar fasciitis. Patients between the ages of 8 and 80 years are affected, but it is most common in middle-aged women and younger male runners. An appropriate diagnosis must be made by the doctor to allow enough time for the condition to run its course. Most patients can be cured within 6 weeks if treatment is begun soon after the onset of symptoms.

Etiology.—Usually that patient's symptoms are the worst when just getting out of bed or just after prolonged sitting. Because limited dorsiflexion of the foot strains the plantar fascia, tightness of the Achilles tendon will predispose to plantar fasciitis. During the night, the foot tends to remain in an equinus position and the fascial tissues contract. The plantar fascia is put under tension in the morning when weight is put on the foot, and this aggravates the pain. Exercise that stretches the heel cord and night splints can interrupt this cycle. Heel spurs are found in half of the patients with plantar fasciitis, and the inflamed, thickened fascia may be more painful if it abuts against a heel spur.

Diagnosis.—Initially, the pain is migratory or diffuse, but with time it is localized at the medial calcaneal tuberosity. Heel pain can decrease during the day and then worsen with increased activity. Plantar fasciitis typically causes worse pain in the morning. Nocturnal pain may raise suspicions of neuropathic pain, such as tarsal tunnel syndrome, infections, or tumors. Risk factors in plantar fasciitis include unaccustomed walking or running, sudden gain in body weight, or obesity, increase in running distance, shoes with poor cushioning, tightness of Achilles tendon, change in the walking surface, and an occupation involving prolonged weight-bearing.

Treatment.—Doctors should recommend that patients wear shoes with arch supports and soft heels. Early treatment should include oral anti-inflammatory drugs, Achilles tendon stretching exercises, shoe inserts, and night splints. Steroid injections are no longer recommended for first-line management. The night splint would consist of a molded ankle-foot orthosis to hold the plantar fascia and Achilles tendon in a relative position of stretch during the night. Usually, the condition is self-limiting.

▶ The authors stress the importance of Achilles tendon stretching exercises and the use of night splints to reduce the symptoms of plantar fasciitis. They recommend stretching the gastrocnemius and soleus individually. Care should be taken to avoid overstretching of the peroneals when doing these exercises. The plantar fascia should also be stretched.

F.J. George, A.T.C., P.T.

Open Lateral Retinacular Lengthening Compared With Arthroscopic Release: A Prospective, Randomized Outcome Study
O'Neill DB (St John Sport Medicine Ctr, Nassau Bay, Tex)
J Bone Joint Surg (Am) 79-A:1759–1769, 1997   3–50

Purpose.—Many adolescents and young adults have pain in the anterior peripatellar aspect of the knee, often with no apparent anatomical or traumatic cause. In 15% to 20% of patients, surgery becomes necessary. Good results have been reported with both open lateral retinacular lengthening and arthroscopic lateral retinacular release, each of which has its own advantages. The outcomes of these 2 approaches were compared in patients with anterior peripatellar pain and lateral patellar tilting.

Methods.—Eighty-six patients with pain in the anterior peripatellar aspect of the knee were studied. In addition, all patients had lateral patellar tilting, or rotational malalignment, demonstrated on Merchant tangential patellofemoral radiographs. The patients did not respond to at least 6 months in a structured quadriceps and hamstrings rehabilitation program. The patients were randomly assigned to arthroscopic lateral retinacular release (group 1) (Fig 1) or open lateral retinacular lengthening (group 2) (Fig 2). The patients were followed up for a mean of 46 months.

Results.—At last follow-up, 93% of group 1 and 100% of group 2 patients had returned to their presymptomatic level of athletic activity. No significant difference between the 2 treatments was present in terms of range of motion, thigh atrophy, complication rate, or the need for subsequent surgery. Neither was there any difference on open- or closed-chain testing on an isokinetic dynamometer. Using the Tegner and Lysholm modification of the Lysholm and Gillquist knee rating system, a score of 80 or better was achieved for 77% of knees in group 1 vs. 88% in group 2.

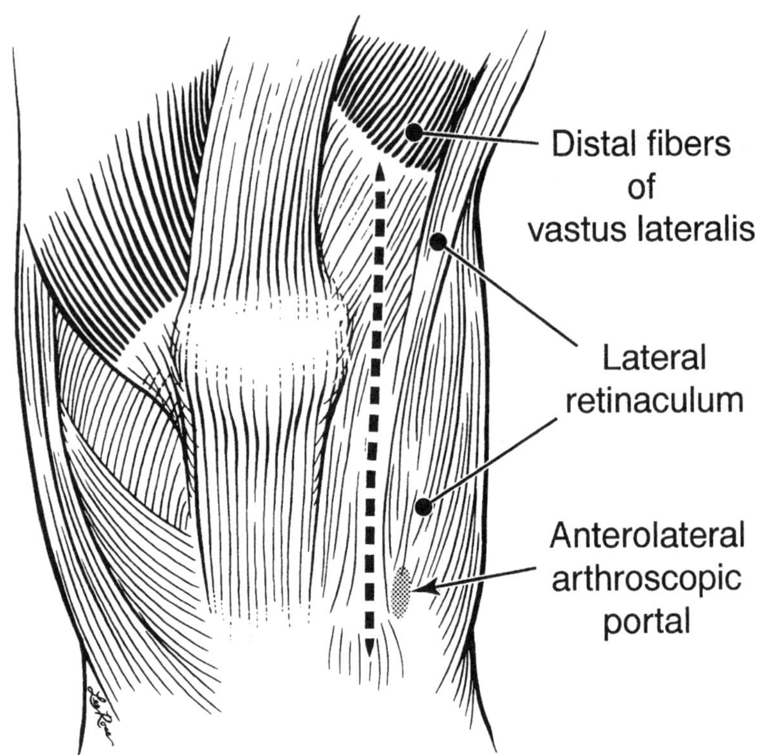

FIGURE 1.—Drawing showing the operative technique for arthroscopic lateral retinacular release. With use of an anterolateral arthroscopic portal, the entire thickness of the lateral retinaculum, capsule, and synovial tissue is incised longitudinally 1 cm from the lateral border of the patella. The incision extends from the vastus lateralis muscle fibers to just beyond the tibial joint line. (Courtesy of O'Neill DB: Open lateral retinacular lengthening compared with arthroscopic release: A prospective, randomized outcome study. *J Bone Joint Surg Am* 79A:1759–1769, 1997.)

The percentage of knees scoring less than 70 points was 14% vs. 0%, respectively. The difference in knee rating scores was significant. The duration of follow-up was not significantly related to outcome in either group, although knee function tended to improve with time.

Conclusions.—Compared with arthroscopic lateral retinacular release, open lateral retinacular lengthening appears to provide significantly better knee scores in patients with anterior peripatellar pain and lateral patellar tilting. Open surgery tends to provide better results in other outcome measures as well, including return to sports. The open procedure also provides somewhat better performance on open-chain testing of the knee extensor mechanism.

▶ Although there was no significant difference between the 2 groups with regard to range of motion, thigh atrophy, operative complications, or the need for subsequent surgery, it was the author's observation that more patients who had have open lateral retinacular lengthening were able to

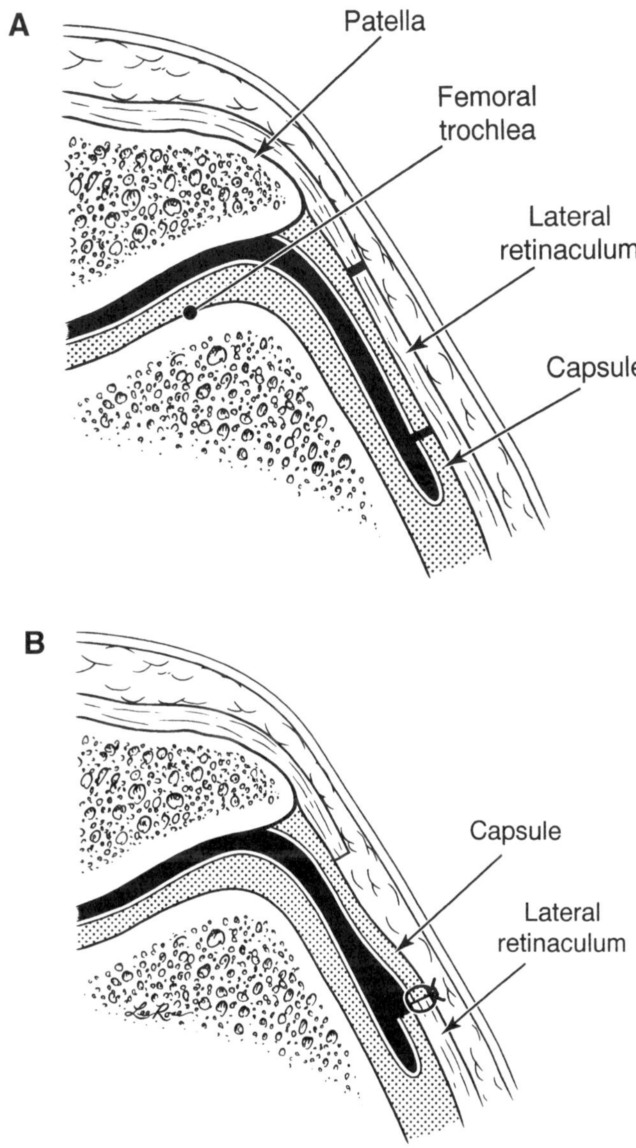

FIGURE 2.—Drawings showing the operative technique for open lateral retinacular lengthening. **A,** the lateral retinaculum is incised longitudinally 1 cm lateral to the lateral patellar border. The dissection is carried laterally 2 cm, keeping superficial to the deep retinaculum and the lateral aspect of the knee capsule. The deep retinaculum and the capsule are incised longitudinally 2 cm lateral to the overlying retinacular incision. **B,** the medial free edge of the knee capsule and the deep retinaculum is sutured to the lateral free edge of the superficial lateral retinaculum, effecting the lateral retinacular lengthening. (Courtesy of O'Neill DB: Open lateral retinacular lengthening compared with arthroscopic release: A prospective, randomized outcome study. *J Bone Joint Surg Am* 79A:1759–1769, 1997.)

return to the previous level of athletic activity and had better results with isokinetic dynamometer testing than those who had arthroscopic lateral retinacular release. In my view, the most important determinate with regard to either open or closed lateral retinacular release is the presence of tight retinacular structures as demonstrated clinically by a positive Sage sign. From the technical standpoint, less than optimum results occur with arthroscopic release in which the surgeon fails to section both the lateral retinaculum and underlying joint capsule. Also, violation of the lateral geniculate artery with subsequent hematoma formation can adversely effect prompt recovery from the procedure.

J.S. Torg, M.D.

4 Exercise Physiology, Biomechanics, Fitness, and Training

Convection as One of the Limiting Factors of Human Respiration During Normoxic Exercise
Heller H, Schuster K-D (Univ of Bonn, Germany)
Am J Physiol 272:R1874–R1879, 1997   4–1

Introduction.—Each has been suspected, but it is not known which of the various components of the oxygen conducting pathways becomes the predominantly limiting one during increasing oxygen consumption (VO_2). A novel method is introduced for examining respiratory conditions by use of the naturally occurring stable isotopic oxygen molecules $^{16}O_2$ and $^{16}O^{18}O$. The lighter molecule, $^{16}O_2$, diffuses 3% quicker and passes the respiratory chain 1.3% faster than $^{16}O^{18}O$. Within convective pathways, $^{16}O_2$ is transported as quickly as $^{16}O^{18}O$ (and can be quantified using the overall fractionation factor α_o. The more that oxygen is confined by diffusion and/or mitrochondrial function, the more the isotopic composition of oxygen changes during transport from the environment to the mitochondria. Isotopic composition of oxygen changes less with growing limitation by convective pathways.

Methods.—Six healthy, sedentary research subjects participated in normoxic exercise on a cycle ergometer. Isotopic analysis was undertaken during rest and at work rates of 50, 100, 150, 200, and 250 W by respiratory mass spectometry.

Results.—A decrease in α_o was observed in all volunteers from 1.0072 at rest to 1.0033 at 250 W.

Conclusion.—Oxygen transport was increasingly influenced by convection but was decreasingly limited by diffusion. The relative contribution of convection to the entire resistance to respiratory oxygen flow varied from $\geq 44.6\%$ at rest to $\geq 74.6\%$ at 250 W. The diffusive pathways decreasingly contributed to resistance to oxygen flow by $\leq 24\%$ at rest and $\leq 11\%$ at 250 W (Fig 2).

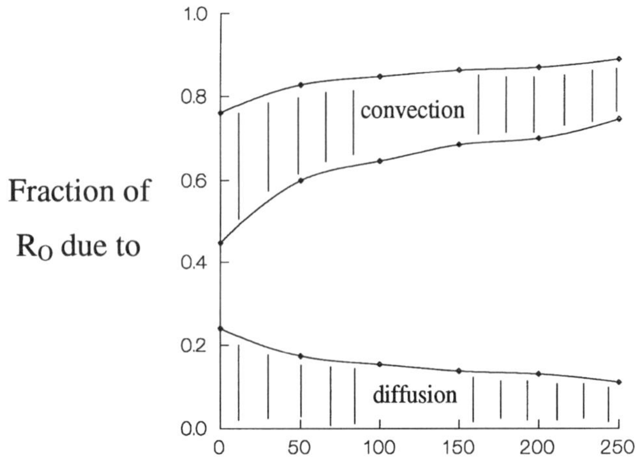

FIGURE 2.—Ranges in fraction of overall resistance of respiration to oxygen flow (R_o) as a result of convective and diffusive oxygen pathways with increasing levels of exercise loads as obtained from all subjects. (Courtesy of Heller H, Schuster K-D: Convection as one of the limiting factors of human respiration during normoxic exercise. *Am J Physiol* 272:R1874–R1879, 1997, copyright The American Physiological Society.)

▶ The idea of representing oxygen transport as a conductance process is not new,[1, 2] and use of this approach has for some 30 years provided apparently irrefutable evidence that the dominant "resistance" to oxygen transport lies within the cardiorespiratory system (principally, the peak cardiac output) rather than in pulmonary diffusion or tissue utilization of oxygen. The new elements in the present study are the "lumping" of convective and diffusional processes, and the use of isotopic oxygen (with its slower rate of diffusion) to separate the 2 components.

R.J. Shephard, M.D., Ph.D., D.P.E.

References

1. Shephard, R.J: *Physiology and Biochemistry of Exercise*. New York, Praeger, 1982.
2. Shephard, R.J: *Aerobic Fitness and Health*. Champaign, Ill, Human Kinetics Publishers. 1994.

Intense Exercise Impairs the Integrity of the Pulmonary Blood-Gas Barrier in Elite Athletes

Hopkins SR, Schoene RB, Henderson WR, et al (Univ of California, San Diego; Univ of Washington, Seattle)

Am J Respir Crit Care Med 155:1090–1094, 1997   4–2

Introduction.—The thinness of the blood-gas barrier in mammals allows gas exchange. This makes it susceptible to mechanical stresses when capillary pressure is elevated. The stresses can be so large in thoroughbred racehorses during intense exercise that the capillaries fail and bleeding occurs. Anecdotal evidence exists regarding exercise-induced pulmonary hemorrhage in elite human athletes. Elite athletes with a history suggestive of lung bleeding underwent bronchoalveolar lavage (BAL) after intense exercise to determine whether capillary permeability increased to the extent of causing mechanical failure and lung bleeding.

Methods.—The 6 athletes participated in a 7-minute cycling race simulation 1 hour before BAL. The 4 controls did not exercise before BAL. The BAL fluid underwent analysis for cell counts, fluid proteins, eicosanoid radioimmunoassays, inflammatory markers, and surfactant proteins.

Results.—Athletes had significantly higher concentrations of red blood cells, total protein, albumin, and leukotriene B_4 in BAL, compared to controls who did not exercise (Figure 1). White blood cell concentrations and differential counts were within normal limits for both groups, but athletes had significantly lower levels of lymphocytes in BAL fluid, compared to controls. There were no between-group differences in surfactant apoprotein A, tumor necrosis factor bioactivity, lipopolysaccharide, or interleukin-8.

Conclusion.—Brief, but intense, exercise in athletes with a history suggestive of lung bleeding changes blood-gas barrier function, causing higher

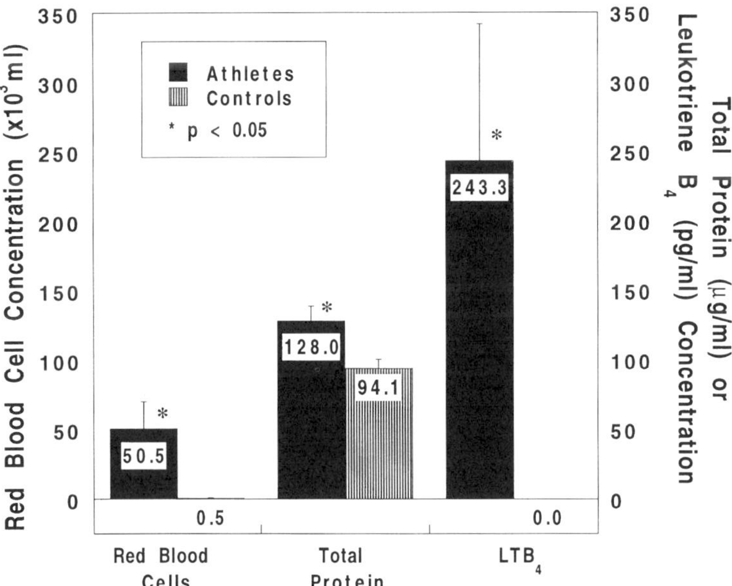

FIGURE 1.—Red blood cell, total protein, and leukotriene B_4 concentration in the bronchoalveolar lavage fluid of athletes compared with control subjects. Values are mean ±SEM. *Abbreviation: LTB₄,* leukotriene B_4. (Courtesy of Hopkins SR, Schoene RB, Henderson WR, et al: Intense exercise impairs the integrity of the pulmonary blood-gas barrier in elite athletes. *Am J Respir Critical Care Med* 155:1090–1094, 1997.)

concentrations of red cells and protein in BAL fluid. In the absence of activation of proinflammatory pathways (except leukotriene B_4) in the airspaces, it is likely that mechanical stress is the mechanism for altered blood-gas barrier function.

▶ A number of reports over the years suggesting that a prolonged bout of intensive exercise such as a marathon run induces a transient reduction in pulmonary diffusing capacity, and it has been questioned whether this functional change reflects the development of a short-lived pulmonary edema. Studies of racehorses have suggested that the problem arises from a substantial increase in pulmonary capillary pressure, with resulting structural damage and leakage of protein and red cells through the capillary walls.[1] A possible alternative explanation would be a response to inflammation, induced by muscle damage, as in the acute respiratory distress syndrome.

The exercise-induced rise in pulmonary vascular pressures is less dramatic in humans than in racehorses, but nevertheless West and colleagues show here that a relatively brief bout of exercise can cause an increase in protein and red cell content in the BAL fluid of endurance athletes. The absence of inflammatory cytokines (interleukin-8 and tumor necrosis factor-alpha) might seem to point to a mechanical rather than an inflammatory explanation of the pulmonary changes, although cytokines act at very low concentrations and have a short half-life, so they are not always easy to detect.

R.J. Shephard, M.D., Ph.D., D.P.E.

Reference

1. West JB, Mathieu-Costello O, Jones JH, et al: Stress failure of pulmonary capillaries in racehorses with exercise-induced pulmonary hemorrhage. *J Appl Physiol* 75:1097–1109, 1993.

Restricted Postexercise Pulmonary Diffusion Capacity and Central Blood Volume Depletion
Hanel B, Teunissen I, Rabøl A, et al (Univ of Copenhagen)
J Appl Physiol 83:11–17, 1997
4–3

Introduction.—After exercise of various durations and intensities, pulmonary diffusion capacity for carbon monoxide is impaired. A decrease in membrane diffusion capacity and pulmonary capillary blood volume is reflected by the postexercise reduction in pulmonary diffusion capacity for carbon monoxide. There may be a reduction in the central blood volume after exercise. In rowers and controls at rest before exercise and during postexercise recovery, measurements were taken of pulmonary diffusion capacity for carbon monoxide, regional electrical impedance, the distribution of ^{99m}Tc-labeled erythrocytes, and total blood volume. This was done to test the hypothesis that the decrease in pulmonary diffusion capacity for carbon monoxide during recovery from exercise is caused by a redistribution of the blood volume from the central vascular bed to more distal regions.

Methods.—Before and after a 6-minute "all-out" row, pulmonary diffusion capacity for carbon monoxide, regional electrical impedance, and the distribution of ^{99m}Tc-labeled erythrocytes, together with the concentration of plasma atrial natriuretic peptide, were determined in 9 oarsmen and in 6 controls.

Results.—Pulmonary diffusion capacity for carbon monoxide was reduced by 6%, the thoracic-to-thigh electrical impedance ratio rose by 14%, thoracic blood volume decreased by 7%, and thigh blood volume increased by 3% at 2½ hours after exercise in the upright seated position. A decrease in plasma atrial natriuretic peptide concentration from 15 to 12 pmol/L also resulted. The thoracic-to-thigh electrical impedance ratio increased by 10% and pulmonary diffusion capacity for carbon monoxide decreased by 12% in the supine position. In the control group, the pulmonary diffusion capacity for carbon monoxide remained stable in the supine position.

Conclusion.—About one half of the postexercise reduction in pulmonary diffusion capacity for carbon monoxide is explained by a decrease in the pulmonary blood volume, as was evidenced by the increase in the thoracic-to-thigh electrical impedance ratio and the corresponding redistribution of the blood volume in the seated and supine positions. The lower plasma atrial natriuretic peptide, which helps upregulate the blood volume after exercise in athletes, underscored the role of a reduced postexercise central blood volume.

▶ There have been repeated reports of impaired pulmonary diffusing capacity after sustained bouts of exercise, but it is unclear whether such changes have reflected an exposure to air pollutants, a transient decrease in cardiac function, or a harbinger of acute respiratory distress syndrome induced by muscle damage. Those who have envisaged such dire possibilities may be relieved to learn of a much simpler and less disturbing explanation of the change. Diffusing capacity is a composite number that reflects gas transfer across the alveolar-capillary membrane plus a second term that results from the product of pulmonary blood volume and the rate of reaction between carbon monoxide and blood. Thus, if the central blood volume falls, there will automatically be a decrease in the measured pulmonary diffusing capacity.

R.J. Shephard, M.D., Ph.D., D.P.E.

Respiratory Muscle Work Compromises Leg Blood Flow During Maximal Exercise

Harms CA, Babcock MA, McClaran SR, et al (Univ of Wisconsin, Madison)
J Appl Physiol 82:1573–1583, 1997   4–4

Background.—The metabolic cost of breathing may represent a significant proportion of total oxygen consumption and total blood flow during strenuous exercise. Although the respiratory muscles' need for perfusion may theoretically decrease the blood flow available for muscles of locomotion, such a competition phenomenon between chest and limb muscles has not been established. The effects of increased work of breathing (Wb) on blood flow and oxygen consumption of locomotor muscles during maximal exercise were determined.

Methods.—Seven non-smoking, male competitive cyclists performed 14 rounds of exercise, each of 2.5-minutes duration and at maximal oxygen consumption, on a cycle ergometer. The work of inspiration was either increased by the application of resistive loads, reduced through the use of a proportional-assist ventilator, or unaltered during the exercise session, with each participant receiving each ventilatory intervention. Samples of arterial and venous blood were taken, and oxygen consumption, esophageal pressure, arterial blood pressure, and blood flow to the leg were monitored. Work of breathing was estimated from the area of the ventilatory pressure volume loops.

Results.—Work of breathing was increased 128.2% ± 25.2% and was decreased by 36.7% ± 26.6% relative to controls by application of resistive load or by inspiratory assist, respectively. Work of breathing was significantly and inversely associated with blood flow to the legs and oxygen consumption in the legs ($r = -0.84$ and -0.77, respectively). Total oxygen consumption did not increase with increased Wb, but decreased by 9.3% when Wb was decreased by inspiratory assist (Fig 7). The propor-

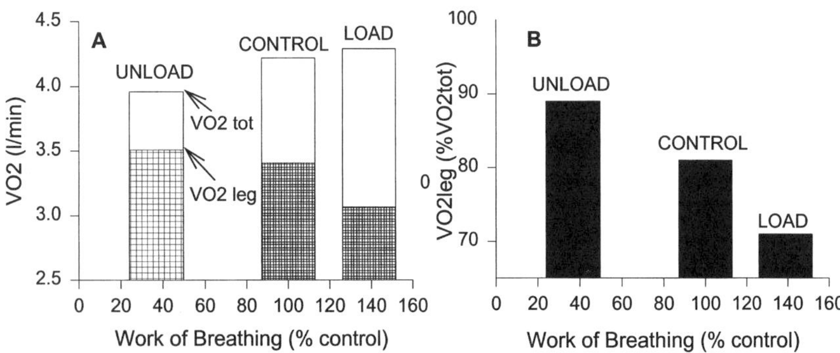

FIGURE 7.—**A**, $\dot{V}_{O_{2tot}}$ was significantly lower with unloading and unchanged with loading, whereas $\dot{V}_{O_{2legs}}$ was significantly increased with unloading and decreased with loading. **B**, respiratory muscle unloading increased and respiratory muscle loading reduced the fraction of total O_2 consumed by the legs. *Abbreviations:* $\dot{V}_{O_{2tot}}$, total oxygen consumption; $\dot{V}_{O_{2legs}}$, oxygen consumption by the legs. (Courtesy of Harms CA, Babcock MA, McClaran SR, et al: Respiratory muscle work compromises leg blood flow during maximal exercise. *J Appl Physiol* 82:1573–1583, 1997.)

tion of total oxygen use directed toward the legs was 71%, 89%, and 81% during the respiratory loading, respiratory unloading, and control tests, respectively. The association between Wb and leg vascular resistance was significant and positive ($r = 0.73$), and leg vascular resistance was significantly associated with norepinephrine spillover ($r = 0.71$), an indicator of sympathetic stimulation of leg vessels.

Conclusions.—Increased Wb commonly encountered during maximal exercise decreases perfusion and oxygen use in locomotor muscles. It is likely that this effect is mediated by vasoconstriction in these muscle groups.

▶ Early studies suggest that in healthy young adults, Wb accounted for at least 5% to 10% of the total observed oxygen consumption during exercise at 80% of maximal oxygen intake.[1] Moreover, because the oxygen cost of breathing was rising in exponential fashion as peak effort was approached, Wb would account for a substantial fraction of the total oxygen consumption during all-out effort. A point of diminishing returns could be envisaged, where the added cost of extra ventilation was greater than the resulting increase in oxygen intake. Implicit in this argument would be a corresponding redistribution of cardiac output as respiratory work increased. Harms et al. have now made an elegant test of this hypothesis, demonstrating that leg metabolism accounts for a larger percentage of total oxygen consumption when respiratory work is reduced by ventilatory assistance, and a greater percentage when respiratory effort is increased by external loading.

R.J. Shephard, M.D., Ph.D.

Reference

1. Shephard, RJ: Oxygen cost of breathing during vigorous exercise. *Quart J Exp Physiol* 51:336–350, 1996.

Cardiac Output Estimated Noninvasively From Oxygen Uptake During Exercise

Stringer WW, Hansen JE, Wasserman K (Univ of California, Los Angeles)
J Appl Physiol 82:908–912, 1997   4–5

Introduction.—A noninvasive method for estimating cardiac output (CO) is needed. It is possible to achieve this through measurement of oxygen uptake $\dot{V}O_2$ because almost all CO passes through the lungs. Both CO and stroke volume (SV) might be able to be estimated from $\dot{V}O_2$ and heart rate if the behavior of arteriovenous oxygen content difference ($C[a\text{-}vDO_2]$) were known. The $C(a\text{-}vDO_2)$ was measured during progressive ramp pattern cycle ergometric exercise to exhaustion while continuously measuring $\dot{V}O_2$ and sampling arterial and mixed venous blood.

Methods.—Five healthy research subjects underwent 10 exercise tests to exhaustion while arterial and mixed venous blood were sampled. A CO-oximeter was used to evaluate samples for blood gases and oxyhemoglobin

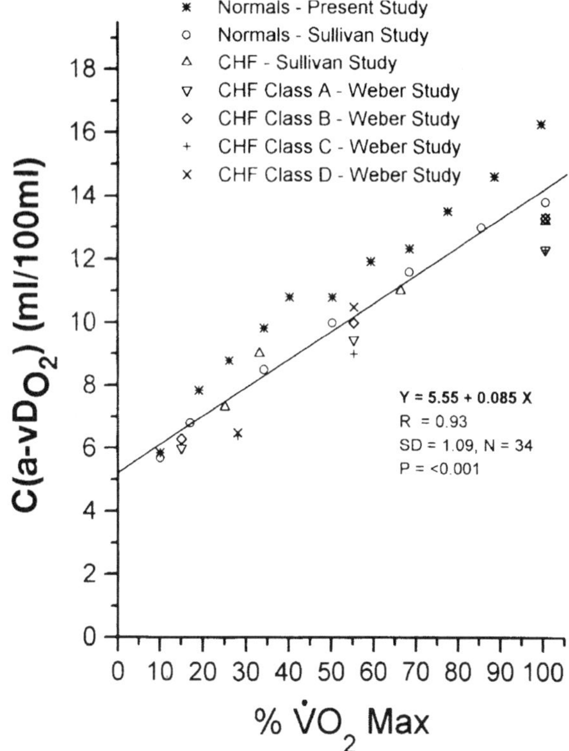

FIGURE 6.—Regression of C(a-vDo$_2$) values. If C(a-vDo$_2$) values from studies of Weber and Janicki and Sullivan et al. (both congestive heart failure and normal subjects) are plotted with present study as a function of %$\dot{V}O_{2max}$, a similar regression with a similar intercept and slope to those in Fig 2 is obtained, despite a wide variation in cardiac function. *Abbreviations: C(a-vDo$_2$)*, arteriovenous oxygen content difference; $\dot{V}O_{2max}$, maximum oxygen consumption. (Courtesy of Stringer WW, Hansen JE, Wasserman K: Cardiac output estimated noninvasively from oxygen uptake during exercise. *J Appl Physiol* 82:908–912, 1997.)

and hemoglobin concentration. A linear regression was used to estimate CO from the C(a-vDO$_2$).

Results.—Correlation was good between CO estimated from C(a-vDO$_2$) and CO determined by the direct Fick method. There was a small coefficient of variation of the estimated CO between the lactic acidosis threshold and peak $\dot{V}O_2$. When compared with similar measurements from investigations performed in patients who were normal and those with congestive heart failure, the behavior of C(a-vDO$_2$), as it related to $\dot{V}O_2$, was similar regardless of heart function (Figure 6).

Conclusion.—Cardiac output may be accurately estimated from $\dot{V}O_2$ during exercise in normal research subjects and patients with heart failure. This approach gives a simple and cost-effective determination of cardiac output in response to exercise, independent of disturbed lung physiology and acid-base changes during exercise.

▶ The indirect measurement of CO by such methods as carbon dioxide or acetylene rebreathing is fraught with many problems, and it is thus an attractive idea to infer the CO from measurements of oxygen consumption. Indeed, the decline in maximal oxygen intake with age has previously been adduced as evidence that older adults have difficulty in sustaining their cardiac stroke volume during maximal effort. It is plain from the Fick equation that the prediction of CO from oxygen consumption depends on the assumed $C(a-vDo_2)$. As the authors' figure demonstrates, the $C(a-vDo_2)$ increases in relatively linear fashion from a resting value of about 50 ml/L to about 140 ml/L in maximal effort. The limits of $C(a-vDo_2)$ during maximal effort probably extend from 120 to 160 ml/L, so that for occasional subjects with an unusual a-v difference, the error in prediction of CO could be as large as 14%. However, the stated error of 7% to 9% seems a realistic average, and is better than can be claimed for many alternative methods of estimating CO.

R.J. Shephard, M.D., Ph.D., D.P.E.

Cardiovascular Response to Sudden Strenuous Exercise: An Exercise Echocardiographic Study
Chesler RM, Michielli DW, Aron M, et al (SUNY Health Science Ctr, Brooklyn, NY)
Med Sci Sports Exerc 29:1299–1303, 1997   4–6

Background.—Sudden strenuous exercise (SSE), necessary in certain occupations and as a reaction to some life-threatening situations, has been associated with ischemic-like responses and a decrease in left ventricular (LV) function. The underlying mechanism may be a mismatch between myocardial oxygen supply and demand, resulting in transient subendocardial ischemia. The response of LV internal dimensions and posterior wall thickness during SSE without warm-up and SSE with warm-up was studied.

Methods and Findings.—Fifteen healthy, untrained men, with a mean age of 26 years, participated. Continuous 2–D targeted on M–mode echocardiography was performed. Continuous EKG and blood pressure were recorded at rest and during the last 10 seconds of SSE. Men engaging in SSE with and without warm-up did not differ significantly in LV internal dimensions, maximal heart rate, maximal rate pressure product, ECG, or maximal mean arterial pressure.

Conclusions.—Reduced LV function was not correlated with SSE without warm-up. These findings contradict data from previous studies, in which SSE has been associated with transient global LV dysfunction.

▶ This study has implications for all of us who race to catch a bus, train, or plane. Earlier research suggests that sudden, strenuous exercise without warm-up can cause transient left ventricular dysfunction from transient global ischemia. This study, in 15 healthy, untrained college men free of coronary heart disease, finds no such ventricular dysfunction or ischemia. Based on this study (using echocardiography and EKG and blood pressure monitoring), sudden strenuous exercise without warm-up is safe, provided of course, you don't have coronary heart disease. The authors speculate that transient ischemia in the earlier research came from handgripping (of handle bars or front bars of treadmills). Handgripping, which these authors prevented, will boost afterload and might thus provoke transient left ventricular dysfunction. So it's safe to run for your plane, but not carrying your suitcase.

E.R. Eichner, M.D.

Effect of Venous Obstruction of Lower Extremities on Exercise Tolerance
Ben-Dov I, Morag B, Farfel Z (Tel-Aviv Univ, Tel-Hashomer, Israel)
Chest 111:506–508, 1997   4–7

Background.—The effect of venous occlusion on extremity exercise capacity has not been well characterized. This report describes a patient with bilateral iliofemoral and inferior vena cava thrombosis with significant exercise intolerance.

Case Report.—Male, 63, was active until occurrence of iliofemoral deep thrombophlebitis and pulmonary emboli. Contrast venography was performed, which was complicated by iliofemoral thrombophlebitis. Following this, the patient experienced persistent leg edema and marked exercise intolerance. There were no signs of pulmonary hypertension or heart failure. Peripheral pulse and leg muscle strength were normal. Neither ECG nor thallium dipyridamole myocardial scan demonstrated any ischemic zones. Doppler echocardiogram revealed normal left and right ventricular function, without pulmonary hypertension. The values of FEV_1, FVC, and total lung capacity were within the normal range. It was hypothesized that lower body venous obstruction might be the cause of the exercise intolerance experienced by this patient. The patient performed upper and lower extremity incremental maximal cycle ergometry, with a cardiopulmonary exercise system. Lower extremity exercise capacity was significantly reduced, whereas upper extremity peak oxygen uptake was normal (Fig 1). Bilateral iliofemoral vein study demonstrated severe obstruction of the right common iliac vein and complete occlusion of the left common iliac vein and the inferior vena cava.

Conclusions.—This case report describes a patient with a severe peripheral venous occlusion that caused marked exercise intolerance, in the absence of abnormal heart or lung function. Venous disease can lead to exercise intolerance.

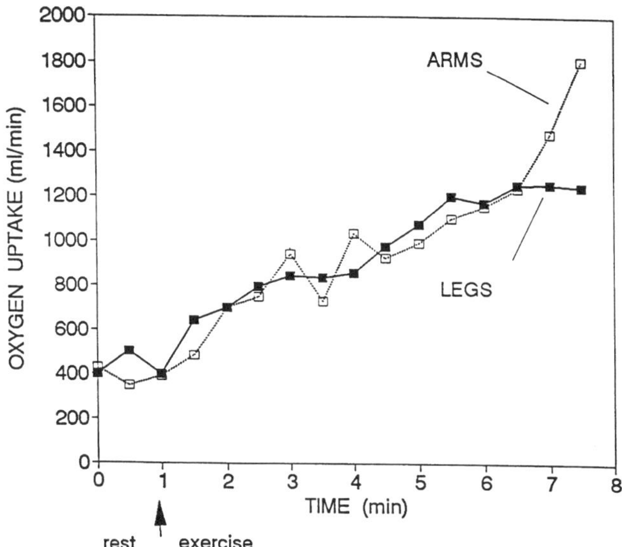

FIGURE 1.—Oxygen uptake in a patient with severe lower body venous occlusion during an incremental maximal lower extremity (-) and upper extremity (--) cycle ergometry exercise. Peak O_2 uptake during the arm exercise exceeds that during the leg exercise. (Courtesy of Ben-Dov I, Morag B, Farfel Z: Effect of venous obstruction of lower extremities on exercise tolerance. *Chest* 111:506–508, 1997.)

▶ Venous obstruction can cause substantial volumes of blood to accumulate in the limbs. I first became acutely aware of this problem when I was testing partial pressure suits at the RAF Institute of Aviation Medicine. Although sitting in a fighter-pilot's seat, doing no more than manipulating a few controls, the loss of blood was enough to cause a loss of consciousness within 5–10 minutes. In my case, the venous obstruction was caused by a torso pressure suit, which had been inflated to 80–100 mm Hg. However, as in the case described by Ben-Dov, et al, a similar situation can arise with thrombosis of the major vessels. Diastolic filling of the heart is impaired, stroke volume decreases, and there is a rapid decline in peak oxygen intake. It is interesting that peak oxygen intake for the upper limbs was unaffected by the venous obstruction. I do not agree with Ben-Dov that this necessarily indicates that peripheral factors such as a local venous back-pressure were limiting leg performance. In my view, it tends to substantiate an alternative hypothesis that because of a smaller volume of active muscle, the limitation for some types of arm work is peripheral rather than central.[1] Given a peripheral limitation, arm work is less affected by limited preloading of the ventricles.

R.J. Shephard, M.D., Ph.D., D.P.E.

Reference

1. Shephard RJ, Bouhlel E, Vandewalle H, et al: Muscle mass as a factor limiting physical work. *J Appl Physiol* 64:1472–1479, 1988.

The Effect of Warm-up Intensity on Range of Motion and Anaerobic Performance

Stewart IB, Sleivert GG (Univ of British Columbia, Vancouver, Canada; Univ of Otago, Dunedin, New Zealand)
J Orthop Sports Phys Ther 27:154–161, 1998   4–8

Introduction.—Athletes commonly warm up to improve performance and reduce the incidence of injuries. Both submaximal exercise and stretching exercises are often performed. There have been inconclusive results on the effects of warm-up on more intensive exercise performance. The role of warm-up intensity on range of motion and anaerobic performance was examined.

Methods.—There were 9 men aged 21.7 ± 1.6 years, weighing 80.2 ± 6.8 kg, with a height of 1.77 ± 0.04 m who completed 4 trials. Each trial involved using an electronic inclinometer and anaerobic capacity test on the treadmill with a time to fatigue at 13 km/hr and 20% grade to evaluate hip, knee, and ankle range of motion. The men either had a warm-up of 15 minutes running at 60%, 70% or 80% maximum oxygen consumption ($\dot{V}O_{2max}$) followed by a series of lower limb stretches or no warm-up.

Results.—Little effect on range of motion was seen with a change in the intensity of warm-up because ankle dorsiflexion and hip extension significantly increased in all warm-up conditions. Knee flexion did not change after any warm-up but hip flexion significantly increased only after the 80% $\dot{V}O_{2max}$ warm-up. Before anaerobic performance for each of the warm-up conditions, heart rate and body temperature were significantly increased. After warm-up at 60% $\dot{V}O_{2max}$, anaerobic performance improved by 10% and after 70% $\dot{V}O_{2max}$, anaerobic performance improved by 13%. Within 5–10 minutes of initiation of exercise, rapid increases in muscle temperature occur, and core temperature increases more gradually over a 30-minute period.

Conclusion.—To improve range of motion and enhance subsequent anaerobic performance, a 15-minute warm-up at an intensity of 60% to 70% $\dot{V}O_{2max}$ is recommended. Performance will not be improved by too high a warm-up intensity.

▶ The effects of warm-up were also commented on in the 1996 YEAR BOOK.[1] The authors of this study recommend a 15-minute warm-up at 60% to 70% $\dot{V}O_{2max}$. In large team situations, this may be difficult to control accurately. Warm-up activities that increase $\dot{V}O_{2max}$ above 70% should be avoided.

F.J. George, A.T.C., P.T.

Reference

1. 1996 YEAR BOOK OF SPORTS MEDICINE, p 219.

A Physiological Review of American Football

Pincivero DM, Bompa TO (Univ of Pittsburgh, Pa; York Univ, Toronto)
Sports Med 23:247–260, 1997   4–9

Introduction.—The high incidence of injury and the physical demand for preparation are 2 of the biggest concerns regarding participation in American football. The physiologic systems are heavily taxed as football combines the physical qualities of nearly all other sports, including size, strength, power, speed, agility, and endurance. For development of optimal training programs, a basic understanding of the physiologic systems used in the sport of football is necessary.

Energy Systems.—It was previously assumed that football relied on an anaerobic source of energy for adenosine triphosphate resynthesis, and that the energy contribution from the anaerobic glycolytic pathway has been underestimated. This hypothesis became doubtful after the elevated blood lactate levels were noticed after a game. This sport primarily uses the phosphocreatine system for its energy supply with secondary involvement of anaerobic glycolysis.

Body Composition.—Defensive and offensive linemen are usually larger, have greater absolute strength scores, and higher levels of percent body fat. The lowest percentage of body fat, lower absolute strength scores, fastest times, and the highest relative $\dot{V}O_{2max}$ values were displayed by offensive backs, defensive backs, and wide receivers. A transition group midway between the backs and linemen appeared to be linebackers.

Conclusion.—Strength training has been the cornerstone of football player development, but the game also depends on a player's speed and power. A hindrance to performance may be a lack of cardiovascular development of university and professional football players with regard to thermal regulation. The performance would also be enhanced by additional aerobic conditioning and a reduction of percent body fat. These would also help prevent injuries and allow a smoother transition into life after football. Reduction of body weight and improvement of cardiovascular endurance would also reduce the risk of coronary artery disease, hypertension, stroke, and diabetes. Because cardiovascular training increases the use of free fatty acids for energy production, aerobic conditioning assists with the problem of excessive weight.

▶ The authors have hypothesized that a lower level of percent body fat has the potential for improving the efficiency of movement, ultimately enhancing muscular activation and, therefore, strength performance. They also state that the reduction of percent body fat along with additional aerobic conditioning would not only enhance performance but also might play a key role in injury prevention.

F.J. George, A.T.C., P.T.

An Investigation Into the Relation Between Step Height and Ground Reaction Forces in Step Exercise: A Pilot Study

Maybury MC, Waterfield J (Good Hope Hosp, Sutton Coldfield, West Midlands, UK; Coventry Univ, UK)
Br J Sports Med 31:109–113, 1997   4–10

Introduction.—Claimed to be a high-intensity, low-impact aerobic workout, step aerobics has a low injury risk and conditions the lower body. Little is known about the effects of step aerobics on ground reaction forces. A previous study found that riser height had a profound effect on all moments. Injuries such as low back pain, stress fractures and osteoarthritis can occur with this exercise. The relationship between step heights and ground reaction forces was investigated.

Methods.—Twelve volunteers with no previous step aerobics experience participated in this study, which required the volunteers to perform at 3 different step heights of 6, 8, and 10 inches. At a cadence of 120 beats/min, the participants performed a basic step. Ground reaction force was measured during 3 1-minute trials. Measurements were taken of peak impact force, time to achieve peak impact, and total time of foot contact, as well as the impulse of the force.

Results.—Between the 6- and 8-inch and the 6- and 10-inch step heights, statistically significant differences were found in the peak impact force, but not between the 8- and 10-inch conditions. The other parameters did not reveal any significant differences. At the various step heights, there were no significant differences for duration of foot contact, for time to achieve peak force, or for impulse.

Conclusion.—Low step heights should be used by participants, particularly novices, as peak impact forces increase with step height. In the pathomechanics of injury during aerobics, there is still no conclusive evidence that ground reaction forces are the main culprit. In step aerobics, eccentric muscle work predominates, which can lead to widespread muscle damage.

▶ This study examined the ground reaction forces during step aerobics, in which intensity was altered by increasing step height. Increases in step height increased both moment forces about the knee joint and impact forces on landing. Peak forces increased with increased step height, so the study supported the use of low step heights with novice steppers. A large component of eccentric muscle activity also was found in step exercise, which can produce greater incidence of muscle injury. Other research in this area has suggested that step exercise must be of a reasonable step height to provide stimulus for bone growth and regeneration. Clearly this type of exercise must be graded to meet the skill and activity level of the participants to optimize fitness and gains in bone density.

M.J.L. Alexander, Ph.D.

Analysis of the Sit–Stand–Sit Movement Cycle in Normal Subjects
Kerr KM, White JA, Barr DA, et al (Univ of Nottingham, England; Queen's Univ of Belfast, Northern Ireland)
Clin Biomech 12:236–245, 1997   4–11

Introduction.—The most mechanically demanding functional task performed during daily activities is rising from a chair. Many potentially ambulant patients and elderly patients remain prisoners in their chairs with the inability to rise from a chair. Seven events were identified in each of the rising and descending phases of the movement cycle, with a total of 14 events. These were studied in spatial and temporal terms with healthy participants.

Methods.—There were 50 normal healthy participants, 25 men and 25 women, ranging in age from 20.1 years to 78.3 years. They were divided into 6 groups on the basis of age and sex: young women, mean age 23.7 years; young men, mean age 20.9 years; middle-aged women, mean age 46 years; middle-aged men, mean age 46.1 years; elderly women, mean age 72.5 years; and elderly men, mean age 71.5 years. Within the same temporal framework, linear displacement and acceleration of the trunk and angular displacement of the knee were recorded simultaneously. An electrogoniometer located at the lateral aspect of the knee was used to take the measurements, and a vector stereograph and triaxial accelerometers lo-

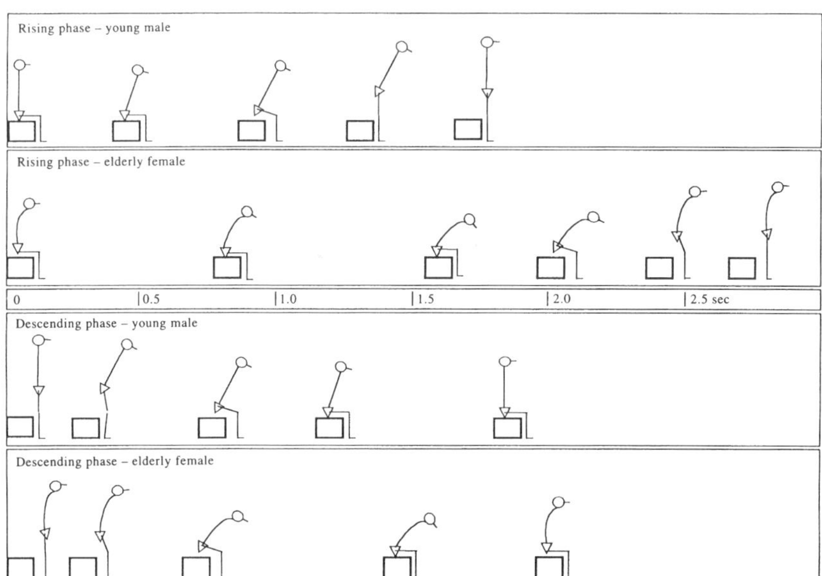

FIGURE 3.—Rising and descending phases of the sit-stand-sit movement cycle (young male subject and elderly female subject. (Reprinted from Kerr KM, White JA, Barr DA, et al: Analysis of the sit-stand-sit movement cycle in normal subjects. *Clin Biomech* 12:236–245, copyright 1997, with kind permission from Elsevier Science Ltd, The Boulevard, Langford Lane, Kidlington OX5 1GB UK.)

cated at the level of C7 also were used. At their own self-selected speed, participants rose and descended to the seated position 6 times.

Results.—To rise, the mean value for the time was 1.91 seconds, and to descend, the mean value was 1.97 seconds. During rising, forward lean velocity was greater than during descending. During descending, recovery velocity was greater than during rising. During the rising phase, elderly women took significant more time during rising than the young and middle-aged groups (Fig 3). With increasing age, the contribution of the forward lean component during the rising phase increased. With increasing age, the percentage contribution of the period of overlap between the forward lean and vertical displacement components tended to decrease during the rising phase.

Conclusion.—For the sit-stand-sit movement cycle, this study has proposed a baseline of descriptive data. These findings should be substantiated with a larger sample.

▶ Rising from a chair is a physically demanding task for many elderly patients and those with arthritis, and these persons often experience difficulty with this task. The older groups in this study experienced increased time to rise from a chair, probably because of decreased ability to generate power from the muscles. The trunk lean during the rising phase served as a means of developing forward momentum and helped position the center of gravity over the base of support during the descending phase in the younger subjects. In the older subjects, the forward lean component moves from a momentum function to a positioning function. The initiation of knee extension is also a critical feature of the movements in rising and occurs later in the movement pattern in women. This timing may be related to the differences in anthropometric variables and the relative position of the center of gravity. This study is unique in recognizing the differences in the sequence of events in sit to stand between genders and age groups.

M.J.L. Alexander, Ph.D.

Energy Absorption of Impacts During Running at Various Stride Lengths
Derrick TR, Hamill J, Caldwell GE (Iowa State Univ, Ames; Univ of Massachusetts, Amherst)
Med Sci Sports Exerc 30:128–135, 1998   4–12

Introduction.—A shock wave is transmitted throughout the skeletal system when the heel contacts the ground during running. The level of shock in the lower extremity is affected by the velocity of progression and by stride length. Alterations in the stride length also influence impact shock. In response to increased impact magnitude, the body appears to increase shock attenuation, but the mechanisms and location of this increased shock attenuation are largely unknown. The locus of energy absorption during the impact phase of the running cycle was investigated.

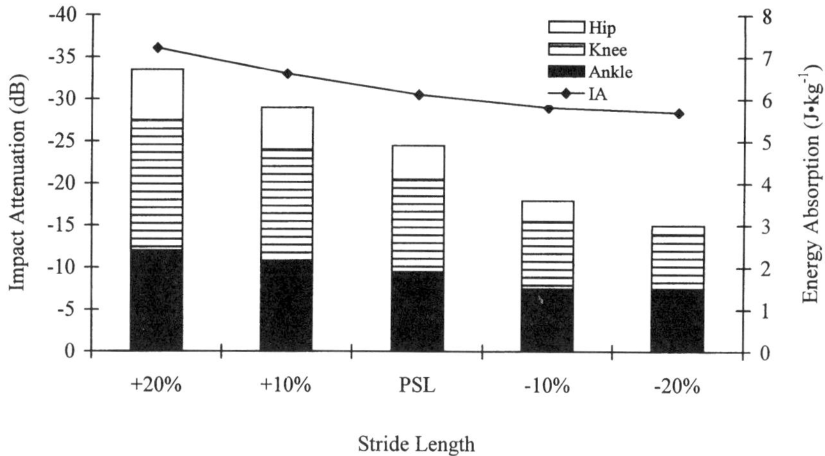

FIGURE 7.—Impact attenuation for each stride length condition is indicated by the line graph. Corresponding impact energy absorption at the hip, knee, and ankle joint is illustrated by the histogram. (Courtesy of Derrick TR, Hamill J, Caldwell GE: Energy absorption of impacts during running at various stride lengths. *Med Sci Sports Exerc* 30:128–135, 1998.)

Methods.—Across 5 stride-length conditions, running speed at 3.83 m.s-1 was kept constant. The 5 conditions were: preferred stride length, plus 10% preferred stride length, minus 10% preferred stride length, plus 20% preferred stride length, and minus 20% preferred stride length. Accelerometers were attached to the leg and head of 10 male runners to generate transfer functions. To estimate the net energy absorbed at the hip, knee, and ankle joints, a rigid body model was used.

Results.—As the stride length increased, there was an increasing degree of shock attenuation (Fig 7). As the stride length increased, the energy absorbed during the impact portion of the running cycle also increased. The greatest adjustment in response to increased shock was shown by the muscles that cross the knee joint.

Conclusion.—The increased perpendicular distance from the line of action of the resultant ground reaction force to the knee joint center played a role in this increased energy absorption. The amount of shock attenuated by some joints may be adjusted by altering the distance between the line of action of the force vector and the joint center, but this mechanism is metabolically costly, as it requires greater muscular effort to counteract.

▶ It is generally believed that stride lengths longer than preferred will produce higher ground reaction forces, and greater magnitude of shock waves through the body. This article reports higher vertical impulses associated with longer stride lengths, produced by larger vertical velocities at landing. Greater impact loads were countered by greater shock attenuation, and greater energy absorption by the muscles which cross the hip, knee, and ankle joints. The knee joint muscles produced the largest amount of shock attenuation, while the ankle joint contributed less energy absorption in longer stride length conditions. Longer stride lengths are related to greater oxygen costs, and to greater eccentric contractions to absorb impact loads. Head accelerations were found to remain relatively constant throughout ranges of increased and decreased stride lengths, while greater eccentric muscle forces were required to absorb impact forces.

M.J.L. Alexander, Ph.D.

Effects of Restricted Knee Flexion and Walking Speed on the Vertical Ground Reaction Force During Gait

Cook TM, Farrell KP, Carey IA, et al (Univ of Iowa, Iowa City; St Ambrose Univ, Davenport, IA; Multicenter Therapy, Spring Lake Park, Minn; et al)
J Orthop Sports Phys Ther 25:236–244, 1997   4–13

Introduction.—The force exerted on the foot by the ground is known as the ground reaction force during gait. The vertical component represents the weight-bearing function of the leg, and it includes the force required to continually oppose gravity as well as the force needed to move the body's center of gravity up and down with each step. Following meniscal and ligamentous repair, debridement, and patellar realignment, it is often necessary to restrict flexion of the knee to allow healing, but when this is done, the normal shock absorption function of the knee is altered. The effects of restricted knee flexion and walking speed were measured on vertical ground reaction force during gait.

Methods.—On 36 healthy men, force plate measurements were taken while they were walking at 3 different speeds when their knee flexion was unrestricted and restricted to 10 degrees and 25 degrees (Fig 2). Walking was done on a level wooden walkway with 1.22 mm inclines at each end. The knee was restricted with a prefabricated adjustable knee orthosis, consisting of medial and lateral uprights.

Results.—In the restricted leg, there were significant increases in 4 characteristics of the vertical ground reaction force during walking with restricted knee flexion. In the unrestricted leg, there were 2 characteristics. Significant speed-knee flexion restriction interactions were seen in the loading rate and unloading rate for the restricted leg and peak force for both legs. There were 2 significant differences between knee flexion restrictions of 10 degrees and 25 degrees at the fast walking speed. The unloading rate with knee flexion restricted to 25 degrees was significantly greater than walking with both a free knee and with knee flexion restricted to 10 degrees at the fast walking speed.

Conclusion.—The force applied to both lower limbs may be significantly altered by restricted knee flexion during gait. To counteract the increases in mechanical stress that result from walking with restricted knee flexion, patients should be instructed to limit their walking speed.

▶ It is sometimes clinically desirable to restrict or completely eliminate flexion of the knee to allow some healing process to occur after meniscal or ligament repair, debridement, and patellar realignment. However, restriction

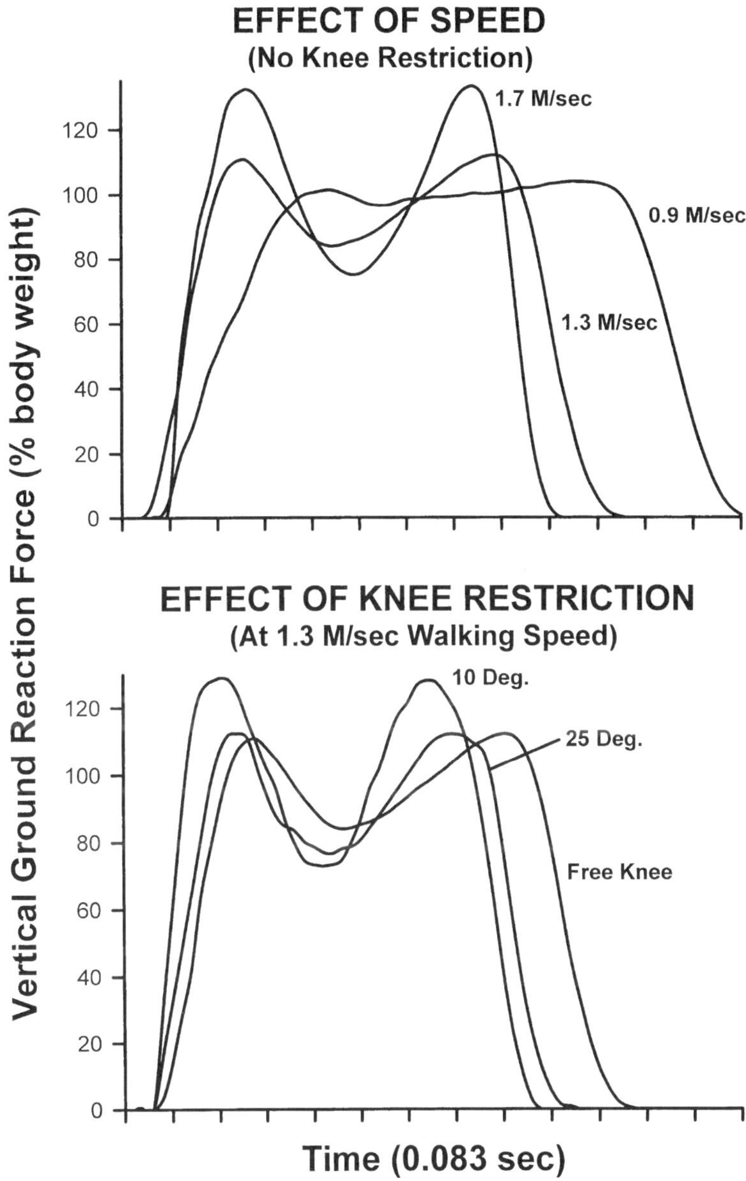

FIGURE 2.—Sample force vs. time recordings from a typical subject showing the effects of walking speed and knee flexion restriction. (Courtesy of Cook TM, Farrell KP, Carey IA, et al: Effects of restricted knee flexion and walking speed on the vertical ground reaction force during gait. *J Orthop Sports Phys Ther* 25:236–244, 1997.)

of knee flexion may alter the shock absorption role of the knee in walking on the restricted side, as well as alter the forces on the unrestricted side. This study examined the effect of restricting knee joint motion with an orthosis on four variables derived from force plate measurements. There were significant differences in loading rates, as well as peak and average forces on both knees when knee flexion was restricted, and when walking speed was increased. One implication of this finding is that if knee flexion restriction devices such as braces or casts are applied to an injured knee, that both the injured and uninjured knees are forced to withstand higher peak and average forces and greater loading rates. This may produce excessive stresses on the joints of both lower extremities, suggesting prudence and caution in the use of these devices, and limitations in walking speed.

M.J.L. Alexander, Ph.D.

Gait Analysis and Bivalved Serial Casting of an Athlete With Shortened Gastrocnemius Muscles: A Single Case Design

Selby-Silverstein L, Farrett WD Jr, Maurer BT, et al (Thomas Jefferson Univ, Philadelphia; Presbyterian/St Luke's Hosp, Denver; Wyeth-Ayerst Research, Radnor, Pa; et al)
J Orthop Sports Phys Ther 25:282–288, 1997   4–14

Introduction.—It was determined whether bivalved serial casting and a positioning program would increase the total dynamic ankle range of motion without increasing the amount of compensatory foot pronation used during gait of an athlete with shortened gastrocnemius muscles.

Methods.—A 21-year-old male athlete ran 25 miles each week and biked 35 miles each week. He complained of uncomfortable toe running, achiness at the base of his heel, and excessive forefoot shoe wear. He had decreased passive range of motion and shortening of the gastrocnemius muscles. To collect functional dynamic ankle range of motion data, a 3-dimensional camera-based kinematic system was used. To determine the relative amount of foot pronation by measuring the pronation-withdrawal phases, the Musgrave Footprint system was used. At baseline and at postintervention and withdrawal phases, data were collected, graphed, and interpreted.

Treatment.—The patient's gastrocnemius muscles were stretched with bilateral bivalved serial casts and a positioning program. The legs and feet were cast in prone position with the knees flexed. The casts were bivalved to permit donning and doffing of the casts (Fig 3). The patient was instructed to don the casts and sit with his knees as extended as possible with his hips flexed to 90 degrees for up to 30 minutes twice a day. An increase in mean total dynamic range of motion without an increase in dynamic foot pronation was seen. The increase in mean total dynamic ankle range of motion was maintained, the pronation measurement had not changed 8 weeks after treatment.

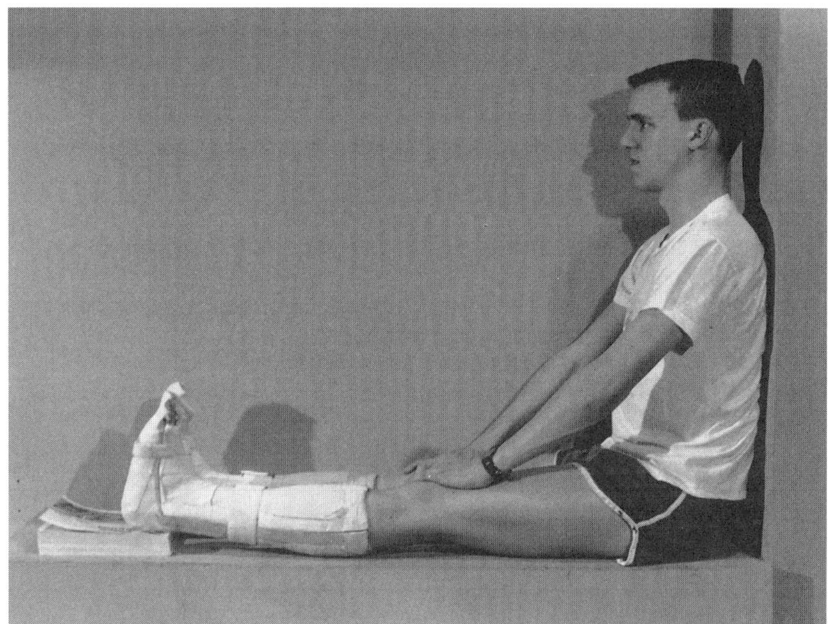

FIGURE 3.—The final pair of bivalved serial casts with the subject demonstrating the final stretch position. (Courtesy of Selby-Silverstein L, Farrett WD Jr, Maurer BT, et al: Gait analysis and bivalved serial casting of an athlete with shortened gastrocnemius muscles: A single case design. *J Orthop Sports Phys Ther* 25(4):282–288, 1997.)

Conclusion.—Lengthening of gastrocnemius muscles resulted for this patient with the use of bivalved serial casting combined with a simple positioning program. Other patients should be considered for this treatment.

▶ Muscle tightness or lack of flexibility may predispose an athlete to muscle strain, tendinitis, or muscle rupture and is commonly treated with flexibility exercises. Stretching exercises can take a variety of forms, including ballistic, static, and neuromuscular techniques. This study examined a form of static stretching using lower leg casts on a subject with chronically shortened gastrocnemius muscles, likely caused by toe running.

After wearing the casts for 40 minutes twice a day for 6 months, the subject increased static ankle range of motion by 5 degrees and dynamic range of motion by 22 degrees. The increased range of ankle motion occurred without an increase in foot pronation. Although this form of static stretching treatment for chronically shortened muscles was somewhat uncomfortable for the subject, its effectiveness should be noted for use by other subjects with chronically shortened muscles.

M.J.L. Alexander, Ph.D.

Sacroiliac Motion for Extreme Hip Positions: A Fresh Cadaver Study

Smidt GL, Wei S-H, McQuade K, et al (Univ of Iowa, Iowa City)
Spine 22:2073–2082, 1997

4–15

Introduction.—There is a poor understanding of the role of the sacroiliac joint in the contexts of low back pain and physical function. The nature and magnitude of joint motion would seem to determine the significance of the sacroiliac joints relative to function and low back pain. Previous studies have reported very small angular and linear motions at the sacroiliac joints. To extend the understanding of the sacroiliac joints, fresh cadavers were used. The 3-dimensional range of motion at the left and right sacroiliac joints was determined. The mechanical structure of the sacroiliac joint was explored.

Methods.—The study included 5 fresh, unembalmed cadavers used less than 24 hours after death, ranging in age from 52 to 68 years and ranging in weight from 66 to 75 kg. Radiopaque markers were placed in the sacrum and in each innominate bone before standardized performance of CT scans at 3-mm intervals, with the fresh cadaver stabilized in the side-lying position on a specially constructed pallet. Coordinates for centroids of the markers were obtained from CT images stored on magnetic tape. Mechanical analysis was performed. To obtain the thickness of the intersubchondral joint space and the general configuration of the sacroiliac joints, the intersubchondral lines on the images were traced and reconstructed. Several positions were analyzed, including the neutral body po-

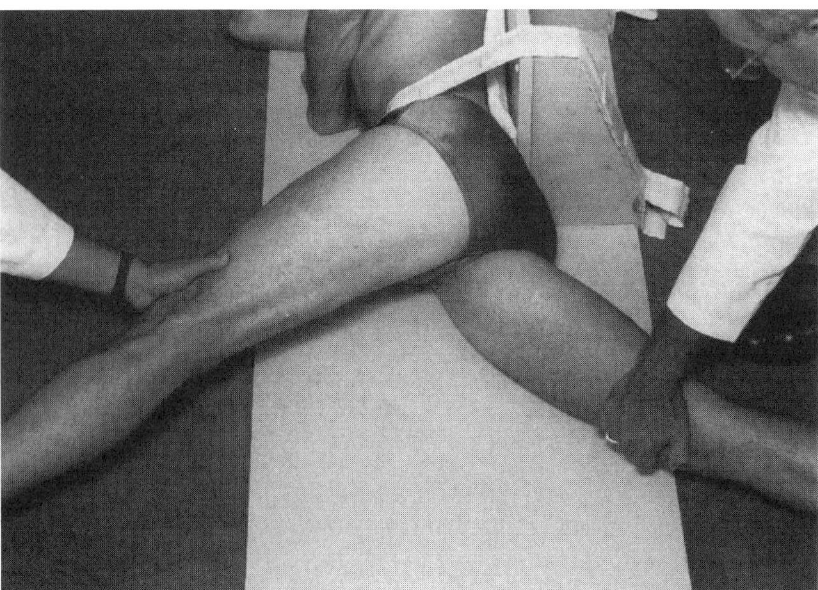

FIGURE 5.—Extreme left hip flexion/right hip extension. (Courtesy of Smidt GL, Wei S-H, McQuade K, et al: Sacroiliac motion for extreme hip positions: A fresh cadaver study. *Spine* 22:2073–2082, 1997.)

sition, the extreme double hip flexion, the extreme double hip extension, the extreme right hip flexion/left hip extension, and the extreme left hip flexion/right hip extension (Fig 5).

Results.—In the sagittal plane (7 degrees on the left and 8 degrees on the right with a range of 3–17 degrees), the largest amount of sacroiliac motion occurred. With respect to both bilateral and reciprocal hip joint positions, definite trends in the direction of angular sacroiliac motion occurred. There was a range of 4–8 mm in the translation or linear motion of the posterior superior iliac spines to the sacrum. With no detectable trends, this motion occurred in all directions. There was a 1.2-mm average intersubchondral thickness of the sacroiliac joint. The joint's shape resembled an airplane propeller.

Conclusion.—Considerable angular and linear motion was seen, even though the subjects were elderly. To elucidate full range of motion at the sacroiliac joint, extreme hip positions are necessary. To complement hip joint motion and influence motion at the lumbosacral junction and, thus, low back pain in both the direct and indirect sense, the magnitude and direction of demonstrated sacroiliac motion appears to be sufficient.

▶ There is some controversy in the literature regarding the amount of motion that occurs in the sacroiliac joint during normal movements. Some authors have reported very small ranges of sacroiliac joint motion during normal activities; however, during extreme hip positions the sacroiliac range of motion was found to be much larger. The use of CT scans in this group of older cadaveric specimens revealed significant amounts of sacroiliac joint motion when the hips were placed in extreme positions.

The authors suggest that athletic activities that require running, jumping, and even throwing may require the full extent of sacroiliac range of motion. However, it is not clear at present whether specific exercises or other means can increase sacroiliac range of motion—or whether excessive sacroiliac range of motion can lead to instability, pain, and joint degeneration. The findings of the study imply that surgical fusion of a problematic sacroiliac joint will place high strains on the contralateral joint, and sacral joint dysfunction may severely restrict hip joint range of motion.

M.J.L. Alexander, Ph.D.

The Strain Behavior of the Anterior Cruciate Ligament During Bicycling: An In Vivo Study

Fleming BC, Beynnon BD, Renstrom PA, et al (Univ of Vermont, Burlington)
Am J Sports Med 26:109–118, 1998   4–16

Introduction.—The rehabilitation protocol prescribed after surgery has bearing on the long-term success of reconstruction of the anterior cruciate ligament. There is still controversy over the optimal knee rehabilitation program, as the optimal levels of muscle activity and joint motion that are beneficial to graft healing are still unknown. Most clinicians consider stationary bicycling to be a safe rehabilitation activity for the healing of the anterior cruciate ligament graft, but the literature has little direct evidence to support this. The strain in the anterior cruciate ligament and the pedal forces during bicycling in vivo were measured to examine the effects of resistance and pedaling speed on anterior cruciate ligament strain values.

Methods.—Ligament strain was measured on 8 patients who had arthroscopic meniscectomy with the use of local anesthesia. The evaluation included 6 different riding conditions: 3 power levels (75, 125, 175 W), which were each performed at 2 cadences of 60 rpm and 90 rpm.

Result.—For the 175-W, 90-rpm condition, the peak ligament strain value was 1.2% and for the 125-W, 60 rpm condition, the peak ligament strain value was 2.1%. Changes in power level of cadence did not produce any significant differences in peak strain values. The strain values were then pooled across the 6 riding conditions. There was 1.7% mean peak strain value, which, when compared to other rehabilitation activities, is considered to be relatively low.

Conclusion.—This selection of power and cadence levels can be included in knee rehabilitation programs without significantly changing ligament strain values. The patient can increase muscle activity by increasing the power level or decreasing the cadence without subjecting the ligament or ligament graft to higher strain values through stationary bicycling as a rehabilitation exercise.

▶ Stationary bicycling is often used in postoperative anterior cruciate ligament (ACL) rehabilitation programs. This study indicates that strain values in the ACL are relatively low in the 6 conditions tested. It appears to be a safe method of increasing muscle strength and protecting the integrity of the ACL graft.

F.J. George, A.T.C., P.T.

Flexibility and Its Effect on Sports Injury and Performance
Gleim GW, McHugh MP (Lenox Hill Hosp, New York)
Sports Med 24:289–299, 1997   4–17

Introduction.—Static flexibility is defined as the range of motion available to a joint, and dynamic flexibility refers to the ease of movement within the obtaining range of motion. When the athlete is instructed to relax, measurements of static flexibility are taken, whereas dynamic flexibility is measured by the amount of stiffness or the resistance of a structure to deformation. Fundamental concepts about flexibility and its measurements were reviewed.

Measurements.—The toe touch is used to measure flexibility, as is the sit-and-reach, because they are indicative of vertebral and hip flexion extensibility. Range of motion can be measured by goniometers. Dynamic flexibility or stiffness is measured passively or actively, with passive stiffness involving quantification of joint angle at the same time as passive torque generation. In animal experiments, repeated submaximal contractions can decrease passive stiffness and provide protection against external mechanical strain injury.

Injuries.—Rates of strains, sprains, or overuse injuries have not been associated with flexibility or stretching. As yet undefined interactions between physiologic, psychological, environmental, and random factors are involved in sports injury. Submaximal contractions (active warm-up) have been found to decrease passive stiffness and increase the force and length at which the muscle fails, Those findings provide a scientific basis for low-intensity warm-up exercises. It can be assumed that fatigued muscles are more susceptible to strain injury.

Conclusions.—Flexibility and injury cannot be scientifically associated in all sports and all levels of play. In some sports that rely on extremes of motion for movement, flexibility is important for performance. In sports which use only the mid portion of range of motion, decreased flexibility may actually increase economy of movement. Accurate definitions of injury and exposure must be found in future studies.

▶ The controversy regarding flexibility and its effects on performance and injury prevention are addressed in this article. More questions have arisen than are answered. Some guidelines to follow are:

1. Develop a stretching program suitable to the needs of the sport.
2. The stretching program should be included as part of the warm-up and done at least 15–20 minutes before exercising and again thereafter. Warm-up exercises before stretching also help to increase tissue extensibility.
3. Apply a low static stretch and avoid bouncing movements at the end of range to reduce the risk of injury.
4. Do not overstretch into pain but rather feel a stretch in the muscles within one's level of tolerance.
5. Hold the stretch for 15–20 seconds.
6. Each muscle group should be stretched 3 or 4 times for maximum benefit.
7. Stretch throughout the season and in the off-season to maintain flexibility. Improved flexibility can be achieved only through a long-term stretching program.
8. Only stretch a warm muscle; a good deal of stretching should be done at the end of the workout, as part of the cool-down phase.[1]

F.J. George, A.T.C., P.T.

Reference

1. George, F: The athletic trainer's perspective. *Clin Sports Med* 16:363–364, 1997.

Shoulder Muscle Firing Patterns During the Windmill Softball Pitch

Maffet MW, Jobe FW, Pink MM, et al (Centinela Hosp, Inglewood, Calif)
Am J Sports Med 25:369–374, 1997   4–18

Background.—Although fast-pitch softball is a popular game, there is a scarcity of data with regard to the muscles involved. This study analyzes the so called windmill delivery used by fast-pitch softball players and characterizes the phases of the pitch and the shoulder muscles involved.

Methods.—Ten female fast-pitch softball pitchers 18 to 29 years old who use the windmill delivery were studied. Maximal muscle testing was performed on 8 shoulder girdle muscles of their pitching arm: anterior and posterior deltoid, pectoralis major, serratus anterior, supraspinatus, infraspinatus, teres minor, and subscapularis. Intramuscular electromyography, high-speed cinematography, and motion analysis were used to assess muscle strength.

Findings.—Six phases of the pitch were identified (Fig 1). In phase 1 (wind-up), the ball is brought from behind the body into a position with the ball next to the leg (i.e., 6 o'clock position). The supraspinatus muscle has the highest activity in this wind-up phase. With the ball between the 6 and 3 o'clock positions, the infraspinatus and supraspinatus muscles are most involved, acting to centralize the humeral head within the glenoid cavity. As the ball moves from the 3 to the 12 o'clock position, the posterior deltoid, infraspinatus, and teres minor are involved in the maximal external rotation. In phase 4, from 12 to 9 o'clock, the subscapularis and pectoralis major are the main muscles involved, providing stability and force, respectively. From 9 o'clock until the ball is released, the pectoralis major and subscapularis muscles are mainly involved in stabilizing the arm and allowing internal rotation and adduction of the humerus. Finally, during follow-through from ball release until forward arm motion ceases, the teres minor is most active. However, the activities of all muscles drop during this last phase because the arm rubs against the lateral thigh just after the ball is released to decelerate the arm.

Several similarities with the baseball pitch were noted. The serratus anterior and pectoralis muscles work in tandem and have similar functions in both pitches. Also, in both pitches, the subscapularis muscle stabilizes the anterior glenohumeral joint and acts as an internal rotator.

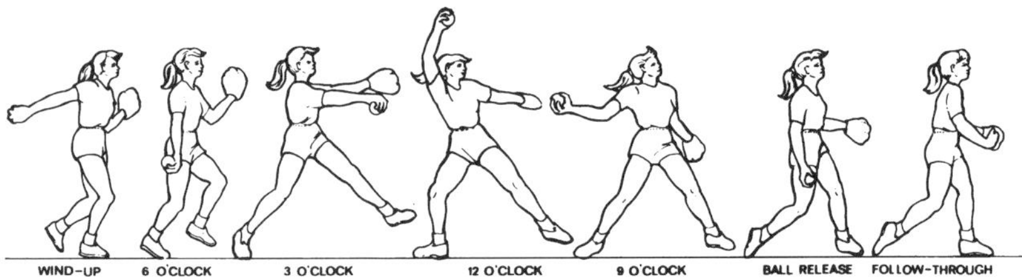

FIGURE 1.—Six phases of the windmill pitch. (Courtesy of Maffet MW, Jobe FW, Pink MM, et al. Shoulder muscle firing patterns during the windmill softball pitch. *Am J Sports Med* 25:369–374, 1997.)

Conclusions.—The windmill pitch occurs with the humerus primarily in the plane of the body. The subscapularis and pectoralis major muscles stabilize the shoulder and arm, while the pectoralis major muscle provides most of the force for throwing the ball. Importantly, the serratus anterior muscle helps synchronize the actions of the scapulohumeral joint. Knowing which shoulder muscles are involved in which phase(s) of the windmill delivery will help in diagnosing injuries and selecting appropriate physical therapy.

▶ With the current popularity of the game of softball, and its recent acceptance into the Olympic Games, there is renewed interest in the technique of windmill pitching. In this analysis of the skill, there were found to be several similarities to the baseball pitch, including the roles of the serratus anterior and pectoralis major. During delivery, the pectoralis muscle performed the powerful adduction and internal rotation of the humerus and is the major force generator in the throw, while the serratus anterior acts simultaneously to stabilize the scapula. Subscapularis is also strongly active to assist with humeral internal rotation and stabilize the anterior capsule. Less activity was seen in the shoulder muscles during the follow-through, as the pitchers contacted the hip after ball release which decreased the forward momentum of the arm. This detailed analysis of the skill will provide sports medicine care providers with a better understanding of the mechanics and muscle firing patterns, and assist with diagnosis of shoulder muscle injuries.

M.J.L. Alexander, Ph.D.

Load Dependence in Carpal Kinematics During Wrist Flexion in Vivo
Valero-Cuevas FJ, Small CF (Queen's Univ, Kingston, Ont, Canada)
Clin Biomech 12:154–159, 1997   4–19

Introduction.—Clinicians would benefit from a simple method for characterizing the in vivo kinematic behavior of the human wrist while moving under load. Such a method would aid particularly in understanding treatment outcomes for conditions such as rheumatoid arthritis. Three-dimensional motion analysis techniques are expensive or invasive; thus a 2-dimensional analysis may be useful. Little is known about the in vivo kinematics of the normal human wrist under load, despite clinical observations of a relationship between motion-loading and pain in wrists affected by rheumatoid arthritis.

Methods.—There were 10 participants with no wrist pathology who participated in an in vivo study of normal wrist kinematics during plantar flexion motion against a constant load. To track the motion of the hand during the task, a custom-designed instrumental apparatus was used. Torques of 0, 1.1. and 2.2 newton-meters were generated in a plaque, unidirectional flexion motion. The Planar Rigid Body Method algorithm and an 8-degree angular step size were used to compute hand kinematics. As indices of changes in the kinematics, the finite radius of motion and the

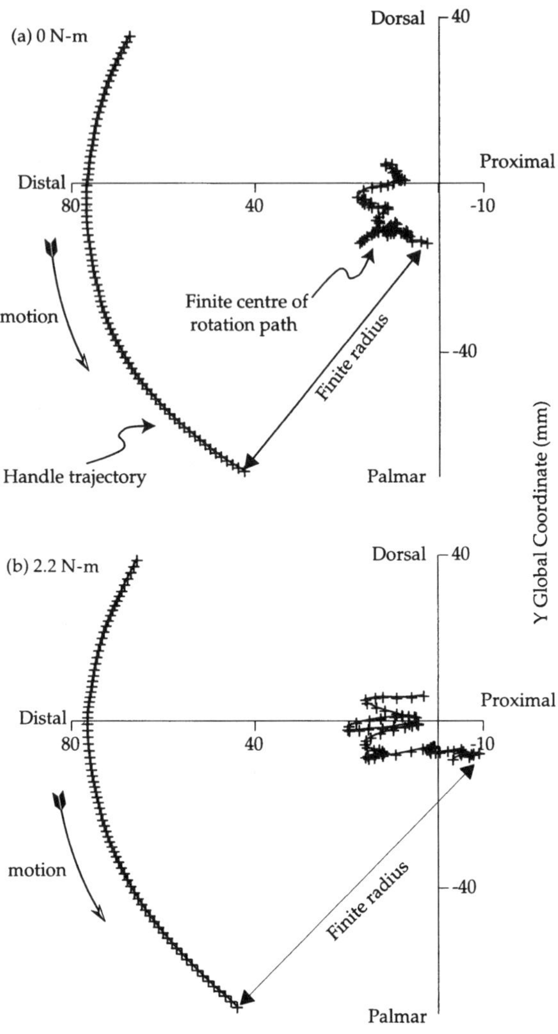

FIGURE 2.—Trajectory and finite center of rotation results at no load (Fig 2, A) and 2.2 newton-meters (Fig 2, B) wrist torque. The Planar Rigid Body Method takes 2 handle positions, calculates their midperpendicular, and locates the finite center of rotation as the distance between the center of rotation and the midpoint between the 2 locations. We define the length of the finite radius of rotation as the distance between the center of rotation and the midpoint between the 2 locations. The finite center of rotation corresponding to the last finite center for each trial is shown. (Reprinted from Valero-Cuevas FJ, Small CF: Load dependence in carpal kinematics during wrist flexion *in vivo*: *Clin Biomech* 12:154–159, Copyright 1997, with kind permission from Elsevier Science Ltd, The Boulevard, Langford Lane, Kidlington OX5 1GB UK.)

range and standard deviation of the residuals to a fitted second-order curve were used.

Results.—With torque, the magnitude of both the range and standard deviation of the residuals increased significantly. A slight increasingly palmarward drift and oscillations in the proximal-distal direction were seen with the path of the finite center of rotation, which corresponded to changes in the length of the finite radius of rotation (Fig 2). Joint forces affect wrist kinematics.

Conclusion.—When generating torque, the wrist does not behave as a smooth mechanism. Carpal kinematics are affected by load. During wrist flexion, fluctuations in the finite radius of motion are the natural kinematic consequence of intercarpal motion. Orchestrated intercarpal motion depends on the soundness of articular and ligamentous structures, so wrist kinematics are particularly sensitive to load and joint integrity. Joint involvement before the onset of gross dysfunction may be evaluated by using simple planar testing of carpal kinematics under reproducible and controlled joint torque conditions. Testing would also help to evaluate treatment outcomes.

▶ Examination of the kinematics of joint motion during wrist flexion revealed that the radius of motion is not constant, but experiences fluctuations in length. This lack of smooth motion is likely due to intercarpal motion. The loaded wrist produced greater fluctuations than the unloaded wrist, and the fluctuations increased with increasing load. The authors concluded that the joint forces which accompany the generation of increased wrist torques induce more irregular carpal motion. Pathological changes in the wrist joint, such as those seen in rheumatoid arthritis, can lead to gross changes in wrist kinematics. An instrumented kinematic analysis of wrist joint motion could be used to evaluate joint dysfunction due to arthritis, ligament tears, or carpal tunnel syndrome.

M.J.L. Alexander, Ph.D.

In Vivo Measurements Show Tensile Axial Strain in the Proximal Lateral Aspect of the Human Femur
Aamodt A, Lund-Larsen J, Eine J, et al (Trondheim Univ, Norway)
J Orthop Res 15:927–931, 1997   4–20

Objective.—The classic theory of Pauwels suggests that the stress pattern for the proximal lateral aspect of the femur involves a bending movement on the femur, causing medial compression and lateral tension. More recently, it has been suggested that muscle forces lead to moment-free loading of the femur, with uniform, axial compressive force throughout the length of the bone. In vivo strain measurements were performing at the proximal lateral aspect of the femur to find out whether this area is subjected to compression or tension during exercise and to measure the magnitude of these strains.

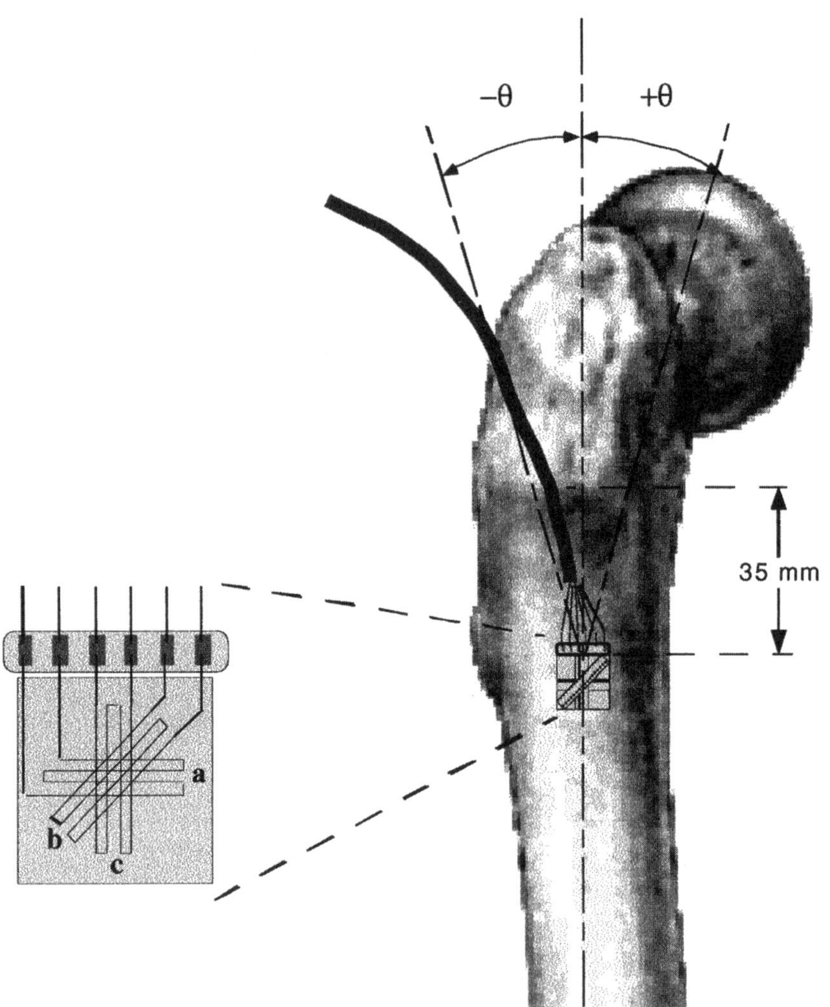

FIGURE 1.—Lateral view of the femur, indicating the site for attachment of the rosette. On the left is a close-up of the rosette with the 3 grid elements (a, b, and c). $+\theta/-\theta$ denotes the angle of the principal tensile strain, zero degree being parallel to the c-element of the rosette. (Courtesy of Aamodt A, Lund-Larsen J, Eine J, et al: In vivo measurements show tensile axial strain in the proximal lateral aspect of the human femur. *J Orthop Res* 15:927–931, 1997.)

Methods.—The measurements were performed in 2 women, aged 24 and 49 years, undergoing surgery for "snapping hip syndrome." Intraoperatively, a strain-gauge rosette was bonded to the lateral aspect of the femur with polymethylmethacrylate adhesive (Fig 1). After the wound was closed, the patients performed a number of maneuvers with the rosette in place, including 2-legged stance, single-legged stance, walking, and stair climbing. The wound was then reopened, the rosette and adhesive removed, and the operation completed.

Results.—Compared with 2-legged stance, principal tensile strain was significantly increased during 1-legged stance, walking, and stair climbing. Under each of the latter 3 conditions, the principal tensile strain was aligned to the longitudinal femoral axis within 22 degrees or less. With each activity, tensile axial strain was observed at the lateral aspect of the femur on dynamic strain measurements.

Conclusion.—This experiment shows that the stance phase of gait places tension on the proximal lateral aspect of the femur. The principal tensile strain increases and becomes more closely aligned to the longitudinal femoral axis during the stance phases than during unloading. Thus, the findings are consistent with the classic bending theory of Pauwels.

▶ There is some controversy regarding the type of loading that occurs on the proximal femur during single-legged stance and during the stance phase of gait. Because of the angle of the femoral neck, the primary loading forces on the lateral proximal femur have usually been described as bending forces. The body weight applied to the superior proximal femur acts medially to the long axis of the femur, producing bending forces on the lateral aspect of the femur. Some recent studies have reported that there are no moments associated with loading of the femur, and that there is uniform axial compression during support as the result of lateral muscle forces resisting the bending forces.

Strain gauges were implanted in 2 patients during hip surgery, and the femoral forces were measured. The strain patterns showed that loading of the femur under normal strain produced tensile forces caused by medial bending of the femur. The results supported the theory that the upper femur is subjected to bending and that there are no muscle forces large enough to overcome these bending forces. Some of the recent mathematical models of the femur have overestimated the lateral muscle forces needed to resist the bending forces caused by body weight.

M.J.L. Alexander, Ph.D.

Muscle, Reflex and Central Components in the Control of the Ankle Joint in Healthy and Spastic Man
Sinkjær T (Aalborg Univ, Denmark)
Acta Neurol Scand 96:1–28, 1997   4–21

Introduction.—In meeting the changing postural and gait requirements around the ankle joint, ankle joint stiffness, defined as a force resisting an angular displacement, is of fundamental importance. The influence of the passive and intrinsic properties of the inactive and active muscle system around the joint, known as the nonreflex component, the mechanical importance of the stretch reflex in the stretched and unloaded muscles, and the supraspinal control of the stretch reflex must be analyzed to understand the control of the ankle joint during different motor tasks.

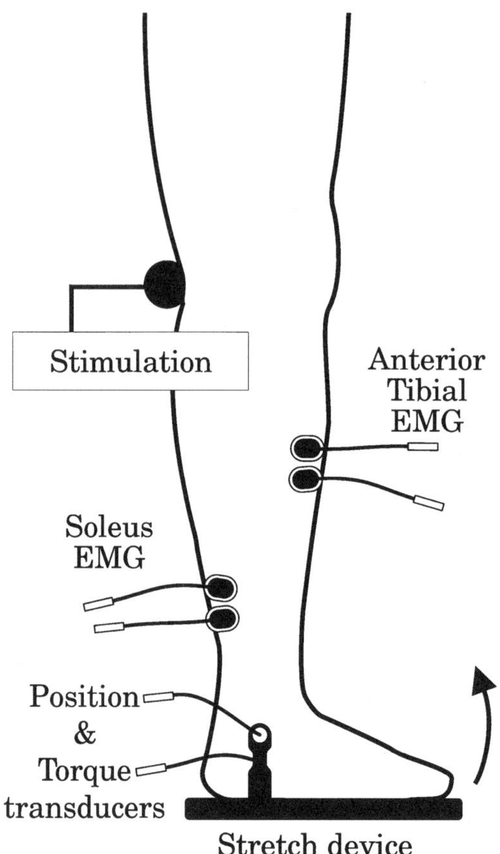

FIGURE 1.—A schematic presentation of the experimental set-up for studying the stretch and H-reflexes during sitting, standing, and walking. The foot was mounted to a platform. In the stretch experiments, torque and position were measured from the platform. To elicit a stretch reflex, the ankle joint was rotated by a motor connected to the platform (not shown). The mechanical importance of the stretch reflex was measured through changes in the joint torque. The stretch reflex was recorded electrically as the compound muscle action potential through bipolar surface electromyogram (*EMG*) electrodes placed above the soleus muscle. During H-reflex experiments, the tibial nerve was stimulated at the popliteal fossa, and the H-reflex recorded over the soleus muscle as during the stretch reflex experiments. Surface EMG electrodes were also placed above the anterior tibial muscle. (Courtesy of Sinkjær T: Muscle, reflex and central components in the control of the ankle joint in healthy and spastic man. *Acta Neurol Scand Suppl* 96:1–28, Copyright 1997, Munksgaard International Publishers Ltd., Copenhagen, Denmark.)

Methods.—Stretch reflex and H-reflex measurements from the ankle extensor muscles were taken during walking, standing, and sitting at matched contraction levels. This stretch was performed by placing the foot on a platform from which the ankle joint torque and the position were measured (Fig 1). An electrical stimulation at the popliteal fossa was applied to elicit the H-reflex, and this method was applied to study the changes in the excitability of the motoneurons during the same motor tasks as studied at the stretch reflex. The intrinsic stiffness of the ankle extensors in healthy subjects was investigated to learn how the contractile properties of a muscle in humans depend on the history of activation. Stretch responses were compared before and after reversible block of the common peroneal nerve and during an attempted, voluntary, fictive dorsiflexion after common peroneal nerve block at matched ankle extensor contraction levels.

Results.—A prolonged contraction increased the intrinsic muscle stiffness by 49% at matched background contraction in sitting participants. Nonreflex stiffness was found to be a prominent factor in normal movements of the ankle joint as there was a general lack of muscle yield and a mechanically important nonreflex stiffness of the ankle extensors. A mechanical strong stretch reflex in the isometric contracted muscles during sitting was found in healthy and spastic individuals. In healthy individuals, the stretch reflex was strongly modulated during a step; however, during standing and walking, no task-specific reflex modulation was seen. The stretch reflex modulation was impaired at least to the extent demonstrated earlier for the H-reflex in spastic patients when the modulation of the short latency stretch reflex during walking was investigated. During the peroneal nerve block investigation, it was found that transmission in the pathways mediating a mechanically important, reciprocal inhibition is facilitated by descending neural control signals.

Conclusions.—It is not always possible to draw conclusions about the stretch reflex based on observations of the H-reflex, at least during walking and standing. Increasing the ankle joint stiffness at those parts of a motor task where the central control allows afferent feedback to add to the muscle activity is the physiologic role of the stretch reflex in man. During the step cycle, this happens to a large extent. A functionally important and integrated part of the locomotor pattern in man is the stretch flex. The transition from stance to swing during walking in spastic patients can be impaired by the mechanically strong stretch reflex and the lack of reflex modulation. To judge the motor skills at the ankle joint in spastic patients, the ability to dorsiflex could be a simple and reliable measure.

▶ This study consisted of a detailed examination of the stretch reflex in the ankle plantarflexor muscles of a group of normal individuals, with some comparisons to spastic individuals. The individuals were perturbed by mounting the foot on a platform and stretching the plantarflexors by moving the foot into dorsiflexion. The stretch reflex was elicited and examined in terms of latency, speed, and electromyogram (EMG) intensity. The H-reflex was also examined by stimulation of the tibial nerve at the popliteal fossa, and the effect on EMG output was measured. The author concluded that the physiologic role of the stretch reflex is to increase ankle joint stiffness by adding to the muscle activity at certain points during the support phase of walking. In spastic patients there was found to be impaired stretch reflex modulation and increased nonreflex stiffness in the ankle plantarflexors during gait. This study emphasizes the importance of a healthy stretch reflex in the ankle joint muscles to produce skilled locomotion in normal individuals.

M.J.L. Alexander, Ph.D.

Jump Distance of Dance Landings Influencing Internal Joint Forces: I. Axial Forces

Simpson KJ, Kanter L (Univ of Georgia, Athens)
Med Sci Sports Exerc 29:916–927, 1997   4–22

Introduction.—Among dancers, lower extremity injuries are common, accounting for up to 86% of reported injuries to ballet dancers. Repetitive axial and shear loading that occurs during dance is involved in the etiology of osteoarthritis, as is evidenced by joint degeneration and arthritic changes appearing in dancers by 25–37 years of age. Knowledge of the

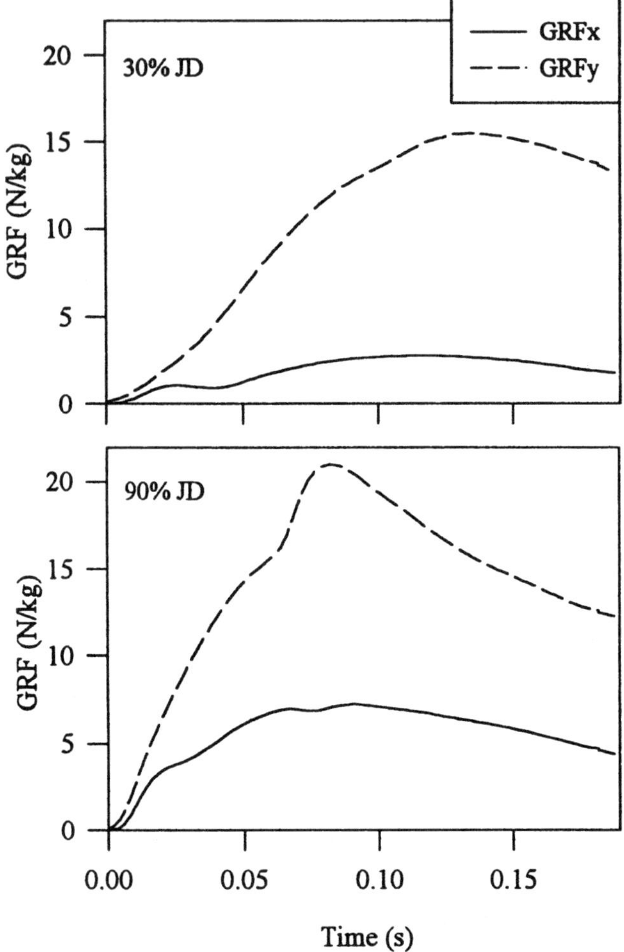

FIGURE 2.—Horizontal (GRF_x) and vertical (GRF_y) ground reaction force curves of a single trial of a representative participant at 30% and 90% jump distance. *Abbreviation: GRF*, ground reaction force. (Courtesy of Simpson KJ, Kanter L: Jump distance of dance landings influencing internal joint forces: I. Axial forces. *Med Sci Sports Exerc* 297:916–927, 1997.)

influences of ground reaction and muscle forces of the generation of joint forces that act on articular surfaces would be helpful in understand the mechanisms that contribute to injury. The effect of jumping distance on component ankle and knee joint axial forces generated during the landing phase of traveling jumps was investigated.

Methods.—There were 6 female dancers who each performed 10 jumps at 30%, 60% and 90% maximum jump distance. They also performed 15 jumps at 35% to 100% jump distance. Film was taken of a sagittal view of the right leg landing onto a force platform.

Results.—At increased jump distance, there was greater ground reaction force maxima, knee and ankle flexion velocity, knee flexion, net ankle and knee joint moment maxima, tibial landing angle, ankle and knee joint reaction axial forces, and quadriceps axial forces peak magnitudes and rates of axial force application (Fig 2). Joint reaction axial force was a less important determinant of knee axial force than quadriceps axial force. For accommodating impact forces, increased quadriceps force was useful; however, increased quadriceps force served to increase its contribution to knee axial force, particularly during the later portion of the impact phase.

Conclusions.—Significant magnitudes and rates of axial force application of muscle axial forces were seen in high impact situations, and these could contribute to excessive joint wear. The joint reaction and muscle axial forces were affected by jump distance, which also influenced the total joint axial forces. When investigating the effect of techniques used to attenuate forces on the lower extremity, the timing of the peak magnitudes and rates of axial forces suggest that the muscle forces occurring after the impact phase should be examined in landing situations.

▶ Dancers have a high incidence of early joint degeneration and arthritic changes, likely caused by the high number of landings they have to perform during practice and performance. This study examined the landing forces at the ankle and knee joints with the use of force plate and electromyogram data. The findings suggest that joint forces are caused by the forces produced at impact as well as the compressive forces resulting from muscle contractions, and that greater jump distance produces higher forces. Greater knee flexion on landing may help to attenuate impact forces, but the greater muscle forces also increase the the total axial forces on the joints. The high magnitudes of the joint axial forces suggest that excessive joint wear may occur in dance athletes, which may be an unavoidable consequence of the number of high-impact landings necessary in the activity.

M.J.L. Alexander, Ph.D.

Ballistic Movement Performance in Karate Athletes

Zehr EP, Sale DG, Dowling JJ (Univ of Alberta, Edmonton, Canada; McMaster Univ, Hamilton, Ont, Canada)
Med Sci Sports Exerc 29:1366–1373, 1997   4–23

Introduction.—Ballistic actions are defined as those movements that are executed with the intent to move as quickly as possible. Enhanced ballistic performance might be expected in athletes who regularly perform these actions if the neuronal mechanisms responsible for and associated with ballistic actions could be amplified by practice or training. Some of the amplified neuronal mechanisms such as more pronounced agonist muscle activation, an altered pattern of antagonist-agonist coactivation, or a greater occurrence of agonist premovement depression might be revealed by electromyography. Ballistic performance and muscle activation were studied in highly trained karate athletes, whose training consisted of punching and kicking.

Methods.—Maximal voluntary isometric and ballistic elbow extension actions were performed by 9 male karate athletes and 13 untrained men. The elbow actions were performed unloaded (L0) and against a load equal to 10% of isometric maximal voluntary contractions (L10). During the isometric and ballistic actions, electromyographic recordings of agonist triceps and antagonist biceps were made. The occurrence and duration of premovement agonist depression were monitored, since ballistic actions (L10) were initiated from a preloaded condition.

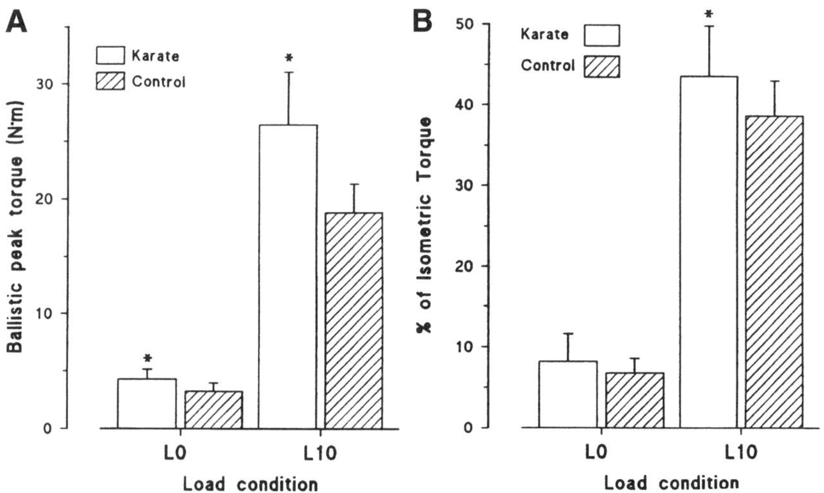

FIGURE 2.—**A panel:** peak torque of ballistic actions in the L0 (no added load) and L10 (added load = 10% maximal voluntary contractions) conditions in karate athletes and control group. **B panel,** ballistic action peak torque expressed as a percentage of the isometric peak torque value. *Asterisk* indicates *P* < 0.05 for between group difference. Values are mean and SD. (Courtesy of Zehr EP, Sale DG, Dowling JJ: Ballistic movement performance in karate athletes. *Med Sci Sports Exerc* 29(10):1366–1373, 1997.)

Results.—Greater isometric (32%) and ballistic action peak torque was achieved by the karate group with L0 (30%) and L10 (40%) (Fig 2). With $L_1 0$ the ratio of ballistic action to isometric action, the peak torque in the karate group was 13% greater, which was indicative of a load-specific training adaptation. The corresponding ratio did not differ significantly between the 2 groups with L0. In the karate group, the ballistic action peak rate of torque development (51%, 51%) and peak acceleration (15%, 9%) with L0 and L10, respectively, were greater. Between the 2 groups, the peak velocity and movement time did not differ significantly. In agonist activation, the ratio of ballistic to isometric action agonist activation, or antagonist coactivation, there were no group differences. In both groups, premovement agonist depression occurred infrequently, and there were no differences between the 2 groups.

Conclusions.—Enhanced elbow extension ballistic performance was seen in the karate athletes. However, this could not be correlated to amplified agonist activation, more frequent occurrence of agonist premovement depression, or altered antagonist activation.

▶ Ballistic movements are defined as those in which the intent is to move as quickly as possible, and are characterized by an agonist burst of activity, followed by an antagonist burst and a second agonist burst. Athletes such as karate athletes who regularly perform ballistic movements were found to be more skilled in some aspects of ballistic movements. Rate of torque development and peak acceleration were greater in the karate group, but differences in the timing of agonist activation and antagonist coactivation were not found. If the most important aspect of ballistic performance is peak velocity attained, the karate athletes were not superior to the control subjects in this measure. However, the loads moved in this elbow extension task were done with the same relative but different absolute loads, and the karate athletes had a 30% greater load. Karate athletes have some enhancement of ballistic movement performance, but the differences in peak velocity are not significant.

M.J.L. Alexander, Ph.D.

A Non-invasive Protocol for the Determination of Lumbosacral Vertebral Angle
Chen Y-L, Lee Y-H (Mingchi Inst of Technology, Taiwan, ROC; Natl Taiwan Inst of Technology, ROC)
Clin Biomech 12:185–189, 1997   4–24

Introduction.—To assess the stresses acting on the low back in lifting, measurements of lumbosacral vertebral angle are important. There may be a relationship between lumbar lordosis and pelvic tilt, but previous studies have found a poor correlation. While the radiographic method is the most accurate for measuring the lumbar spine and pelvic positions, noninvasive techniques are being sought because they may be less costly, have fewer technical difficulties, and have less of a risk of radiation exposure. A

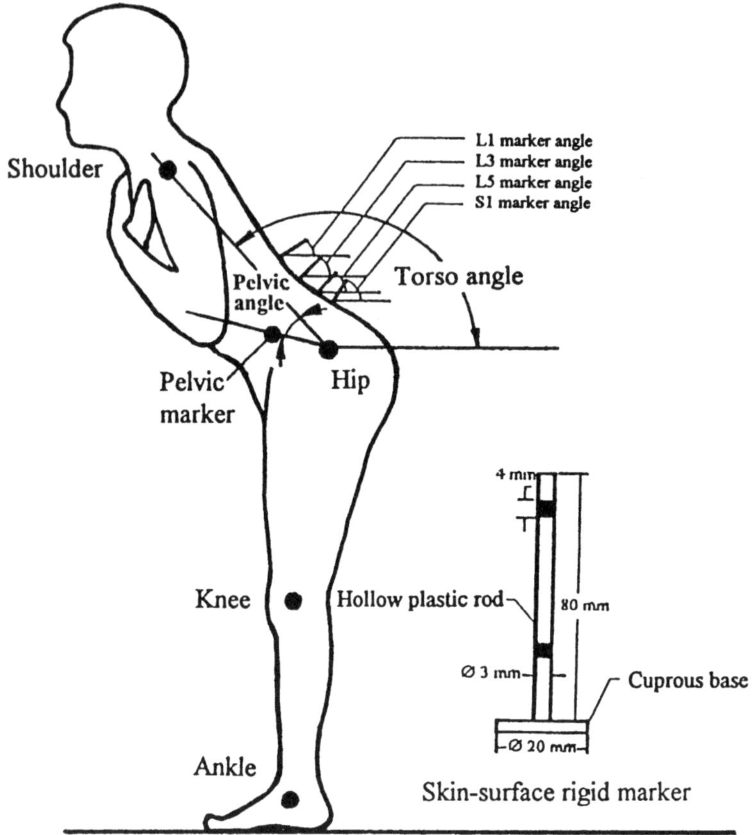

FIGURE 2.—All skin-surface rigid markers and joint markers in the study. (Courtesy of Chen Y-L, Lee Y-H: A non-invasive protocol for the determination of lumbosacral vertebral angle. *Clin Biomech* 12:186–189. Copyright 1997, with kind permission from Elsevier Science Ltd, The Boulvard, Langford Lane, Kidlington OX5 1GB UK.)

noninvasive method to predict the lumbosacral vertebral angles was developed.

Methods.—Measurements of the X-ray and videographic techniques were used, and the 2 measurements were related to each other. In the radiographic and videographic measurements, 16 healthy males participated. For model development, data from 12 of the 16 men were used. For model validation, data from the other 4 men were used. In the videographic technique, surface vertebral rigid markers were attached over the skin at L1, L3, L5, and S1 spinous process (Fig 2). Externally measured marker angle, pelvic angle, and lumbosacral angle were the predicting variables.

Results.—Between the directly measured vertebral angle from the radiographs and the externally measured angles of the surface markers at the L5 and S1 levels, the results showed significant differences. An $R2$ value of

0.97 for the vertebral level of L1 was developed with linear regression models for calculating vertebral angles. An R2 value of 0.98 was found for L2. An R2 value of 0.91 was found for L5. An R^2 value of 0.92 was found for S1. Between the calculated and the radiographic data, there was no significant difference, according to the validation result.

Conclusions.—For the recording of the internal vertebral angle in the sagittal plane, the protocol of using the skin-surface rigid markers and the predicting models is justified to provide a simple and valid noninvasive method. Future investigations should consider the effect of the other body postures, such as the lumbar posture and the knee bend.

▶ The lumbosacral vertebral angle is an important biomechanical landmark for the lumbar spine, because an increased angle will produce higher shear forces between the lumbar vertebrae, and may lead to shear-related injuries such as degenerative changes in the facet joints or spondylolysis. Attachment of skin surface markers over the skin of the lumbar spinous processes and filming the locations provided measurements to estimate the angle, and the measurement was validated by radiographic measurements of the angle. Although there was poor agreement between the 2 methods of measurement, the videographic data could be transformed into linear models that could produce the lumbosacral angle. This method may have some improvements over earlier attempts to estimate this angle noninvasively, but the accuracy is still questionable. As different positions of the spine are assumed, movements of the markers placed over the lumbar spinous processes will produce different landmarks and decrease accuracy.

M.J.L. Alexander, Ph.D.

Neuromuscular Trunk Performance and Spinal Loading During a Fatiguing Isometric Trunk Extension With Varying Torque Requirements

Sparto PJ, Parnianpour M, Marras WS, et al (Ohio State Univ, Columbus)

J Spinal Disord 10:145–156, 1997   4–25

Introduction.—A better indicator of future low back pain may be trunk muscle endurance rather than strength. Various testing protocols have been used by researchers to investigate trunk-muscle endurance, but the predictive value of trunk-muscle endurance tests is still unknown. Little is known about the effect of fatigue on the quality of neuromuscular performance of the trunk. As participants became fatigued while performing an isometric endurance test of varying torque requirements, a novel testing protocol was used to investigate changes in neuromuscular performance, spinal loading, and muscle recruitment.

Methods.—To measure the capability of the trunk musculature to respond to unexpected change in torque demand while the muscles were becoming fatigued, an isometric trunk-extension test was designed. To understand how the neuromuscular system maintains a given torque level during fatigue, the trunk-muscle recruitment patterns and frequency con-

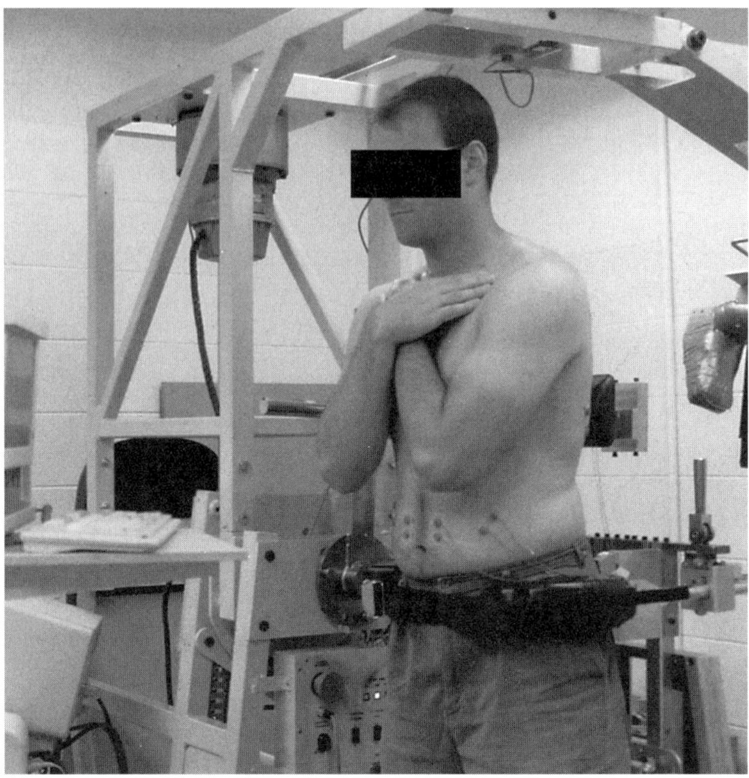

FIGURE 1.—Isometric endurance test experimental setup. (Courtesy of Sparto PJ, Parnianpour M, Marras WS, et al: Neuromuscular trunk performance and spinal loading during a fatiguing isometric trunk extension with varying torque requirements. *J Spinal Disord* 10:145–156, 1997.)

tent of the electromyogram were measured. To examine the effects of the muscle recruitment on the spinal loading and to discern the effect of fatigue on spinal loading, an electromyogram-assisted model of the spine was used. Ten men with a mean age of 25.8 years were instrumented with 10 pairs of bipolar surface electrodes and performed a series of maximal voluntary isometric contractions in the dynamometer (Fig 1).

Results.—There was no change in response time as the participants became fatigued, but there was decreased accuracy in maintaining a reference torque. Significant increases in internal oblique and latissimus dorsi muscle activity were seen in the study of trunk-muscle recruitment. There were changes in spinal loading as a result in this change in recruitment, despite a relatively constant torque output.

Conclusion.—The assumption of a constant maximal stress capacity of the muscle may not be robust when participants are expected to become fatigued during test performance. A potential injury mechanism may be indicated by the observation of a reduction in muscle activity when the torque demand is quite high. This should be studied further.

▶ It is now fairly well documented that trunk muscle endurance performance is a better indicator of future low back pain than is strength. For many manual workers, the ability to maintain a certain trunk position for an extended period is critical for effective job performance. There are questions regarding how trunk muscle recruitment and torque output may change as subjects become fatigued; these were examined in this study.

As trunk muscle fatigue occurred, there were significant increases in activity from other trunk muscles, including the internal oblique and latissimus dorsi. This altered muscle activity produced changes in spinal loading, despite a constant torque output. The study produced no evidence that the response of the trunk extensor muscles to a change in torque requirements would be reduced when fatigued. The observation of a reduction of muscle activity when torque demand is quite high suggests a possible mechanism for some lower back injuries.

M.J.L. Alexander, Ph.D.

Reproducibility of the Kinematics and Kinetics of the Lower Extremity During Normal Stair-Climbing
Yu B, Kienbacher T, Growney ES, et al (Mayo Clinic and Found, Rochester, Minn)
J Orthop Res 15:348–352, 1997   4–26

Introduction.—For patients with disorders of the lower extremity, a clinical evaluation of stair-climbing may be more informative than one of level walking. To assess patients with knee arthritis, stair-climbing has been used as an evaluation procedure. Only one previous study evaluated intrasubject variance and intersubject similarity of kinematic and kinetic stair-climbing data. During normal stair-climbing, the intrasubject reproducibility of the kinematic and kinetic measures of the lower extremity was examined.

Methods.—There were 10 healthy adults who ascended stairs, descended stairs, and walked on level ground. For 3 trials for each participant during each of the 3 conditions, 3-dimensional video and force-plate data were collected. Calculations were made of 3-dimensional angles and moments of the ankle, knee, and hip joints. To determine the intrasubject reproducibility of joint angles and resultant moments, the coefficient of multiple correlation was used. To compare the magnitudes of the coefficients between different steps, different joints, and different joint functions, analysis of variance with repeated measures was conducted.

Results.—When normal participants were climbing stairs, the kinematic and kinetic measures were reproducible. When normal participants were in transition steps from level walking to ascending, and from descending to level walking, the kinetic measures were significantly less reproducible than those during the other steps. The sagittal plane data were more reproducible than data from other planes. Particularly for abduction-adduction and internal-external rotation, the kinetic measures were more

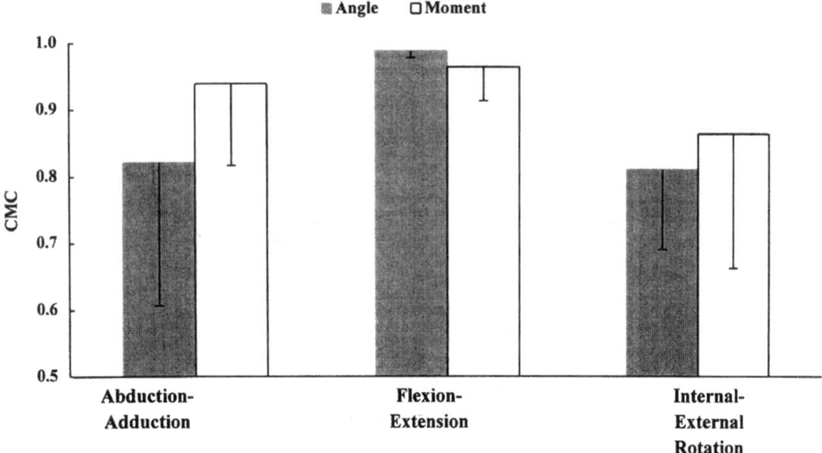

FIGURE 3.—The mean coefficients of multiple correlation (*CMC*) for the joint angles and moments of the lower extremity for different joint functions in steps A₂ (ascending) and D₂ (descending). (Courtesy of Yu B, Kienbacher T, Growney ES, et al: Reproducibility of the kinematics and kinetics of the lower extremity during normal stair-climbing. *J Orthop Res* 15:348–352, 1997.)

reproducible than the kinematic measures. For the flexion-extension angles, the coefficients of multiple correlation were significantly greater than those for abduction-adduction (including inversion-eversion) and internal-external rotation angles (Fig 3).

Conclusions.—The peak-to peak range in values of these measures may account for the difference in the reproducibility of the kinematic and kinetic measures between different joint functions. The major cause of the decreased reproducibility of the internal-external angles and moments was the small peak-to-peak range in values.

▶ Stair-climbing is an important functional activity that requires accurate evaluation for patients with disorders of the lower extremity, such as knee arthritis, injury to the anterior cruciate ligament, and total hip replacements. Three-dimensional angles and moments of the ankle, knee, and hip joints were calculated for 3 trials, and the test-retest reliability of the results were examined. It was concluded that the reliability of the joint angles and moments were reproducible, and that the data from the sagittal plane were the most reliable. The variation that did occur in the test-retest scores was likely caused by variations in motor performance. The ability to accurately evaluate skill in stair-climbing will be useful in evaluation of rehabilitation and exercise programs for patients with lower limb pathology. Specific pathologies such as knee arthritis or hip degeneration may produce specific compensatory movements that can be described using film and biomechanical techniques.

M.J.L. Alexander, Ph.D.

Neuromuscular Fatigue After Maximal Stretch-Shortening Cycle Exercise

Strojnik V, Komi PV (Univ of Jyvskyl, Finland)
J Appl Physiol 84:344–350, 1998   4–27

Background.—Fatigue is a complex process. During maximal stretch-shortening cycle (SSC) exercise, fatigue is characterized by reduced movement efficiency, a sharp drop in maximal isometric force, and high peak lactase values. Previous studies of fatigue during SSC exercise have focused on submaximal workout intensity levels; however, the mechanism of fatigue in maximal SCC exercise may be different. The authors investigated some possible fatigue events during short-duration, maximally intensive SSC exercise.

Methods.—The study included 12 healthy young men who performed drop jumps on an inclined sledge apparatus. The subjects jumped until they could no longer achieve a jumping height greater than 90% of their maximum. The possible mechanisms of this fatigue were investigated by measuring the contractile characteristics of the muscle, activation analysis, and blood parameters.

Results.—The subjects' blood lactate concentrations and serum creatine kinase activation were increased after exercise. Although significant, these changes were physiologically modest. Analysis of the single twitch showed a reduction in peak torque, time to peak, and half-relaxation time. There was no change in double-twitch torque, although the maximal slope of torque rose more steeply. Torque declined during 20 and 100 Hz stimulation. Maximal voluntary torque did not change significantly, although the maximal slope of torque rise was decreased and the activation level and the electromyogram amplitude were increased.

Conclusion.—These findings suggest 2 distinct mechanisms of fatigue in response to maximal SSC. There is a contractile mechanism, which appears to be potentiated by a reduced CA^{2+} transient and faster cross-bridge cycling. However, the dominant reason appears to be impairment of high-frequency action potential propagation. This factor, combined with faster contraction, may depress the rate of force development as a result of reduced fusion of tension of twitches.

▶ There are many theories regarding the sources of neuromuscular fatigue after intense exercise, including CNS fatigue and fatigue in the peripheral processes, such as action potential propagation and impairment in excitation-contraction coupling. Twelve healthy male subjects were fatigued while performing jumping exercise to exhaustion using the SSC. Fatigue seems to be primarily caused by an impairment in the contractile mechanism, possibly as the result of a reduced calcium release from the sarcoplasmic reticulum and reduced capability of the cross bridges to form strong binding.

Decline in force output is one of the most important signs of fatigue, which is somewhat counteracted by recruitment of new motor units. This was substantiated by an increased EMG amplitude. It is unclear whether these effects of fatigue can be decreased by performing these same high-intensity jump exercises on a regular basis.

M.J.L. Alexander, Ph.D.

Older Adults Can Maximally Activate the Biceps Brachii Muscle by Voluntary Command
De Serres SJ, Enoka RM (Cleveland Clinic Found, Ohio; Univ of Colorado, Boulder)
J Appl Physiol 84:284–291, 1998   4–28

Introduction.—Maximum voluntary contraction (MVC) decreases with aging to an extent greater than that predicted by muscle mass lost. It has been suggested that age-related strength loss may be explained, in part, by impairment of muscle activation. Biceps brachii activation was assessed during MVC in older adults.

Methods.—The study used 2 superimposition techniques: quantification of the activation level achieved during MVC and comparison of measured vs. expected MVC forces, based on extrapolation from submaximal forces. The study included 16 healthy older adults (mean age, 74 years), and a comparison group of 16 younger adults (mean age, 28 years). The subjects performed trials of MVCs in response to an investigator's verbal command. The experimental setup included a force transducer to measure isometric flexion or extension force (Fig 1).

Results.—Both the older and younger groups had incomplete activation of the biceps brachii, with the older group having the greater deficit. The mean activation levels were 95.0% and 97.8%, respectively. However, the measured and expected MVC forces were equivalent in both groups, whether the expected value was extrapolated using a third-order polynomial or linearization of the data.

Conclusion.—In contrast to some previous studies, the results suggest that the ability to achieve maximal activation of the biceps brachii muscle is not impaired with age. Compared with an expected value derived from multiple measurements in the evoked force–voluntary force domain, the MVC force exerted by the elbow flexor muscles is as predicted in younger as well as older adults. Thus, age-related reductions in strength do not appear to arise from impairment of the neural drive to muscle.

▶ It is generally agreed that there is a decline in maximum muscle force with age and, possibly, a decline with age in the ability to maximally activate the muscles to produce peak force output. This study compared the ability of younger and older adults to voluntarily activate the elbow flexor muscles. The subjects were asked to produce an MVC on command, and the force output was measured by a force transducer. Using 2 different techniques of estimating maximum force output, both older and younger subjects were able to elicit maximum forces voluntarily, without the aid of muscle stimulation techniques.

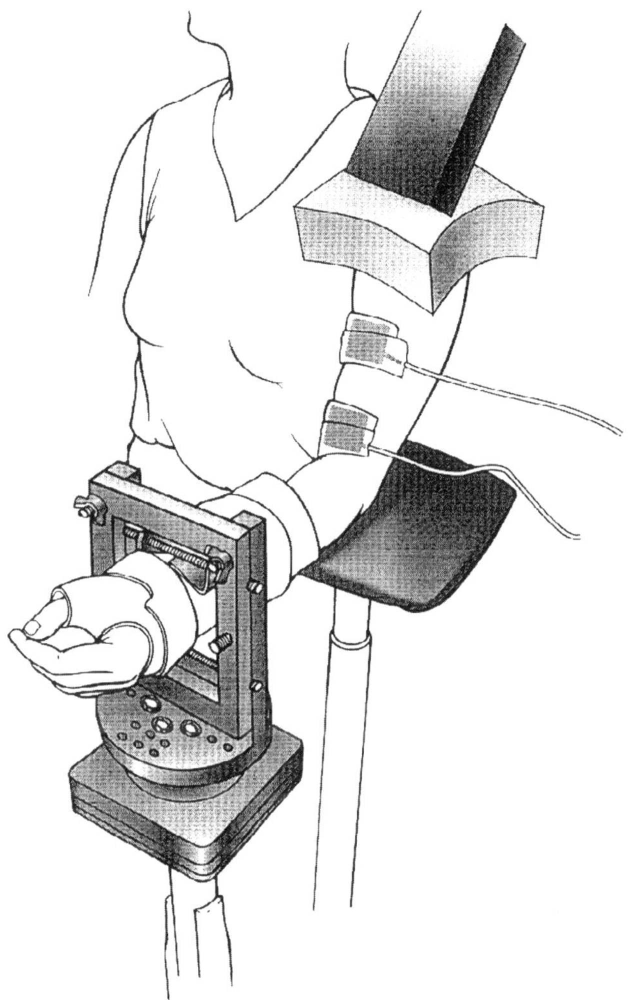

FIGURE 1.—Schematic representation of experimental apparatus with subject's left forearm enclosed in an orthosis. Force transducer is the circular structure located beneath the wrist. (Courtesy of De Serres SJ, Enoka RM: Older adults can maximally activate the biceps brachii muscle by voluntary command. *J Appl Physiol* 84:284–291, 1998.)

The authors conclude that the decline in strength with age does not result from an impairment of the neural drive to the muscle. This finding suggests that the muscular system ages at a more rapid rate than the nervous system, although regular training and conditioning can help to decrease the rate of strength loss in older persons.

M.J.L. Alexander, Ph.D.

An Evaluation of the Length-Tension Relationship in Elderly Human Plantarflexor Muscles

Winegard KJ, Hicks AL, Vandervoort AA (McMaster Univ, Hamilton, Ont, Canada; Univ of Western Ontario, London, Canada)
J Gerontol 52A:B337-B343, 1997   4–29

Introduction.—The length at which a muscle is held determines the amount of isometric tension that can be produced during a muscle contraction. A previous study examined the length-tension relationship of the ankle dorsiflexor muscle group in participants aged 20–80 years and found no differences in the torque-angle relationships between the various age

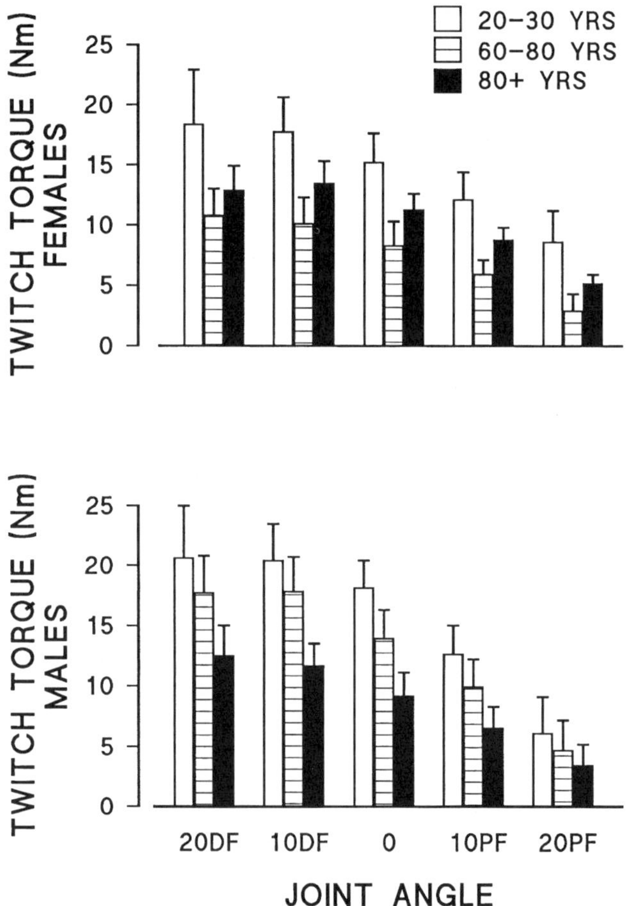

FIGURE 3.—Twitch torque values for 15 females (**A**) and 15 males (**B**) in 3 age groups: 20–30 years (*open bars*), 60–80 years (*hatched bars*), and 80+ years (*filled bars*), at 5 ankle joint angles. Values are means ± SD. (Courtesy of Winegard KJ, Hicks AL, Vandervoort AA: An evaluation of the length-tension relationship in elderly human plantarflexor muscles. *J Gerontol* 52A:B337–B343. Copyright 1997, The Gerontological Society of America.)

groups. No similar studies have been conducted on the antagonist ankle muscles, the plantarflexor group. The effect of aging on the muscle length-tension relationship in the plantar flexor muscles was determined.

Methods.—There were 10 participants aged 20–30 years, 20 who were aged 60–80 years, and 10 who were older than 80 years. At 5 different joint angles, isometric twitch properties, maximum voluntary strength, passive tension, and range of motion were measured. The 5 joint angles were 20-degrees dorsiflexion, 10-degrees dorsiflexion, 0-degrees dorsiflexion, 10-degrees plantarflexion, and 20-degrees plantarflexion.

Results.—For all 3 age groups, active (evoked and voluntary) and passive torque production were maximal when the ankle was rotated into the dorsiflexion positions. When the ankles were rotated into the 20-degree plantarflexion position, the lowest values were recorded. At all joint angles, males were stronger than females (Fig 3). Both elderly adult groups were weaker than the young adults

Conclusions.—The optimal angle for torque production remains the same for younger and older adults, despite the considerable age-associated loss in both voluntary and evoked strength in the plantarflexors. In the muscles crossing the ankle joint, the expected changes in stiffness and flexibility are not so evident. To determine whether any changes in the length-tension relationship with age exist, future studies should examine a less-used muscle group, such as elbow flexors or extensors.

▶ It has been hypothesized that aging has an effect on the length-tension relationship of skeletal muscles, because aging produces a loss in skeletal muscle elasticity and possibly the length at which peak tension is developed. A less elastic muscle may tend to reach the angle of peak torque sooner in the range of motion than a more elastic muscle, which may also be related to loss of joint flexibility in older individuals. Higher rates of torque development were recorded for the younger groups as compared with the 2 older groups, and the peak torque values were higher for the younger groups. A notable finding was that although there were losses in muscle function with age, the optimal angle for torque production remained the same for younger and older adults. This may be related to the function of the plantarflexors, which are one of the main antigravity muscle groups and are used on a regular basis for balance and ambulation. The plantarflexors produce the highest muscle power output of any muscle group during gait and 1–foot balance skills. This muscle group will likely undergo fewer age-related functional changes because of its use and importance in activities of daily living.

M.J.L. Alexander, Ph.D.

Dynamic Trunk Strength of Canadian Football Players, Soccer Players, and Middle to Long Distance Runners

Williams CA, Singh M (Univ of Brighton, Eastbourne, East Sussex, UK; Univ of Alberta, Edmonton, Canada)
J Orthop Sports Phys Ther 25:271–276, 1997   4–30

Background.—Different sports make different demands on the body, and thus muscle strength can be expected to differ for athletes involved in different sports. These investigators tested trunk strength in 3 different groups of athletes to determine how the groups differed.

Methods.—Male varsity athletes participating in soccer (n = 16), Canadian football (n = 15), and middle and long-distance running (n = 16) were studied. A control group consisted of 15 subjects who were recreationally active but were not participating in a systematic training program. None of the subjects had experienced a low-back injury within the previous 12 months, and all refrained from vigorous physical activity for 24 hours before testing. A trunk-testing dynamometer was used to assess peak torque, measured as the greatest torque that developed on 1 of 6 alternating contractions. Six alternating and continuous concentric and eccentric contractions were measured through a range of 60 degrees at a preset angular velocity of 30 degrees/sec. Subjects were encouraged to exert their maximal effort.

Findings.—Peak torques of the eccentric flexors and extensors were significantly greater than those of the concentric flexors and extensors. Both eccentric and concentric flexor torque was significantly greater for soccer and football players compared with runners and the control group. Peak extensor torque for both contraction types was significantly greater for football players compared with runners. Soccer players had significantly greater peak eccentric flexor torque compared with runners or the control group. The angle of peak torque did not differ between any of the 4 groups.

Conclusions.—Training for football players emphasizes upper body muscle groups, and they showed the greatest flexor and extensor torque. Soccer players must twist and turn their torsos; thus, they also exhibit enhanced flexor and extensor torque. Runners may depend less on trunk muscle strength and more on muscle endurance, and thus their torque measurements were sometimes even less than those of recreational athletes. These data confirm that muscle strength differs for participants in different sports.

▶ The trunk strength of elite athletes in most sports is important to optimize performance. Since the limb-muscle pull is stabilized by the muscles and structures of the trunk, trunk strength needs to be emphasized in the training of athletes. Because sports have unique demands on trunk muscle strength, differences between different athletic groups is to be expected. This study reported that football and soccer players had significantly stronger trunk musculature than did runners and recreational athletes. This may

Subscribe to the related journal in your field!

Yes! Begin my one-year subscription to *Journal of Shoulder and Elbow Surgery* (6 issues).

Name ____

Institution ________________________________

Address ____________________________________

City __________________________ State ________

ZIP/PC __________ Country ________________

Specialty __________________________________
(Students/residents, please list Institution)

Subscription prices (through 9/30/98)

		USA	Canada*	Int'l
Individuals	❏	$111.00	$147.66	$138.00
Institutions	❏	134.00	172.27	161.00
Students, residents	❏	55.00	87.74	82.00

Method of payment

Enclose payment (check or credit card number) and we'll send an extra issue FREE!

❏ **Check** (in U.S. dollars, drawn on a U.S. bank, and payable to *Journal of Shoulder and Elbow Surgery*)

❏ VISA ❏ MasterCard ❏ Discover
❏ AmEx ❏ Bill me   Exp. date__________

Card #_______________________________________

Signature ____________________________________

*Includes Canadian GST

Individual/student subscriptions must be in the name of, billed to, and paid for by the individual.

Canada/Int'l prices include airmail postage.
Prices subject to change without notice.

J032983YC

Reservation Card for the Year Book

Yes! I would like my own copy of *Year Book of Sports Medicine*® at the price of **$74.95** plus sales tax, postage, and handling. Please begin my subscription with the current edition according to the terms described below.* I understand that I will have 30 days to examine each annual edition.

Name ____

Address _____________________________________

City ______________________________ State __________ ZIP____________

Method of Payment

Check (in U.S. dollars, drawn on a U.S. bank, payable to *Year Book of Sports Medicine*®)

❏ VISA   ❏ MasterCard   ❏ Discover   ❏ AmEx   ❏ Bill me

Card number _________________________________ Exp. date: __________

Signature ____________________________________

Prices are subject to change without notice.

PMC-033

---

*Your Year Book service guarantee:

When you subscribe to the *Year Book*, you will receive advance notice of future annual volumes about two months before publication. To receive the new edition, you need do nothing—we'll send you the new volume as soon as it is available. If you want to discontinue, the advance notice allows you time to notify us of your decision. If you are not completely satisfied, you have 30 days to return any *Year Book*.

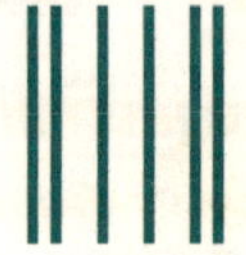

BUSINESS REPLY MAIL

FIRST-CLASS MAIL   PERMIT NO 135   ST LOUIS MO

POSTAGE WILL BE PAID BY ADDRESSEE

SUBSCRIPTION SERVICES
MOSBY–YEAR BOOK, INC.
11830 WESTLINE INDUSTRIAL DRIVE
ST. LOUIS   MO 63146-9988

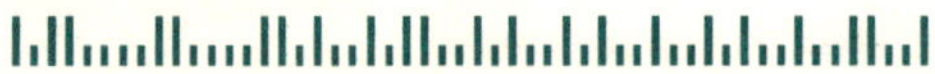

BUSINESS REPLY MAIL

FIRST-CLASS MAIL   PERMIT NO 135   ST LOUIS MO

POSTAGE WILL BE PAID BY ADDRESSEE

Ｍ Mosby

PAT NEWMAN
11830 WESTLINE INDUSTRIAL DRIVE
PO BOX 46908
ST. LOUIS   MO 63146-9934

Want to speed up the process?

To order the *Year Book*,
you also may call 1-800-426-4545

To subscribe to the journal today,
call toll-free in the U.S.:
1-800-453-4351
or fax 314-432-1158
Outside the U.S., call: 314-453-4351

Visit us at:
www.mosby.com/Mosby/Periodicals

Mosby–Year Book, Inc.
Subscription Services
11830 Westline Industrial Drive
St. Louis, MO   63146 U.S.A.

Ｍ Mosby

be because of greater need for endurance in runners, rather than absolute strength. Flexor muscle strength was found to be proportionally higher in the football and soccer players, whereas extensor strength was only slightly higher than in the other groups. There were no significant differences between groups for the angle of peak torque. possibly because of the slow testing speed of 30 degrees/sec. This study provides useful reference data for trunk strength in several athletic groups.

M.J.L. Alexander, Ph.D.

Muscle-specific Creatine Kinase Gene Polymorphism and VO$_{2max}$ in the HERITAGE Family Study
Rivera MA, Dionne FT, Simoneau J-A, et al (Laval Univ, Québec; Univ of Puerto Rico, San Juan; Univ of Minnesota, Minneapolis; et al)
Med Sci Sports Exerc 29:1311–1317, 1997   4–31

Background.—The maximal oxygen intake response to endurance training differs significantly between individuals, probably because of genetic differences. To determine the reasons for this variability, the authors investigate a panel of genes involved in the process of adenosine triphosphate regeneration and in other metabolic pathways related to aerobic performance. A DNA polymorphism in the muscle-specific creatine kinase (*CKMM*) gene is studied for its effects on maximal oxygen intake before and after endurance training.

Methods.—The study included 160 unrelated white subjects and 80 unrelated sedentary adult offspring selected randomly from the HERITAGE Family Study. A polymerase chain reaction assay with digestion by the *NcoI* restriction enzyme was used to detect *CKMM* polymorphism. Maximal cycle ergometer tests were performed to determine the subjects' maximal oxygen intake in both the sedentary state and in response to a standardized, 20-week endurance training program. The effects of genotype on maximal oxygen intake at these 2 points were analyzed.

Results.—The subjects had a mean maximal oxygen intake of 2,119 mL/min. The mean increase of maximal oxygen intake in response to endurance training was 283 mL/min for women and 363 mL/min for men. Men and women were comparable in their allele and genotype frequencies. Parents were shown to have a significant association between maximal oxygen intake, adjusted for age and sex, and *CKMM* genotype; however, offspring had no such association. Both parents and offspring had genotypic differences in the maximal oxygen intake response to training, after adjustment for age, sex, baseline maximal oxygen intake, and body mass. The response to endurance training was significantly reduced in parents and offspring who were homozygous for the rare allele. Nine percent of the variance in response to training was explained by genotype.

Conclusion.—A DNA polymorphism in the *CKKM* gene has a significant impact on the response of maximal oxygen intake to endurance training. For subjects homozygous for the rare allele, the response to training is 1.5 to 3 times lower than for subjects with other genotypes. The study provides the first strong evidence that a genetic polymorphism could affect the individual response to endurance training.

▶ Sports scientists have argued for many years about whether athletes are individuals who have chosen their parents wisely or whether their superb performance has been achieved mainly through rigorous training. The issue is important to team managers because it influences tactics for obtaining gold medals. If parentage is the key factor, the stress should be on talent scouting, but if training is the answer, much more effort needs to be spent on perfecting training schedules. Common sense suggests a substantial genetic component to performance. For example, training is unlikely to increase aerobic power by more than 20% to 30%, yet the top endurance competitors have an aerobic power that is 100% larger than that of the average fit young adult; the remaining 70% advantage in fitness is the result of finding someone who has a baseline aerobic power 3–4 standard deviations above the population average.

Laboratory investigations have attempted to apportion variance between environmental factors (including training) and inheritance by looking at differences of interindividual variance between monozygotic and dizygotic twins, occasionally supplemented by findings on other close relatives. Unfortunately, the number of available twins has usually been rather small, and estimates of heritability have been correspondingly unstable.

The human genome project is now offering the prospect of uncovering the precise genes responsible for the inherited portion of various functional characteristics. The original estimate that all of the mysteries of the human genome would be clarified within 10 years is proving grossly overoptimistic, but it is encouraging to see the identification of genes that describe a significant fraction of the variance in aerobic power.

R.J. Shephard, M.D., Ph.D., D.P.E.

The Reproducibility of the Bruce Protocol Exercise Test for the Determination of Aerobic Capacity in Older Women
Fielding RA, Frontera WR, Hughes VA, et al (Tufts Univ, Boston; Boston Univ; Pennsylvania State Univ, Univ Park; et al)
Med Sci Sports Exerc 29:1109–1113, 1997   4–32

Introduction.—The Bruce protocol appears to be reproducible in young men, but middle-aged and older women with reduced exercise tolerance may not achieve their true maximal oxygen intake or exercise time to exhaustion at a single test. Because reliable determinations of maximal oxygen intake are important for clinical and research purposes, the reproducibility of the Bruce protocol was examined in middle-aged and older women.

Methods.—Study participants were 17 healthy women age 51–68 years. None engaged in any program of regular physical activity. Over an average

TABLE 3.—Pearson's Product Correlation Coefficients Between Variables

		T1 vs T2	T2 vs T3	T2 vs T4	T2 vs T5
$\dot{V}O_{2max}$ (mL·kg^{-1}·min^{-1})	r	0.75	0.88	0.89	0.76
	P	0.0005	<0.0001	<0.0001	0.0006
$\dot{V}_{Emax}$ (L·min^{-1}·STPD)	r	0.70	0.82	0.70	0.72
	P	0.0017	<0.0001	0.0026	0.0017
Heart rate max (beats·min^{-1})	r	0.85	0.81	0.85	0.77
	P	<0.0001	<0.0001	<0.0001	0.0004
Exercise time (s)	r	0.81	0.88	0.85	0.82
	P	<0.0001	<0.0001	<0.0001	<0.0001

(Courtesy of Fielding RA, Frontera WR, Hughes VA, et al: The reproducibility of the Bruce protocol exercise test for the determination of aerobic capacity in older women. *Med Sci Sports Exerc* 29:1109–1113, 1997.)

period of 7 weeks, each woman performed 5 exercise tests separated by at least 1 week. The tests consisted of a modification of the Bruce protocol on a motor driven treadmill. The women were instructed to exercise to their own volitional fatigue. Oxygen intake, heart rate, blood pressure, and ratings of perceived exertion (RPE) were recorded during the tests.

Results.—Average values of maximum oxygen intake during the 5 trials were not significantly different (27.5, 28.3, 28.4, 29.6, and 28.2 mL/kg^{-1}/min^{-1}). Twenty-one (25%) tests met criteria for a plateau in oxygen intake. Overall, the mean coefficient of variation in maximum oxygen intake in the 5 tests was 6.5%. There was agreement among repeated tests, as indicated by significant Pearson's correlation coefficients for the study variables (Table 3). Within subject variance was lower than between subject variance. Variables that did not differ significantly between trials included mean maximal ventilation, the maximal respiratory exchange ratio, peak systolic and diastolic blood pressure, RPE, and exercise time to exhaustion.

Discussion.—The Bruce protocol yielded highly reproducible measures of maximal oxygen intake, maximal heart rate, blood pressure, RPE, and ventilation in these sedentary older women. The best agreement for maximal oxygen intake was between trials 2 and 3, with a mean difference of 0.1 mL/kg^{-1}/min^{-1}. Results suggest that a single test is adequate to assess aerobic power in middle-aged and older women.

▶ How low is low? The present authors found a test–retest variance of 4.2 (mL/[kg/min])^2 in women age 51–68 years during performance of the Bruce treadmill test. This sounds quite attractive until we read that the average aerobic power was only 28 mL/[kg/min]. Thus, the coefficient of variation for repeat testing of the same subject was 7.3%, rather more than the 4% to 5% that many authors have reported for repeated measurements of younger individuals.[1] Perhaps the most useful feature of this article is the demonstration that there is little systematic increment of aerobic power when a series of treadmill measurements are performed by elderly individuals.

R.J. Shephard, M.D., Ph.D., D.P.E.

Reference

1. Wright GR, Sidney KH, Shephard RJ: Variance of direct and indirect measurements of aerobic power. *J Sports Med Phys Fitness* 18:33–42, 1978.

Dynamic Loading Affects the Mechanical Properties and Failure Site of Porcine Spines

Yingling VR, Callaghan JP, McGill SM (Univ of Waterloo, Ont)
Clin Biomech 12:301–305, 1997
4–33

Background.—To optimize rehabilitation and injury prevention programs, it is necessary to understand the mechanical properties of biological tissues. In this study, the effect of a range of physiologic loading rates on the stored energy, stiffness, ultimate load at failure, and the deformation at failure were examined in porcine spinal motion segments.

Methods.—The cervical spines of 26 healthy domestic pigs were excised at death with all soft tissue. Within 20 hours, all testing was accomplished. Each cervical spine was separated into 2 specimens, each consisting of 3 vertebral bodies and 2 intervening intervertebral discs (C2–C4) and (C5–C7). The outside vertebrae were fixed so that the middle was loaded in an unconstrained, physiologic manner. All loading was performed in an artificial abdomen chamber to simulate in vivo pressures of the abdominal cavity. The spines were loaded to failure at 5 loading rates: 100, 1,000, 3,000, 10,000, and 16,000 N/s with a servohydraulic dynamic testing machine. Failed specimens were dissected to determine the type of failure. Load deformation curves were sampled at 50 Hz.

Results.—Dynamic loading increased the ultimate load compared to quasistatic loading (100 N/s). The actual magnitude of the dynamic loading (1,000–16,000 N/s) did not appear to have a significant effect on ultimate load. These results were the same for stiffness, as well. The displacement to failure decreased as load rate increased, although this effect was less important at high load rates. Failure at low load rates occurred in the end plates, but at higher load rates, failure was more common in the vertebral body.

Conclusions.—The effect of load rate on the mechanical characteristics of spinal motion segments was investigated in a porcine model. Both the mechanical characteristics and the injuries of porcine spines were affected as the loading rate changed from quasistatic to dynamic. The shifting of the site of injury and the decreased deformation at failure as loading rate increased suggests a change in the mechanisms of injury as dynamic loading occurs, but the mechanism remains unknown.

▶ It is well known that loading rate affects the mechanical properties of tissues subjected to various rates of loading, which is related to the types of injuries that occur in high-speed sports activities and car crashes. This study examined the types of failure that occur in porcine cervical spinal units under various loading rates. As seen in other biological tissues, ultimate load to failure, displacement to failure, and stiffness increased with increased loading rates. As well, increasing loading rate produced different types of injuries, as the injury site changed from the end-plate to the vertebral body as loading rate increased. Many previous studies have been limited to examination of cervical vertebrae only, without the intervening disk, which alters the mechanical properties and injury types. This study confirms that failure load, stiffness, and displacement to failure will increase with high rates of dynamic loading, and it adds to our limited knowledge of the failure modes of the cervical spine.

M.J.L. Alexander, Ph.D.

The Effect of Lifelong Exercise on Canine Articular Cartilage
Newton PM, Mow VC, Gardner TR, et al (Columbia Univ, New York; Univ of Iowa, Iowa City)
Am J Sports Med 25:282–287, 1997 4–34

Background.—Osteoarthritis, or degenerative joint disease, is a common cause of pain and disability in older people, but its cause in normal, uninjured joints is not known. One hypothesis is that regular joint use over many years causes repetitive articular cartilage damage, which eventually leads to tissue degeneration. A canine model was used to examine whether lifetime exercise with increased mechanical demands on the synovial joint results in joint degeneration or changes.

Methods.—Male beagle puppies were randomly assigned, with 11 animals in the experimental and 10 in the control group. The only difference between these 2 groups was that the experimental group exercised 5 days a week for 75 minutes a day on a motor-driven treadmill with an average speed of 3.3 km/hr while carrying a load of about 130% of body weight. The control group was limited to normal activity in a dog run. All animals were sacrificed at 550 weeks. All left hindlimbs were used for mechanical testing and all right hindlimbs were used for light microscopic studies.

Results.—None of the joints examined in this study had ligament or meniscal injuries, cartilage erosions, or osteophytes. There were no differences in safranin O staining or cartilage fibrillation between these 2 groups. The thickness of tibial articular cartilage and the mechanical joint properties were not significantly different between the 2 groups.

Conclusions.—A lifetime of weight-bearing exercise did not cause cartilage fibrillation and erosion, osteophytes, changes in cartilage thickness or changes in articular surface mechanical properties in canine joints. This suggests that load-bearing exercise does not necessarily lead to joint degeneration. Further work is necessary to examine the effects of more intense loading on the joint articular cartilage.

▶ It has been suggested that repetitive, high-intensity exercise causes articular cartilage changes that increase the probability of joint degeneration, such as that commonly seen in older football and basketball players. This study examined the effect of lifelong, high-intensity weight-bearing exercise on the articular cartilage of the canine knee joint. One group of dogs exercised 5 days a week for 10 years with weights on their backs, whereas the others remained in their cages for the same period. This study provides the first evidence from a randomized controlled study that regular lifelong increased joint use does not produce joint degeneration in the articular cartilage of dogs. In fact, the cartilage of the exercised dogs was slightly stronger and thicker. The authors suggested that this increased strength of cartilage was caused by the greater fluid pressurization that occurs with higher joint loading. Further studies should be conducted to examine the effects of higher levels of joint loading on articular cartilage characteristics, because the loads carried by the dogs during running were not comparable to those that may be experienced by athletes such as football players during play.

M.J.L. Alexander, Ph.D.

Flexion Relaxation of the Hamstring Muscles During Lumbar-Pelvic Rhythm

Sihvonen T (Univ Hosp of Kuopio, Finland)
Arch Phys Med Rehabil 78:486–490, 1997   4–35

Background.—During trunk flexion with straight knees, the activity of the erector spinae muscle suddenly decreases as the flexion of the trunk and the pelvic rotation increase (lumbar-pelvic rhythm) and the back muscles relax in the bent posture. This sudden activity decrease in the erector muscles of the spine, or flexion relaxation (FR), occurs at 40–70 degrees of body flexion. Similar studies have not been performed on the dynamic behavior of the hip extensor muscles or hamstrings in lumbar-pelvic rhythm. The activity of the back and hamstring muscles were simultaneously monitored during sagittal forward body flexion and extension in healthy volunteers.

Methods.—The study group included 21 healthy men and 19 healthy women, age 17–48 years, without back pain. Surface recordings of the electrical activity in the back and hamstring muscles were performed on both sides at the L4–L5 lumbar level and the upper part of the hamstring muscles. Electromyography (EMG) and motion signals were recorded during flexion and extension with straight knees and feet 15 cm apart. The cycle of bending and extension lasted about 4 seconds and was repeated 4 times in 30 seconds. Simultaneously, lumbar and pelvic motion were assessed in real time with a 2-inclinometer method with electronic, magnetoresistive movement sensors fixed at the sacrum and the thoracolumbar area.

Results.—Back flexion relaxation occurred at an average lumbar flexion of 79 degrees. Hamstring activity persisted and only halted as nearly complete lumbar flexion was attained. The last part of lumbar and pelvic flexion was completed without either back muscle activity or hamstring bracing.

Conclusions.—This study of lumbar-pelvic rhythm in healthy volunteers demonstrated that lumbar-pelvic rhythm is controlled by the back and hamstring muscles, but with different timing. Several functional parameters can be measured during this activity, which may be useful in documenting functional back pain syndromes and the effects of therapeutic interventions.

▶ It is generally accepted that during forward trunk flexion, the erector spinae muscles are relaxed as the trunk approaches full flexion. The trunk extensors and hamstrings are active eccentrically during initial trunk lowering, but as the muscles reach an elongated position the weight is taken by the posterior spinal ligaments. The sudden decrease in trunk muscle activity (the flexion relaxation phenomenon) occurs at 40–70 degrees of trunk flexion and may be a factor in lower back injury during lifting and bending in the workplace. This study reported that the hip extensors (the hamstring muscles) also relax during forward flexion but are active further into the range of motion than the back extensors. As full lumbar flexion is approached, there is no back muscle activity or hamstring bracing occurring in healthy subjects. In some low back pain subjects, only the hamstrings relax in full trunk flexion, whereas the back extensors remain active. Some lower back injuries may be the result of poor timing of the relaxation of the hamstring and lumbar muscles, and may be a motor control issue rather than a lower back strength deficiency.

M.J.L. Alexander, Ph.D.

Lumbar Mobility in Former Élite Male Weight-Lifters, Soccer Players, Long-Distance Runners and Shooters
Räty HP, Battié MC, Videman T, et al (Univ of Helsinki; Research Ctr for Sport and Health Sciences, Jyväskylä, Finland; Univ of Alberta, Edmonton, et al)
Clin Biomech 12:325–330, 1997   4–36

Introduction.—Although full spinal range of motion (RoM) is thought to reflect a healthy back, prospective studies in adults and adolescents indicate that spinal flexibility does not predict back injury. Even in sports requiring spinal mobility, athletes and controls may exhibit small differences, especially in lumbar extension. Lumbar mobility was investigated in former elite athletes who had participated in 4 different types of sports.

Methods.—The athletes, all men, had represented Finland at least once in international competitions between 1920 and 1965. A questionnaire was sent to selected surviving athletes in 1985. Of the 147 athletes chosen from respondents, 38 were long-distance runners, 35 were shooters, 37 were soccer players, and 37 were weight lifters. Results of clinical examinations and interviews were available for 117 of these athletes. Data

TABLE 2.—Unadjusted Mean Lumbar Flexion, Extension, and Total Range of Motion in Degrees (SD)

	Flexion	Extension	RoM
Disc-height narrowing (*)			
≤2	19 (6)	39 (10)	57 (10)
≤3	17 (5)	36 (7)	53 (7)
≤5	18 (6)	36 (10)	54 (11)
>5	18 (8)	30 (5)	49 (10)
P†	0.62	**0.015**	**0.043**
Athlete group			
Weight-lifters	18 (7)	35 (8)	54 (10)
Soccer players	19 (7)	36 (8)	54 (10)
Runners	17 (5)	37 (8)	55 (10)
Shooters	17 (6)	35 (10)	52 (10)
P	0.19	0.66	0.99
Work			
Light $n = 75$	18 (6)	36 (8)	54 (8)
Mixed $n = 24$	19 (6)	40 (8)	59 (11)
Heavy $n = 15$	15 (5)	31 (9)	46 (11)
P	0.13	**0.0033**	**0.0002**
LBP/12 months			
No $n = 61$	17 (7)	37 (8)	55 (10)
Yes $n = 53$	18 (6)	34 (9)	53 (10)
P	0.52	0.061	0.25
LBP episodes/lifetime			
≤10 $n = 89$	18 (6)	37 (8)	55 (10)
>10 $n = 25$	18 (7)	33 (9)	51 (10)
P	0.96	**0.035**	0.083

*Quartiles of the distribution of all subjects used as cutoff points for categories.
†P value for differences between the groups. Bold print, P values less than 0.05.
RoM range of motion; LBP, low back pain.
(Reprinted from Räty HP, Battié MC, Videman T, et al: Lumbar mobility of former élite male weight-lifters, soccer players, long-distance runners and shooters. *Clin Biomech* 12:325–330, 1997. Copyright 1997. Reprinted with kind permission from Elsevier Science Ltd, The Boulevard, Langford Lane, Kidlington OX5 1GB UK.)

collected included sports experience, occupational history, back pain history, anthropometric characteristics, and lumbar MRI scans.

Results.—The former elite athletes ranged in age from 45 to 68 years. No differences were observed between groups in lumbar sagittal mobility. Flexion, extension, and RoM declined with increasing age in univariate analysis, although not to a significant degree, given the study participants' age range. There was an association between high body mass index (BMI) and low flexion and low RoM in the lower parts of the lumbar spine. Flexion, extension, and total RoM showed no association with body mass, height, or straight leg raising. There was lower mobility among athletes with heavy occupational physical loading, but there was greater mobility among those whose work involved some lifting and working in a variety of positions. Decreased extension was associated with a history of low back pain (Table 2). After adjusting for age and work, there was a tendency for shooters to be less mobile than the other athletes.

Conclusion.—The sports represented in this group of athletes involve different loading patterns, but none emphasize spinal mobility to a great extent. Runners, shooters, weight lifters, and soccer players did not differ significantly in back mobility in middle age and beyond. There does appear to be a relationship, however, between both heavy work and disk height narrowing and reductions in spinal mobility.

▶ Sarna, et al have conducted some fascinating analyses of function in former international athletes in recent years. The present report differs from an earlier report[1] in that a comparison is drawn between different classes of competitor, rather than between athletes as a group and the general population. Mobility of the spine and other joints often can be important to functional capacity when the elderly attempt the activities of daily living. The present report looks at sagittal mobility of the lumbar spine in athletes 45–68 years of age. At this stage in life, there was surprisingly little difference between soccer players and weight lifters (where adverse effects might have been anticipated from the high-compression forces that are exerted on the spine) and pistol shooters (a group whose general activity patterns are more typical of the general public). However, the soccer players and weight lifters did experience their first episodes of back pain at an earlier age than the pistol shooters. Thus, it is hoped that the authors will repeat their observations when the same subjects range in age from 65 to 88 years, and flexibility of the major joints is becoming more critical to quality of life.

R.J. Shephard, M.D., Ph.D., D.P.E.

Reference

1. Sarna S, Salci T, Koskenvuo M, et al: Increased life expectancy of world-class male athletes. *Med Sci Sports Exerc* 25:237–244, 1993.

Energy Cost of Stair Climbing and Descending on the College Alumnus Questionnaire
Bassett DR, Vachon JA, Kirkland AO, et al (Univ of Tennessee, Knoxville)
Med Sci Sports Exerc 29:1250–1254, 1997   4–37

Background.—Stair climbing is reported to require an energy expenditure of 0.40 kcal/step (0.30 kcal/step to ascend and 0.10 kcal/step to descend). Moreover, these figures are critical to estimates of energy expenditure in a college alumnus questionnaire. The present authors quantified oxygen uptake during stair stepping to obtain a more precise estimate of energy expenditure.

Methods.—Eighteen subjects (10 men and 8 women, mean age 25 years) who exercised ≥30 min/session for ≥3 sessions/week were recruited. The goal was to recruit subjects who could maintain a metabolic steady state during the stair-stepping exercise. Peak oxygen uptake and maximal heart rate were determined by treadmill testing, and oxygen uptake, peak oxygen uptake, and carbon dioxide production were calculated. Stair stepping involved a motorized escalator with 0.203 in (8 inch) tall steps presented at a rate of 70 steps/min. Subjects walked up the down escalator for 7 minutes, and then they walked down the up escalator for 7 minutes. In each instance, expired air from 5 to 7 minutes was collected in a Douglas bag. Oxygen uptake and carbon dioxide production were measured in air from the Douglas bag, and oxygen uptake was converted by use of the respiratory exchange ratio into kilocalories per minute values. In all subjects, oxygen uptake during stair stepping was <80% of peak oxygen uptake as measured on the treadmill.

Results.—After adjustment for body mass, both men and women used 62% of their peak oxygen uptake while walking up the stairs. This equates to an energy cost of 8.6 METs (metabolic equivalents), or about 0.6 kJ/step (0.15 kcal/step) for a 70-kg person. While walking down the stairs, the energy cost was 2.88 METs, or about 0.2 kJ/step (0.05 kcal/step) for a 70-kg person. The overall energy expenditure for going up and down 1 step was 1.63 MET/min.

Conclusions.—The total measured energy expenditure for ascending and descending steps was 0.8 kJ/step (0.20 kcal/step). This number is half the 1.6 kJ/step (0.40 kcal/step) adopted by the college alumnus questionnaire. Furthermore, an individual's energy expenditure can be estimated even more closely by considering body mass (the above energy expenditures were based on a 70-kg person). Thus, studies that estimate a physical activity index based on responses to the college alumnus questionnaire should be modified to reflect the more accurate, measured estimate of energy expenditure of 0.8 kJ/step (0.20 kcal/step).

▶ Paffenbarger's concept[1] that one needs to spend 8 MJ/week of energy to avoid various chronic diseases is widely quoted, and, indeed, it is a lynch pin of those opposed to exercise. "Who is going to be willing to spend 8 MJ/week for the rest of their lives?" they have argued. However, the estimation of energy expenditures from questionnaires is always very imprecise. Now Bassett et al. show that at least 1 important element in the equation, the energy cost of climbing stairs, may be out by a factor of 2. If other elements in the equation such as the energy cost of walking a city block are similarly flawed, it may be that we have to spend much less energy than Dr. Paffenbarger has been telling us in order to maintain health. And this will be good news for those who have to advise ordinary people who are not very interested in spending an hour or more per day in deliberate physical activity.

R.J. Shephard, M.D., Ph.D., D.P.E.

Reference

1. Paffenbarger RS, Hyde RT, Wing AL, et al: Some inter-relationships of physical activity, physiological fitness, health and longevity. In: C Bouchard, RJ Shephard, T Stephens (eds.). *Physical Activity, Fitness & Health.* Champaign, IL: Human Kinetics Publishers, 1994, pp. 119–133.

A New Approach to the Assessment of Anaerobic Metabolism: Measurement of Lactate in Saliva

Segura R, Javierre C, Ventura JLL, et al (Univ of Barcelona)
Br J Sports Med 30:305–309, 1996   4–38

Introduction.—In experimental and routine studies of physical performance, serial determinations of plasma or blood lactate are considered to be very useful. Pricking procedures are generally preferred because samples obtained from the earlobe or the fingertip are virtually identical to those obtained by arterial or venous catheterization. Nevertheless, even a pricking procedure requires some technical expertise, and may cause stress and anxiety. A new procedure that uses saliva rather than blood has been developed.

Methods.—Nine individuals were tested on their performance of a maximum graded exercise test on a cycle ergometer at increasing workrates that ranged from 25 to 300 W. Every 3 minutes, parallel determinations were made of lactate in saliva and in capillary blood samples. Using 25-µL samples in both types of fluids, lactate determinations were performed with an electroenzymatic method.

Results.—The concentration of lactate in saliva was approximately 15% of that in plasma for each situation, and during the exercise test, it

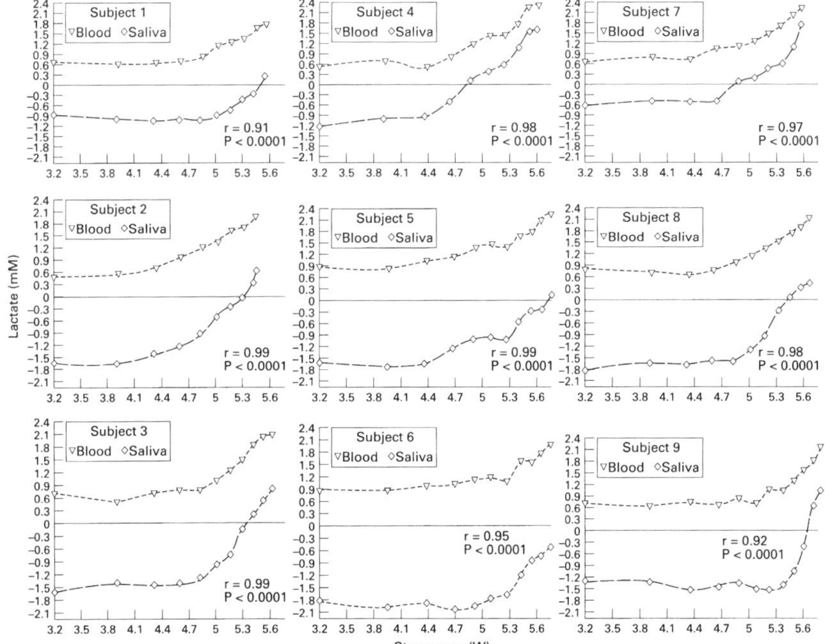

FIGURE 1.—Ln of the concentration of lactate in blood (*dotted line with triangles*) and in saliva (*dashed line with diamonds*) vs. the ln of the power output (ln-ln model) for each of the 9 individuals studied. (Courtesy of Segura R, Javierre C, Ventura JLL, et al: A new approach to the assessment of anaerobic metabolism: Measurement of lactate in saliva. *Br J Sports Med* 30:305–309, 1996.)

had the same pattern of evolution (Fig 1). There was a good correlation between lactate concentrations in saliva and blood. When kept at 4°C, lactate appeared to be very stable in saliva during a period of 40 days after collection. The values of the 40-day samples were compared with those of the fresh samples, and they were virtually identical.

Conclusion.—As an alternative to determination of lactate in blood, determination of lactate in saliva can be used. Because the collection of the samples required no special expertise, saliva samples overcame most of the drawbacks of the procedures being used currently.

▶ Repeat lactate measurements are commonly needed both by the exercise scientist and the top-level coach or trainer. However, frequent finger pricks are unpopular with the individuals concerned, and sometimes a temptation to squeeze the finger when sampling distorts the relative mix of blood and serum in the specimen. The possibility of making determinations on saliva specimens thus has its attractions. The volume of saliva required for analysis is small. Moreover, the lactate content of the saliva not only has a similar time course to blood concentrations, but remains stable for periods as long as 40 days. The crucial variable is, of course, the constancy of the rate of saliva secretion. It is necessary to stimulate maximum secretion by use of a dilute solution of citric acid. Mechanical stimulation (for example, by chewing gum) yields very erratic results.

R.J. Shephard, M.D., Ph.D., D.P.E.

Lactate and Ammonia Concentration in Blood and Sweat During Incremental Cycle Ergometer Exercise
Ament W, Huizenga JR, Mook GA, et al (Univ of Groningen, The Netherlands)
Int J Sports Med 18:35–39, 1997   4–39

Objective.—Lactate and ammonia are byproducts of muscle cell metabolism, and they increase in blood and sweat during exercise. Whether sweat ammonia is produced by the sweat gland itself or originates from blood plasma is unknown. The physiologic response of lactate and ammonia in blood and sweat during exercise of increasing intensity was measured during an incremental exercise test in 10 individuals.

Methods.—Ten healthy individuals (1 woman), aged 21 to 45 years, cycled for 3.5 minutes at 0, 50, 100, 150, and 200 W; 7 also cycled at 175 W. At the last 0.5 minutes of each step, blood was collected from the right earlobe snd sweat was collected in a bag attached to the individual's back. Lactate was analyzed enzymatically, ammonia in sweat was measured by the indophenol method, and ammonia in blood was determined using the Blood Ammonia Checker.

Results.—During increased work, both ammonia and lactate concentrations in blood increased disproportionately, whereas ammonia and lactate

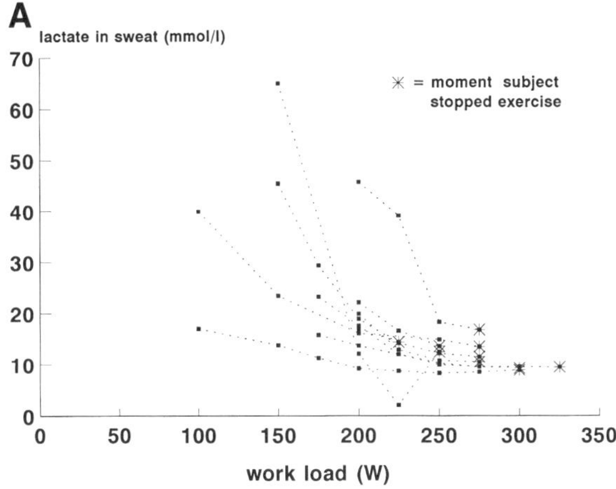

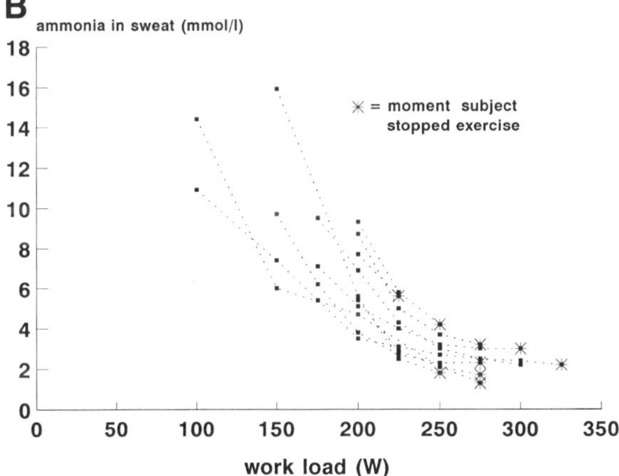

FIGURE 2.—Concentration of lactate (**top**) and ammonia (**bottom**) in sweat of all subjects during incremental exercise. (Courtesy of Ament W, Huizenga JR, Mook GA, et al: Lactate and ammonia concentration in blood and sweat during incremental cycle ergometer exercise. *Int J Sports Med* 18:35–39, 1997. George Thieme Verlag.)

concentrations in sweat were high at exercise onset and decreased as the work rate increased (Fig 2).

Conclusion.—Lactate, apparently produced in the clear cells of the eccrine gland, acidifies sweat and leads to the diffusion of ammonia from the eccrine duct cell to the duct lumen. The source of ammonia in sweat is still unclear, but it could arise from ammonia in plasma or from urease activity of skin bacteria.

▶ The presence of substantial quantities of lactate in human sweat has been recognised for quite a long time, and, indeed, if a subject is sweating hard, this lactate has the potential to contaminate specimens of capillary blood drawn from the finger tip. This study shows rather nicely that there is a decrease in the lactate content of sweat as the work rate (and presumably the rate of sweat production) increases. It also suggests that sweat lactate may have a functional role in clearing ammonia from the body; the sweat content of ammonia moves more or less in parallel with sweat lactate.

R.J. Shephard, M.D., Ph.D., D.P.E.

Comparison of the Testosterone-to-Cortisol Ratio Values Obtained From Hormonal Assays in Saliva and Serum

Obmiński Z, Stupnicki R (Inst of Sport, Warsaw, Poland)
J Sports Med Phys Fitness 37:50–55, 1997   4–40

Background.—Overtraining can upset the balance between anabolism and catabolism. This metabolic equilibrium is often assessed by determining the testosterone-cortisol ratio (T/C) in serum. However, measuring the T/C ratio in saliva may be a better approach, because testosterone and cortisol levels in saliva reflect the biologically active fraction of these hormones rather than the total concentrations in serum. These authors evaluated whether the T/C ratio in serum or saliva offers a better measure of metabolic equilibrium in athletes.

Methods.—The subjects were elite athletes involved in karate (n = 12; body mass index 25.0 ± 1.6) or triathlons (n = 5; body mass index 22.0 ± 0.4). Serum and saliva samples were collected simultaneously and were assayed for levels of testosterone and cortisol.

Findings.—Cortisol levels in serum increased more steeply after reaching a concentration of 600 nmol/L, perhaps because corticosteroid binding globulin became saturated at this point. Thus, serum cortisol data are compared as 2 subsets: <600 and ≥600 nmol/L. Not surprisingly, given the lower serum cortisol levels between subsets, the mean T/C ratio differed significantly between the 2 subsets. When the 2 subsets were combined, however, saliva and serum levels of testosterone (r = 0.963) correlated significantly better than the saliva and serum levels of cortisol (r = 0.874). The mean T/C ratio in serum (4.87 ± 1.86) was 3 times higher than the mean T/C ratio in saliva (1.67 ± 0.85), although the T/C ratio in saliva and serum correlated highly (r = 0.831).

Conclusions.—Serum levels of cortisol increased more steeply after reaching 600 nmol/L. Thus, the T/C ratio will differ depending on the cortisol serum concentration, with a serum cortisol concentration ≥600 nmol/L giving a lower T/C ratio. Overall, however, the T/C ratio measured in saliva correlated very well with the ratio measured in serum. Furthermore, saliva samples are less invasive to obtain than serum samples. Thus, the authors recommend the use of saliva to measure the ratio of biologically active testosterone to cortisol.

▶ The testosterone/cortisol ratio reflects the balance of anabolism to catabolism and is thus one indicator of overtraining in an athlete. One problem in making such measurements is that most biochemical tests measure the total quantities of hormone in the plasma, whereas what the body sees is the free concentration of each hormone. There is a striking difference of T/C ratio between plasma and saliva, and if it is confirmed that the salivary values provide a better indication of free hormone ratio, this will be important to the future assessment of overtraining.

R.J. Shephard, M.D., Ph.D., D.P.E.

Comparison of Single Versus Multiple Lifestyle Interventions: Are the Antihypertensive Effects of Exercise Training and Diet-induced Weight Loss Additive?
Gordon NF, Scott CB, Levine BD (Presbyterian Hosp of Dallas; Univ of Texas, Dallas; Candler Hosp, Savannah, Ga)
Am J Cardiol 79:763–767, 1997   4–41

Background.—Lifestyle modifications are widely used as definitive or adjunctive therapy for high blood pressure (BP). Separately, aerobic exercise training and diet-induced weight loss have been shown to reduce BP. However, the possible additive effect of their combined use is unknown. This issue was addressed in a 3-way randomized trial.

Methods.—Fifty-five sedentary, overweight adults with high-normal blood pressure or stage 1 or 2 hypertension participated in the study. The patients were assigned into 3 intervention groups, each intervention to last 12 weeks. One group was assigned aerobic exercise only—they exercised for 30–45 minutes 3–5 days/week at 60% to 85% of maximal heart rate. Another group was assigned to dietary modification only, with reduction of energy intake and dietary fat for the purpose of weight loss. The third group was assigned to both exercise training and dietary modification. Outcome measures included BP, body mass, and maximal graded treadmill testing.

Results.—Seven patients dropped out of the study for various reasons, leaving 48 patients for analysis. Mean reduction in body mass was 7 kg with exercise plus diet, compared to 6 kg with diet only and 1 kg with exercise only (Table 3). Patients assigned to both diet and exercise also had a greater improvement in maximal oxygen intake: 4.3 mL/(kg-min), compared with 1.9 mL/kg/min with diet only and 2.5 mL/[kg-min] with exercise only. However, there was no significant difference between groups in the mean blood pressure reduction achieved: 12.5/8 mm Hg with exercise plus diet, 11/7.5 mm Hg with diet only, and 10/6 mm Hg with exercise only.

Conclusions.—Although each is effective in reducing hypertension, aerobic exercise training and diet-induced weight loss do not have additive effects on blood pressure. In terms of BP only, no greater effect is to be expected when both diet and exercise are prescribed for patients with high-normal BP or stage 1 or 2 hypertension. However, both interventions have important benefits besides their antihypertensive effect.

TABLE 3.—Changes in Outcome Measures After 12 Weeks of Lifestyle Intervention

| | Change from Baseline | | |
Outcome Measures	Exercise Only (n = 14)	Diet Only (n = 15)	Exercise Plus Diet (n = 19)
Weight (kg)	−1.0 ± 1.8	−5.8 ± 3.9*‡	−7.1 ± 2.9*‡
Body fat (%)	−0.5 ± 1.0	−1.6 ± 1.3*	−2.4 ± 1.7*‡
Maximal oxygen uptake (ml/kg/min)	2.5 ± 2.6†	1.9 ± 2.0†	4.3 ± 2.6*§
Maximal oxygen uptake (ml/min)	223 ± 242†§	49 ± 146	208 ± 227*
Systolic BP (mm Hg)	−9.9 ± 6.4*	−11.3 ± 12.1†	−12.5 ± 6.3*
Diastolic BP (mm Hg)	−5.9 ± 4.6*	−7.5 ± 4.3*	−7.9 ± 4.3*

Note: Values are expressed as mean ± SD.

*$P \leq 0.001$, changes from baseline statistically significant where indicated.

†$P \leq 0.01$; changes from baseline statistically significant where indicated.

‡$P \leq 0.001$; differences between interventions were statistically significant vs. exercise only.

§$P \leq 0.05$; differences between interventions were statistically significant vs. diet only.

Abbreviation: BP, blood pressure.

(Reprinted by permission of the publisher, from Gordon NF, Scott CB, Levine BD: Comparison of single versus multiple lifestyle interventions: Are the antihypertensive effects of exercise training and diet-induced weight loss additive? *Am J Cardiol* 79:763–767, Copyright 1997 by Excerpta Medica, Inc.)

▶ Many of those who are involved with health promotion either come from a nutritional background, or have a strong grounding in this discipline. Thus, there is a tendency to regard exercise mainly as a means of bringing the body into energy balance, a task that can be accomplished more readily by a combination of exercise and dieting than by exercise alone. However, dieting imparts a negative element to the health promotional "message," and a number of recent articles have demonstrated that for several goals of preventive medicine, dieting plus exercise offers no advantage of outcome over exercise alone. The article by Gordon and associates echoes this finding. Although combined therapy achieved a larger weight loss than exercise alone, the decrease in systemic BP was very similar for exercise, dieting, or exercise plus dieting. One limitation of the study is that it continued for only 12 weeks, and advocates of combined therapy may argue that a longer study would have demonstrated some advantage to combined treatment. This latter position is supported by a recent study of Katzel et al.,[1] where an advantage was shown for combined treatment over a 9-month study.

R.J. Shephard, M.D., Ph.D., D.P.E.

Reference

1. Katzel LJ, Bleecker ER, Colman EG, et al: Effects of weight loss vs. aerobic exercise training on risk factors for coronary disease in healthy, obese middle-aged and older men. *JAMA* 24:1915–1921, 1995.

Seasonal Variations in the Body Composition of Lightweight Rowers

Morris FL, Payne WR (Univ of Melbourne; Univ of Ballarat)
Br J Sports Med 30:301–304, 1996   4–42

Introduction.—During the competitive season, lightweight rowers often reduce their body mass to meet the weight criteria and regain weight in the off-season. Little is known about the effects of seasonal body-mass fluctuations on body composition, specifically fat and lean mass. Weight-loss techniques employed throughout the rowing seasons were documented. The effect of energy restrictions on the body composition of the lightweight rower was evaluated. Whether intense training provided the necessary stimulus to increase or maintain lean tissue was also determined.

Methods.—There were 18 rowers, 12 men and 6 women. The women had an average age of 23.1 years and a height of 1.71 m. The men had an average age of 23.5 years and 1.81 m. Dual energy x-ray absorptiometry and skin-fold techniques were used to assess body mass, fat mass, and

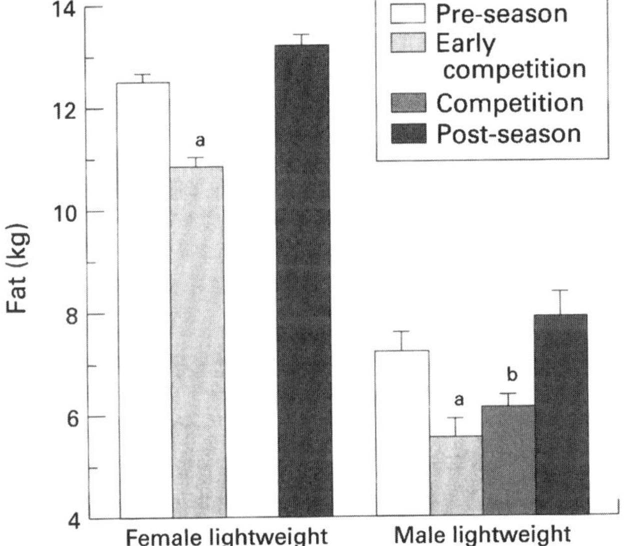

FIGURE 2.—Seasonal comparison of body fat estimate (kg) of female (n = 6) and male (n = 12) lightweight rowers, as measured by dual energy x-ray absorptiometry. Values are means. Errors bars = standard error of the mean. (Courtesy of Morris FL, Payne WR: Seasonal variations in the body composition of lightweight rowers. *Br J Sports Med* 30:301–304, 1996. Official Journal of the American Thoracic Society. Copyright American Lung Association.)

fat-free mass. A questionnaire was used to document weight control techniques before major regattas.

Results.—There was a reduction in body mass preseason to competition among both the men and the women (Fig 2). The women decreased from 61.3 to 57 kg (5.9%), and the men decreased from 75.6 to 69.8 kg (7.8%). A significant reduction in fat mass mirrored the body-weight reductions. The women's measurements of skin folds decreased from 80.9 to 68.2 mm and the men's measurements decreased from 54.2 to 41.8 mm. The women's percentage of body fat decreased from 22.1% to 19.7% and the men's percentage of body fat decreased from 10% to 7.8%. The total fat in women decreased from 12.5 to 10.9 kg and the men's total fat decreased from 7.3 to 5.6 kg. Despite a season of intensive rowing training, no changes were seen in fat-free mass. Reduced total energy and dietary fat intakes accounted for seasonal body-mass changes. In 73.3% of the participants, acute body-mass reductions were achieved by exercise. In 71.4%, participants achieved reductions through food restrictions, and in 62.9%, they achieved reduction through fluid restrictions.

Conclusion.—A significant reduction in fat mass accounts for seasonal body-mass alterations in lightweight rowers. An increase in fat-free mass was limited by the weight restrictions, which may be beneficial to rowing performance.

▶ Lightweight rowers adopt many of the techniques of wrestlers in an attempt to achieve their desired weight category. However, it is always difficult to lose fat without some loss of lean tissue, and the rowers often face a resulting decrement in their physical performance.[1] In the present study, the rowers were somewhat fatter preseason than in other published series, and no lean mass was lost as they prepared for competition. Nevertheless, rigorous training failed to achieve the increase of lean mass that would have been expected if their energy balance had been maintained.

R.J. Shephard, M.D., Ph.D., D.P.E.

Reference

1. Koutedakis Y, Pacy PJ, Quevedo RM, et al: The effects of two different periods of weight-reduction on selected performance parameters in elite lightweight oarswomen. *Int J Sports Med* 15:472–477, 1994.

"Living High-Training Low": Effect of Moderate-altitude Acclimatization With Low-altitude Training on Performance

Levine BD, Stray-Gundersen J (Presbyterian Hosp of Dallas; Univ of Texas, Dallas)
J Appl Physiol 83:102–112, 1997   4–43

Introduction.—Altitude training is frequently used by competitive athletes to improve sea-level performance. However, there are controversies over the objective benefits. The interpretation of most previous studies of

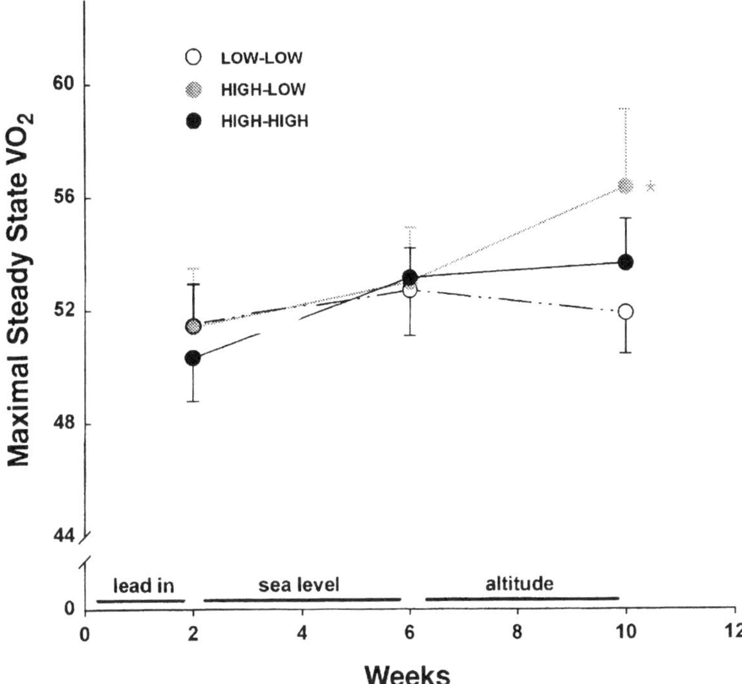

FIGURE 4.—Oxygen uptake (Vo$_2$) at maximal steady state, determined from ventilatory threshold, at baseline, after sea-level training in Dallas (sea level), and after altitude training camp or sea-level control (altitude). *$P < 0.05$ compared with previous time point. (Courtesy of Levine BD, Stray-Gunderson J: "Living high-training low": Effect of moderate-altitude acclimatization with low-altitude training on performance. *J Appl Physiol* 83:102–112, 1997.)

altitude training has been complicated by incomplete characterization of athletic performance, lack of appropriate controls, and small participant numbers. The hypothesis of this study was that athletes who live at moderate altitude and train at low altitude would acquire the physiologic advantages of altitude acclimatization of maximizing their oxygen transport and not go through the detraining associated with hypoxic exercise.

Methods.—Thirty-nine competitive runners, 27 men and 12 women, were randomly assigned to 3 groups: 13 were "high-low," living at a moderate altitude of 2,500 m and training at a low altitude of 1,250 m; 13 were "high-high," living and training at a moderate altitude of 2,500 m; and 13 were "low-low," living and training in a mountain environment at sea level of 150 m. They had a 2-week lead-in phase, then 4 weeks of supervised training at sea level, and then 4 weeks of field training camp, at which point they were assigned into the 3 groups. Measurements were taken for O$_2$ intake, anaerobic capacity, maximal steady state, running economy, velocity at maximal O$_2$ uptake (VO$_{2max}$), and blood compartment volumes.

Results.—There was a significant increase of VO$_{2max}$ of 5% in both altitude groups; this was in direct proportion to an increase in red-cell mass volume of 9%. Neither of these variables changed in the control group. Only in the high-low group was 5-km time improved during the field training camp (13.4 ± 10 seconds), and this was in direct proportion to the increase in VO_{2max}. The high-low group was the only group that had an improvement in velocity at VO_{2max} and maximal steady state (Fig 4).

Conclusion.—In trained runners, 4 weeks of living at high altitude and training at low altitude improved sea-level running performance because of the altitude acclimatization, which involved an increase in VO_{2max} and red-cell mass volume. Improved performance was also attributable to maintenance of sea-level training velocities, which may have also accounted for the increase in maximal steady state and velocity at VO_{2max}.

▶ Debate over the advantages of altitude training dates back to the early days (at least) of preparation for the Mexico City Olympic Games of 1968. There were some attempts at experimentation, but views for and against high-altitude camps were based mainly on the strong opinions of coaches and individual competitors. The consensus seemed to be that such training did not help the well-trained competitor. Although a small increase of hemoglobin level might develop with prolonged residence at altitude, this was offset by problems from disruption of the normal training schedule, learning of an inappropriate competitive pace, and psychological problems of living in an unfamiliar environment. However, many of the problems associated with high-altitude training might be avoided if the athletes lived at a high altitude but carried out their training sessions at an altitude much closer to sea level (the "living-high, training low" regimen). A careful, small-group comparison of this approach is described here. Both living high and training high and living high and training low augmented aerobic power in the present study, but the living high and training low regimen had the clear advantage in terms of track performance. One weakness that will be noticed immediately by those who have conducted research in this area is that the participants were not particularly fit initially (an aerobic power of only 50–51 mL/[kg·min] in endurance competitors). An equally careful study of top-level international-standard athletes is needed.

R.J. Shephard, M.D., Ph.D., D.P.E.

Aquatic-based Rehabilitation and Training for the Elite Athlete
Thein JM, Brody LT (Univ of Wisconsin, Madison)
J Orthop Sports Phys Ther 27:32–41, 1998   4–44

Introduction.—Athletes frequently have overuse injuries, such as tendinitis, bursitis, and stress fractures, and 3 weeks of inactivity can lead to a significant loss of cardiovascular fitness. A decrease of as much as 16% of maximal oxygen consumption can occur after 6 weeks of rest. During an active rest period of recovery, athletes often resort to a water-based program. The pool may be used to regain strength, or improve cardiovascular endurance while resting the injury. Aquatic-based rehabilitation and training was reviewed.

Water Properties.—To maintain equilibrium in the pool, buoyant equipment may be necessary on the trunk or at various points along the limb. In rehabilitation, buoyancy may be used as assistance, support, and resistance. To reduce effusion or allow the athlete to exercise an injured extremity without an increase in effusion, hydrostatic pressure may be used. Regardless of buoyancy, there is resistance to most movement in water because water is more viscous than air.

Exercise.—For intense training of the elite athlete, temperature recommendations should be between 26°C and 28°C. The rate of perceived exertion in deep-water running and the heart rate-$\dot{V}O_2$ relationship is skill dependent. Exercises to be performed in water can help maintain or improve cardiovascular function and the athlete should train at a heart rate about 20 beats/min lower than on land. Exercises include deep water running, deep water cross-country skiing, vertical kicking, hamstring stretching, resistive tubing, rapid alternating shoulder internal and external rotation, duplicating sports-specific activities such as the tennis swing, closed chain activities such as an overhead push-pull, resisted seated knee flexion and extension, side-to-side jumping, abdominal strengthening, sport-specific core activities such as the golf swing, and balance activities.

Transition.—Returning too quickly to land after injury is the biggest mistake made by most athletes, followed by training too hard, too soon, and failing to allow adequate time for recovery. The lower extremity- or spine-injured athlete should be put through a battery of sports-specific tests in shallow water to assess readiness for impact before resuming land impact activities. As long as the athlete and clinician feel necessary, land-based programs may continue to be complemented by pool programs. Even after returning to preinjury status, the athlete may enjoy training in the pool for variety and to give extremities a needed break from impact.

▶ Cross-training of athletes has been accepted in training programs to prevent overuse injuries and for the rehabilitation of injuries. The authors have outlined a general aquatic-based program to serve these purposes. These concepts may also be used with the not-so-elite athlete. Many athletes appear to enjoy these programs and they certainly help to break the tedium of year-round training programs.

F.J. George, A.T.C., P.T.

Influence of Strength Training on Sprint Running Performance: Current Findings and Implications for Training
Delecluse C (Katholieke Universiteit Leuven, Belgium)
Sports Med 24:147–156, 1997   4–45

Introduction.—It is accepted that, by means of strength training, sprint speed can be improved, but excessive hypertrophy is not necessary for successful sprint results. Training must be individualized to match the mixture of ingredients to the requirements of the event. There is an interrelationship between strength and speed, and the athlete must accelerate body mass when velocity is low and apply forces to the ground when moving at more than 11 m/sec. There must be a multidimensional view of strength training for sprinting.

Sprint Running.—The best pacing strategy is an all-out effort for a 100-m sprint. Three phases in a 100-m sprint begin with a phase which requires high initial acceleration over the first 10 m. In the second, or transition, phase, the athlete attains high velocities of 10 to 36 meters; the third phases involves the extent to which an athlete can achieve and maintain high running velocities between 36 and 100 meters. The muscles of the hip, knee, and ankle joints are used to accelerate the body and propel it in the horizontal direction in sprinting. Strength training methods are said to improve sprint times.

Strength Training.—Strength-training methods include hypertrophy training, which increases the mean cross-sectional area of muscle fibers and is characterized by many sets of repetitions with submaximal loads of 60% to 80%. Neuronal activation training makes use of short-term and extremely fast maximal actions against near maximum loads of 90% to 100%. Stretch-shortening cycle exercises are part of speed-strength training, which demands loads that the athlete can manage in a reactive ballistic way and with a high velocity in movement execution. Overspeed training involves using downhill running, high speed treadmill running, and towing using a motorized device or another runner to achieve changes in the nervous system with long-term supramaximal sprint training. Uphill running is the classic overload training technique.

Conclusion.—No specific mechanism is solely responsible for speed, endurance, or strength. A sprinter aims partly for selective hypertrophy of fast twitch fibers and specific adaptations of the neuromuscular system. Strength training effects seem to be movement and velocity specific, thus adequate use of stretch-shortening cycle and sprint-associated exercises are essential. An improved explosive force production and probably faster sprint times can result with prolonged strength and power training.

▶ When developing a strength-training program for sprinters, an individualized strength-training approach is necessary. Specific areas of the sprint which need improvement must also be evaluated. The author gives the example of athletes with high proportions of slow twitch fibers needing more speed-strength training and plyometrics, with a goal of selective hypertrophy.

F.J. George, A.T.C., P.T.

Comparison of Nonballistic Active Knee Extension in Neural Slump Position and Static Stretch Techniques on Hamstring Flexibility
Webright WG, Randolph BJ, Perrin DH (Univ of Virginia, Charlottesville; Walter Reed Army Med Ctr, Washington, DC)
J Orthop Sports Phys Ther 26:7–13, 1997   4–46

Background.—There are various stretching techniques to improve hamstring flexibility. The effectiveness for improving hamstring flexibility of different techniques has been compared, including proprioceptive neuromuscular facilitation relaxation techniques, modifications of these techniques, ballistic stretching, and static stretching. Nonballistic, active range-of-motion exercises have been reported to be more effective than static stretching for increasing range of motion, although there is no published data to support this.

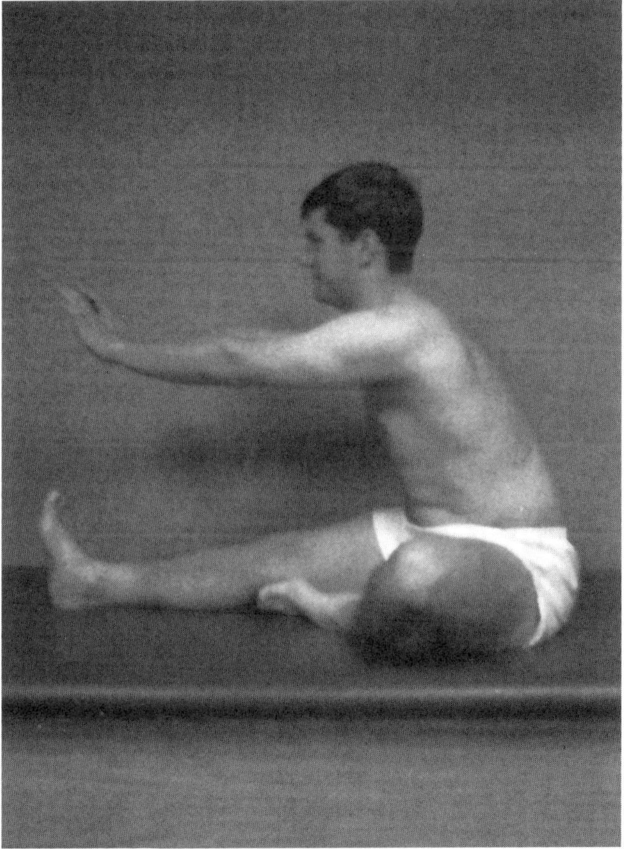

FIGURE 2.—Static hamstring stretch. (Courtesy of Webright WG, Randolph BJ, Perrin DH: Comparison of nonballistic active knee extension in neural slump position and static stretch techniques on hamstring flexibility. *J Orthop Sports Phys Ther* 26:7–13, 1997.)

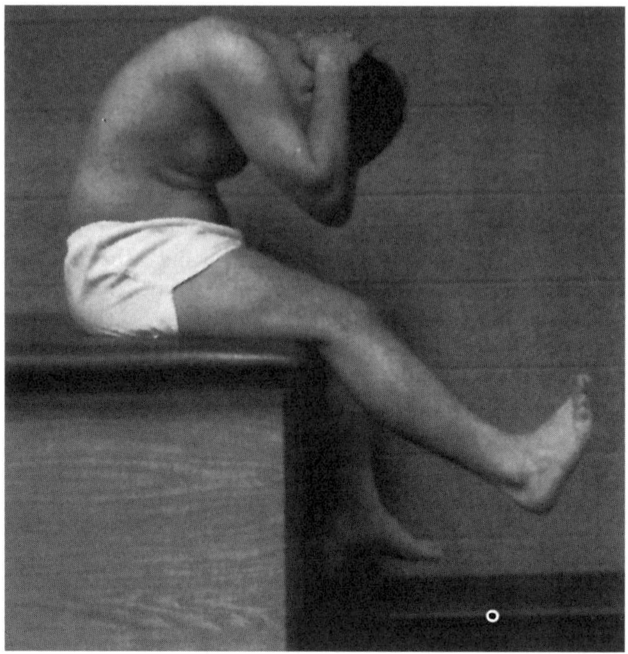

FIGURE 3.—End position for the nonballistic active knee extension stretch in neural slump position. (Courtesy of Webright WG, Randolph BJ, Perrin DH: Comparison of nonballistic active knee extension in neural slump position and static stretch techniques on hamstring flexibility. *J Orthop Sports Phys Ther* 26:7–13, 1997.)

Methods.—The effect of nonballistic, repetitive active knee extension movement performed in a neural slump sitting position was compared to that of static stretching on hamstring flexibility. There were 40 healthy adult subjects with limited right hamstring flexibility. Subjects were assigned to one of three groups. Group 1 was the static stretch group and performed a 30-second stretch twice a day (Fig 2). Group 2 was the active stretch group and performed 30 repetitions of active knee extension in a neural slump sitting position twice a day (Fig 3). Group 3 was the control group. Before and after a 6-week stretching program, hamstring flexibility was measured by an active knee extension test.

Results.—Goniometric measurement of knee joint flexion angle was determined from videotape recordings of the active knee extension test. A 3 (group) × 2 (test) repeated measured analysis of variance and Tukey post hoc testing showed no significant differences in knee joint range of motion improvements between static and active stretch. Knee joint range of motion improved significantly in groups 1 and 2 compared to the control group.

Discussion.—These results indicate that hamstring flexibility in uninjured individuals can be improved by 6 weeks of nonballistic, repetitive active knee extension consisting of 30 repetitions twice a day in a neural slump sitting position. Equal results can be obtained by static stretching for 30 seconds twice a day.

▶ This study demonstrates 2 methods of improving hamstring flexibility in healthy subjects. Both methods improve hamstring flexibility. One method was not significantly superior to the other for improving flexibility. The authors recommend using the static stretch technique because it takes less time to perform. The authors emphasize that when doing the static stretch, the spine should remain neutral by avoiding cervical flexion and moving only from the hips.

F.J. George, A.T.C., P.T.

Rat Tendon Morphologic and Functional Changes Resulting From Soft Tissue Mobilization

Davidson CJ, Ganion LR, Gehlsen GM, et al (Ball State Univ, Muncie, Ind)
Med Sci Sports Exerc 29:313–319, 1997   4–47

Introduction.—Soft tissue mobilization fosters improved tendon action. The mechanism responsible for improvement is not understood. Augmented Soft Tissue Mobilization (ASTM) has been used successfully in the treatment of tendonitis. Instruments, rather than the therapist's fingers or hands, are used in ASTM to introduce a controlled amount of microtrauma into an area of excessive scar or soft tissue fibrosis. The morphologic and functional changes in rat Achilles' tendons were assessed after enzyme-induced injury with collagenase and subsequent ASTM therapy.

Methods.—Four groups of 5 male Sprague-Dawley rats were randomized to either group A, control; group B, tendinitis; group C, tendinitis plus ASTM; group D, ASTM alone. Tendonitis was induced with collagenase injections in Achilles' tendons in group B and C animals. Animals in group C and D were anesthetized and underwent ASTM to the affected Achilles' tendon. Without breaking overlying skin, considerable pressure was applied in a longitudinal plane to the tendon. The instrument was moved distal to proximal and proximal to distal along the length of the tendon. On postoperative days 21, 25, 29, and 33, ASTM was applied to the Achilles tendon for 3 minutes. All animals underwent gait analysis before each treatment. Rats were killed 10 days after final ASTM. Tendons were examined by means of light microscopy, electron microscopy, and immunoelectron microscopy.

Results.—In groups A, B, C, and D, respectively, light microscopy showed collagen fibers aligned in parallel, and few fibroblasts; disrupted and randomly arranged collagen fibers, and numerous fibroblasts; misaligned collagen fibers, and an abundance of fibroblasts; and parallel aligned fibers, and occasional areas with increased numbers of fibroblasts. There was a significant difference in fibroblast counts between group C and all other groups. Significant differences were also detected between groups B and A and groups B and D. Electron microscopy revealed that the rough endoplasmic reticulum was highly developed in the fibroblasts of group C. Immunoelectron microscopy showed appreciable staining with fibronectin antibodies. On postoperative day 21, there was a significant difference in stride length and stride frequency values for animals in group C only.

Conclusion.—Augmented Soft Tissue Mobilization seemed to promote healing of tendon injury and earlier recovery of limb function in rats. This enhanced healing is probably because of increased fibroblast recruitment.

▶ Augmented Soft Tissue Massage involves the use of a solid instrument rather than the hands and fingers. It is certainly easier to perform than traditional soft tissue massage and saves a great deal of wear and tear on the therapist. This study indicates the effectiveness of ASTM in promoting healing via increased fibroblast recruitment. The tendons in this study were massaged in a longitudinal plane. Those animals treated with ASTM also had a significant improvement in gait, compared with the nontreated animals.

F.J. George, A.T.C., P.T.

Articular Cartilage: I. Tissue and Chondrocyte-Matrix Interactions
Buckwalter JA, Mankin HJ (Univ of Iowa, Iowa City; Massachusetts Gen Hosp, Boston)
J Bone Joint Surg Am 79-A:600–611, 1997   4–48

Introduction.—The function and durability of synovial joints is not duplicated with any current prostheses. An arrangement of multiple distinct tissues form these complex structures, including ligament, joint capsule, synovial tissue, subchondral bone, and hyaline articular cartilage. Most people have normal joint function for 80 years or more and this level of performance is not approached by any synthetic material. The design of articular cartilage and the interactions between chondrocytes and their matrix were reviewed.

Composition and Structure.—The macromolecular framework of the tissue matrix is formed by chondrocytes from 3 classes of molecules: proteoglycans, collagen, and noncollagenous proteins. The tissue is given its form and tensile stiffness and strength from types II, IX, and XI collagen. The tissue is given its stiffness to compression and resilience by large aggregating proteoglycans. As a marker of turnover and degeneration of cartilage, cartilage oligomeric protein may have value, and it can influence interactions between the chondrocytes and the matrix. The cells are protected from injury by the matrix, which determines the types and concentrations of molecules that reach the cells.

Interactions.—Continual internal remodeling occurs as the cells replace matrix macromolecules lost through degradation. The ability of chondrocytes to detect alterations in the macromolecular composition and organization of the matrix will influence normal matrix turnover. Mechanical, electric, and physicochemical signals are created by loading of the tissue as a result of use of the joint. The signals help direct the degradative and synthetic activity of chondrocytes. Alterations in the composition of the matrix occur with a prolonged severe decrease in the use of the joint, which eventually leads to loss of tissue structure and mechanical properties. Synthetic activity of chondrocytes is stimulated by use of the joint. Alterations in the composition of the matrix occur with aging as well.

Conclusion.—It is still unknown how mechanical loading of joints influences the function of chondrocytes. Persistent change in the molecular organization of the matrix may be caused by loading, altering the response of the chondrocytes to subsequent loading. The matrix may record the loading history of the tissue, alter the response of the cells on the basis of the loading history, and transduce and transmit signals.

Articular Cartilage: II. Degeneration and Osteoarthrosis, Repair, Regeneration, and Transplantation
Buckwalter JA, Mankin HJ (Univ of Iowa, Iowa City; Massachusetts Gen Hosp, Boston)
J Bone Joint Surg Am 79-A:612–632, 1997   4–49

Introduction.—The most common causes of impairment in middle-aged and older people are joint pain and loss of mobility. The pain and loss of motion are often caused by degeneration of articular cartilage, which usually occurs with idiopathic or primary osteoarthrosis, but can also occur from joint injury or developmental, metabolic, and inflammatory disorders that destroy the articular surface. Because the adult articular cartilage does not have the capacity to repair structural damage resulting from injury or disease, it is thought that adult articular cartilage is an inert bearing surface. If it is inert, little or nothing can be done to prevent the degeneration of articular cartilage and replacement of the articular surface would be the most appropriate treatment for advanced degeneration of cartilage. However, if articular cartilage is not inert, therapeutic approaches that can restore articular cartilage would be appropriate for some patients. A determination of which view is correct is critical for development and implementation of methods of preventing and treating osteoarthrosis.

Degeneration.—The development and progression of osteoarthrosis is influenced by age-related changes in articular cartilage. Lifelong moderate use of normal joints does not increase the risk; however, the mechanism responsible for osteoarthrosis remains poorly understood. The risk of degeneration of normal joints is increased with high-impact and torsional loads. A greater risk of degenerative joint disease is seen with individuals who have an abnormal joint anatomy, joint instability, disturbances of joint or muscle innervation, or inadequate muscle strength or endurance.

Regeneration.—To restore a joint, surgeons will débride and penetrate subchondral bone, and perform an osteotomy to decrease symptoms and restore or maintain a function. There is considerable variance of results.

Loading and motion have an important influence on the healing of articular cartilage and joints. The formation of a new articular surface can be stimulated with transplantation of chondrocytes and mesenchymal stem cells, use of periosteal and perichondrial grafts, synthetic matrices, and growth factors.

Transplantation.—For the treatment of focal defects of articular cartilage in selected patients, transplantation of osteochondral autologous grafts and allografts can be effective. A durable articular surface has not been predictably restored by any of these methods, however. A detailed analysis of the structural and functional abnormalities of the involved joint is necessary to determine future optimum methods. Correction of mechanical abnormalities, débridement, and applications of growth factors, implants, or transplants may be used by the surgeon.

▶ These 2 articles (Abstracts 4–49 and 4–50) present a comprehensive description of the form, function, and biochemistry of articular cartilage. They successfully correlate the current state of knowledge with regard to the biological and mechanical properties and how they relate to both degeneration and approaches to restoring the composition, structure, and function of the cartilage.

J.S. Torg, M.D.

5 Metabolism, Nutrition, and Doping

Deviations From Maximum Weight Predict High-density Lipoprotein Cholesterol Levels in Runners: The National Runners' Health Study
Williams PT (Ernest Orlando Lawrence Berkeley Natl Lab, Calif)
Int J Obes 21:6–13, 1997   5–1

Introduction.—Individual weight history is often not factored into the relationship between adiposity and high-density lipoprotein (HDL) cholesterol levels. Past weight, in addition to current weight, may play a role in HDL cholesterol levels. The elevated HDL cholesterol levels of long-distance runners may be related to their previous weight level. To verify that plasma HDL cholesterol levels were dependent on prior weight and current body mass, data on the weight histories of runners were compared.

Methods.—There were 6,847 men who ran between 0 and 171 km per week. Questionnaires from a national cross-sectional survey were compared to physician-supplied data. Recordings were taken of self-reported current body mass and greatest lifetime mass and body circumferences, and these were compared with data supplied by physicians on plasma concentrations of low-density lipoprotein cholesterol, triglycerides, and HDL cholesterol.

Results.—In runners with the greatest weight loss since their maximum lifetime body mass and the greatest reductions in circumference of their waist, hip, and chest since their maximum mass had the greatest current HDL cholesterol levels. Runners with the greatest decreases in total and regional adiposity since their maximum mass had significantly lower plasma levels of triglycerides, low-density lipoprotein cholesterol, and total cholesterol/HDL cholesterol. When adjustments were made for current body mass index and running distance, the results remained significant.

Conclusion.—Current mass that is relatively high or low within a runner's lifetime range of masses may have an effect on lipoprotein concentrations. Deviation from maximum mass exerts a significant effect on HDL cholesterol levels.

▶ Correction of obesity by dieting is a discouraging process, and any initial loss of fat is quickly regained. It has been hypothesized that an increase of lipoprotein lipase activity in the fat cells of individuals who have lost weight encourages a return of body fat content to its previous set point.[1] It is still unclear why exercise helps to counter this homeostatic process, but the increase of HDL cholesterol and an accelerated catabolism of very low density lipoprotein and chylomicrons in runners who have lost substantial amounts of weight may be a part of the puzzle.

R.J. Shephard, M.D., Ph.D., D.P.E.

Reference

1. Schwartz RS, Brunzell JD: Increase of adipose lipase activity with weight loss. *J Clin Invest* 67:1425–1430, 1981.

Effects of Tennis Training on Lipid Metabolism and Lipoproteins in Recreational Players

Ferrauti A, Weber K, Strüder HK (Univ Cologne, Germany)
Br J Sports Med 31:322–327, 1997   5–2

Introduction.—Physical exercise has a specific lipid modulating effect, and most lipid-lowering sports programs are based on endurance activities such as jogging, swimming, and cycling. To find out if tennis, a popular "lifetime sport," would also have a beneficial effect on lipid metabolism, middle-aged recreational tennis players were examined after tennis training (TT) and running-intensive tennis training (RIT) sessions.

Methods.—Forty-six recreational players entered the study and 38 were included in the data analysis. In an exercise study, 8 men and 8 women took part in a 2-week TT session and in an RIT session designed to examine the short-term metabolic effects of various levels of exercise. Because of a greater increase in lipolysis and greater acceptance by players, the RIT was used in a 6-week longitudinal study designed to assess long-term effects of the program. Twenty-two players (11 men and 11 women) took part in the longitudinal study (3 90-minute sessions per week). Sixteen additional players served as controls. Measurements obtained included body weight, serum lipids and lipoproteins, and endurance capacity.

Results.—The TT sessions involved hitting balls without running and doubles match training; with RIT, players had to run during the ball machine program and participated in singles baseline rallies. Fifteen of 16 players chose the more vigorous RIT as their preferred training method. Participation in the 6-week RIT led to a decrease in body weight and an increase in the anaerobic threshold. These changes differed significantly from findings in controls. The training group had a noticeable rise in the high density lipoprotein$_2$-cholesterol/high density lipoprotein$_3$-cholesterol ratio and a trend toward decreased total cholesterol, triglycerides, and the total cholesterol/-high density lipoprotein cholesterol ratio. Changes in the lipoprotein profile were not significantly different in training and control groups.

Conclusion.—Middle-aged recreational players who participate in a tennis training program can improve their cardiovascular risk factors. After a 6-week training period participants in this study showed a reduction in body weight, an increase in physical performance, and a tendency toward an improved lipid profile. Recommended training requires a high work/rest ratio and maintains an aerobic level of intensity.

▶ This group argues that too many health-oriented and lipid-lowering programs have been based on boring endurance activities like jogging, swimming, and cycling. The authors imply that more people have more fun playing tennis and would be more apt to stick with it. So, they studied whether tennis play would improve health and lipid markers. Sure enough, when middle-aged men and women underwent a 6-week tennis training program, they had fun, lost weight, improved their physical performance, and had a small (nonsignificant) improvement in lipid profile. Tennis can also help maintain bone density in women.[1] But competitive squash play by midlife men can bring a risk of death from coronary heart disease.[2] So let's play tennis, but not so much to win as for fun, fitness, and health.

E.R. Eichner, M.D.

References

1. 1997 YEAR BOOK OF SPORTS MEDICINE, pp 337–340.
2. 1993 YEAR BOOK OF SPORTS MEDICINE, pp 232–233; pp 248–249.

Blood Glutathione Status Following Distance Running
Dufaux B, Heine O, Kothe A, et al (German Sport Univ Cologne, Germany; Medizinal-Untersuchungsstelle, Herford, Germany)
Int J Sports Med 18:89–93, 1997
5–3

Introduction.—The generation of highly reactive oxygen species during exercise has a number of potential causes, including an increase in metabolism and activation of eosinophils. It is difficult to document oxidative stress in physical exercise because of the highly reactive and extremely short-lived nature of most free radicals of interest. The ratio of reduced (GSH) vs. oxidized (GSSG) glutathione is recognized as a sensitive measure of oxidative stress, but studies using this measure during exercise have had conflicting results. To examine further the ratio of GSH to GSSG, glutathione state was investigated in 12 moderately trained men after prolonged exercise.

Methods.—Study participants ranged in age from 22 to 29 years and had a running regimen of 10–20 km/week. During a 2.5 hour race, they covered between 19 and 26 km at a speed between 53% and 82% of that at which blood lactate concentration reached 4 mmol/L lactate (as assessed during a previous treadmill test). Venous blood samples were collected 1 hour before, immediately before and after, 1 and 2 hours after the race,

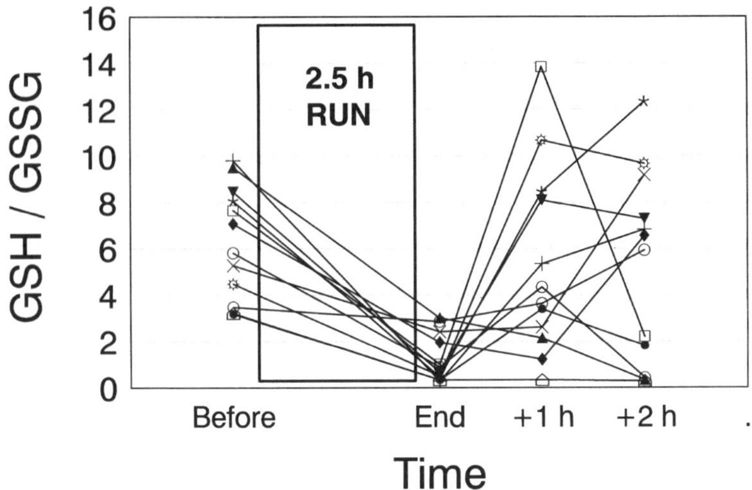

FIGURE 5.—Individual values of the ratio of reduced (*GSH*) to oxidized (*GSSG*) glutathione before and after the first 2 hours after a 2.5 hour run in 12 subjects. (Courtesy of Dufaux B, Heine O, Kothe A, et al: Blood glutathione status following distance running. *Int J Sports Med* 18:89–93, 1997, Georg Thieme Verlag.)

and 1 and 2 days after the race. Samples were analyzed for GSH, GSSG, and thiobarbituric acid reactive substances (TBARS).

Results.—Immediately after exercise, there was a pronounced decline in GSH concentration, but mean GSH values returned to baseline 1 hour after the race. Mean GSSG value was significantly elevated immediately after exercise. Blood samples taken the day after the race yielded GSH and GSSG concentrations that did not differ from baseline. Immediately after completion of the run, the mean ratio of GSH to GSSG fell to 18% of pre-exercise values. From a baseline mean GSH to GSSG ratio of 6.3, the ratio dropped to a value of less than 1.0 in 8 of the 12 participants. Subsequent normalization of ratio values differed considerably among participants (Fig 5) in the early recovery period, a finding not previously reported.

Discussion.—Exhaustive distance running in moderately trained young men led to a pronounced decrease of blood GSH, with a simultaneous increase of GSSG. Concentrations of TBARS did not change significantly with exercise. Findings suggest that a critical shift in the blood glutathione redox status may be reached under such exercise conditions, but the changes are generally short-lived.

▶ One argument against exercise is that it increases the production of highly reactive oxygen species, which can cause cellular damage, aging, and neoplasia. Perhaps for this reason, some observers have found the greatest longevity in sedentary animals, which were provided with only a restricted diet. It is difficult to evaluate the production of reactive species in humans. As might be expected from their name, reactive species react quickly and disappear from the bloodstream in short order. However, glutathione is a major scavenger of free radicals, and the ratio of reduced to oxidized glutathione provides a convenient index of oxidative stress. In the present study, a 2.5 hour run produced a dramatic drop in the glutathione redox ratio to only 18% of its resting value. The problem was quite short-lived, and within an hour the baseline had been regained or even overshot. Although this study suggests some short-lived oxidative stress from a single, prolonged bout of exercise, it does not answer the question of what happens when the exercise is repeated frequently. There is some evidence that training increases the activity of enzymes that metabolize the reactive species, quickly restoring normal or even subnormal levels of free radicals in the regular exerciser.

R.J. Shephard, M.D., Ph.D., D.P.E.

Prolonged Exercise Decreases Serum Leptin Concentrations
Landt M, Lawson GM, Helgeson JM, et al (Washington Univ, St Louis; Mayo Clinic, Rochester, Minn; State Univ of New York, Syracuse)
Metabolism 46:1109–1112, 1997   5–4

Introduction.—Leptin is secreted in a 146-amino acid form and production increases with increasing adiposity. It appears to be involved in the feedback regulation of body (fat) mass. In individuals with non–insulin-dependent diabetes, human immunodeficiency virus infection, or anorexia nervosa, plasma leptin concentrations were similar to normal levels. Previous studies have shown that leptin concentrations are reduced with exercise. In a group of exercisers, plasma leptin concentrations were measured to determine whether a negative energy balance caused by physical exertion alters plasma leptin concentrations.

Methods.—Subjects were 12 men who fasted overnight and pedaled a stationary cycle ergometer for 2 hours and 14 nonfasting ultramarathon runners. Both groups had serum leptin and free fatty acid concentrations analyzed through blood samples collected before exercise, immediately after exercise, and 6 to 24 hours after exercise.

Results.—Mean leptin levels were reduced by 8.3%; free fatty acids were highly increased and correlated well with the decrease in serum leptin levels after 2 hours of strenuous pedaling following an overnight fast. Leptin concentrations recovered to pre-exercise levels and free fatty acid concentrations decreased less than pre-exercise levels after 6 hours of rest and refeeding. In this same group of men, a similar decrease in serum leptin levels (12.4%) was seen. Leptin concentrations were reduced by 32% in the prolonged exercise of an ultramarathon in comparison with prerace levels. There was an increase in free fatty acid concentrations, but these values were not correlated with the change in serum leptin concentrations. In blood samples collected 18 to 24 hours after racing, leptin and free fatty acid concentrations trended toward prerace levels.

Conclusion.—Serum leptin concentrations can be reduced by the negative energy balance of exercise, but only at extremes of the severity and duration of exercise. There is a relationship between fatty acid metabolism and leptin homeostasis, but free fatty acids do not seem to directly modulate serum leptin concentrations.

▶ There has been considerable interest recently in leptin, a hormone that apparently controls body fat stores by suppressing appetite and increasing metabolic rate. This preliminary study suggests that severe exercise, sufficient to create a negative energy balance, may also suppress leptin production. This could be 1 reason why the resting metabolic rate falls and people do not always lose as much weight as we think they should when they become involved in an exercise-based weight loss program.

R.J. Shephard, M.D., Ph.D., D.P.E.

Total Energy Expenditure and the Level of Physical Activity Correlate With Plasma Leptin Concentrations in Five-Year-Old Children
Salbe AD, Nicolson M, Ravussin E (NIH, Phoenix, Ariz; AMGEN Inc, Thousand Oaks, Calif)
J Clin Invest 99:592–595, 1997   5–5

Objective.—Leptin decreases food intake and increases energy expenditure in *ob/ob* mice. Low leptin levels have been detected in Pima Indians who gained weight compared with Pima Indians who did not gain weight. The relation between fasting plasma leptin concentrations and energy metabolism was investigated in 123 5-year-old children prone to obesity.

Methods.—During the summers from 1992 to 1995, fasting plasma leptin concentrations, total energy expenditure (TEE) assessed by the double-labeled water method, resting metabolism rate (RMR) assessed by indirect calorimetry, body composition assessed by isotopic water dilution, and physical activity level (PAL) calculated as TEE:RMR were determined in 123 5-year-old Pima Indian children (67 boys).

Results.—Plasma leptin levels were significantly correlated with percent body fat ($r = 0.84$). After adjusting for percent body fat, leptin levels were similar for boys and girls. Both TEE and PAL were significantly correlated with plasma leptin levels after adjusting for percent body fat ($r = 0.42$ and $r = 0.26$, respectively) (Fig 1). RMR was not correlated with leptin concentrations adjusted for body fat.

Conclusion.—The correlation between leptin levels and total energy expenditures suggests that leptin may mediate energy expenditure and physical activity, perhaps by activating the sympathetic nervous system. In addition to controlling food intake, leptin may also increase total daily energy expenditure. Because elevated physical activity levels increase sympathetic nervous system activity and decrease leptin secretion, it is not likely that energy expenditure increases leptin levels.

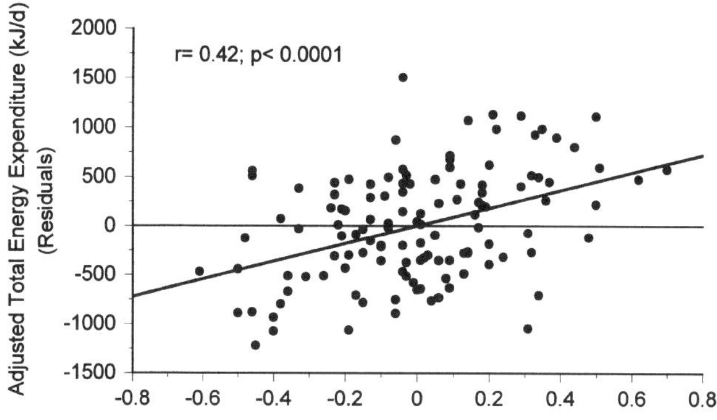

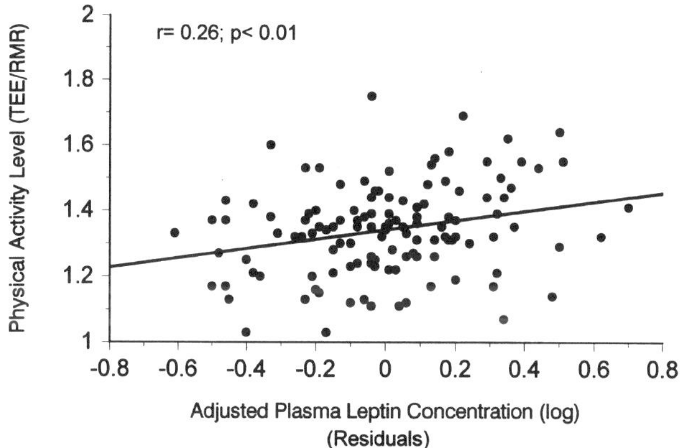

FIGURE 1.—(*Top*) Total energy expenditure, expressed as residuals, plotted against plasma leptin concentrations, also expressed as residuals. Residuals were calculated as the difference between the measured value and the predicted value after adjustment of these variables for their major determinants by multiple linear regression models (on the basis of the entire group of 123 children). The zero point on this graph represents the mean total energy expenditure in this group (5982 ± 961 kJ/d). (*Bottom*) Physical activity level (TEE:RMR) plotted against the residuals of plasma leptin concentration ($\log_{10}$) adjusted for percent body fat. (Courtesy of Salbe AD, Nicolson M, Ravussin E: Total energy expenditure and the level of physical activity correlate with plasma leptin concentrations in five-year-old children. *J Clin Invest* 99:592–595, 1997. Reprinted with permission from the Journal of Clinical Investigation, 1997, 99:592–595, by copyright permission of the American Society for Clinical Investigation.)

► Leptin, of course, is the product of the mouse obese gene. Secreted by fat cells, it decreases food intake by acting on satiety centers in the brain. It also increases metabolic rate and physical activity, perhaps by stimulating the sympathetic nervous system. This cross-sectional study in children shows what has been consistently reported in adults: fasting plasma leptin level best correlates with percent body fat. The new finding is that fasting leptin correlates with physical activity. There is no reason to believe that physical activity elevates leptin, so, most likely, leptin elevates physical activity in children as in mice, perhaps by sympathetic stimulation. And a new study emphasizes that our children need such stimulation. Twenty percent of US children participate in 2 or fewer bouts of vigorous activity a week, while one quarter of all children—and an even higher percentage of minority children—view 4 or more hours of television each day. Boys and girls who view 4 or more hours a day are fatter than those who view less television. This is the fourth cross-sectional national study to link obesity and television viewing among children.[1]

E.R. Eichner, M.D.

Reference

1. Anderson RE, Crespo CJ, Bartlett SJ, et al: Relationship of physical activity and television watching with body weight and level of fatness among children. *JAMA* 279:938–942, 1998.

Effects of Diet and Exercise in Preventing NIDDM in People With Impaired Glucose Tolerance

Pan X-R, Li G-W, Hu Y-H, et al (China-Japan Friendship Hosp, Beijing, China; Da Qing First Hosp, China; NIH, Phoenix, Ariz; et al)
Diabetes Care 20:537–544, 1997   5–6

Background.—Impaired glucose tolerance (IGT) is a significant risk factor for subsequent development of non–insulin-dependent diabetes mellitus (NIDDM). A previous non-randomized study indicated that a 5-year regimen of dietary and exercise interventions may decrease the incidence of NIDDM in patients with IGT. The effects of diet and exercise on the progression of IGT to NIDDM were further explored in this randomized, prospective study.

Methods.—Five hundred seventy-seven patients with IGT from 33 health care clinics in Da Qing, China were assigned to intervention strategies based on their home clinic. Participants from clinics assigned to an intervention based on diet alone who also had body mass indices (BMI) less than 25 kg/m² (lean patients) consumed a diet of 100–120 MJ//kg (25–30 kcal/kg) body mass, 25% to 30% fat, 10% to 15% protein and 55% to 65% carbohydrate. Patients with BMIs greater than or equal to 25 kg/m² (overweight patients) were, in addition, encouraged to restrict food intake with the goal of losing 0.5–1.0 kg body mass per month. Participants from clinics assigned to an intervention based on exercise alone were encouraged to increase their activitiy from 5 to 60 minutes daily, depending on exercise intensity and patient age. Participants from clinics assigned to interventions based on both diet and exercise were encouraged to follow both strategies. Individual counseling by physicians was provided for patients in all 3 intervention groups. Participants from clinics designated as controls received only general information concerning IGT and diabetes mellitus. Patients were studied for 6 years.

Results.—Five hundred thirty of the 577 participants were studied for the full 6 years. The cumulative incidence of NIDDM at the end of the follow-up period was 41.1% in the exercise intervention group, 43.8% in

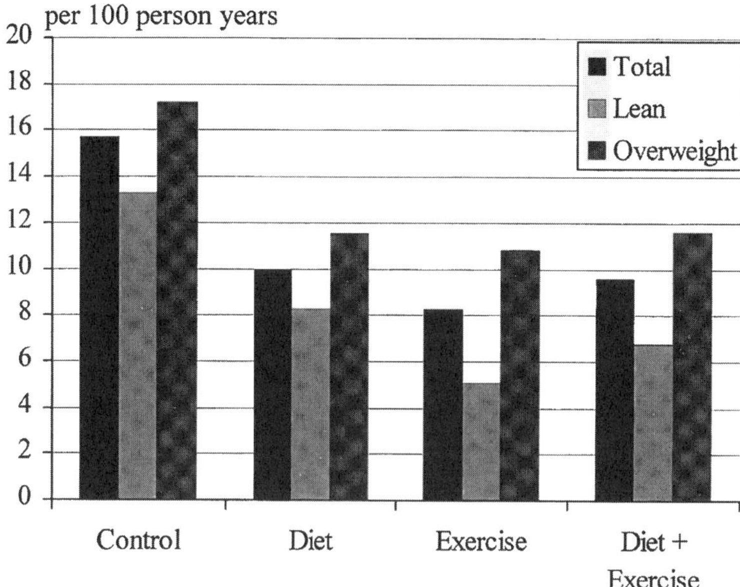

FIGURE 2.—Incidence of diabetes at or before 6-year evaluation. Lean participants constituted 39.2% of the total sample (37.6% of the control group, 42.3% of the diet group, 40.4% of the exercise group, and 39.2% of the diet-plus-exercise group). (Courtesy of Pan X-R, Li G-W, Hu Y-H, et al: Effects of diet and exercise in preventing NIDDM in people with impaired glucose tolerance. *Diabetes Care* 20:537–544, 1997.)

the dietary intervention group, 46.0% in the diet and exercise group, and 67.7% in controls. Differences between intervention and control clinics were statistically significant; however, differences among clinics providing the 3 interventions were not statistically significant. Incidence rates of NIDDM were higher among overweight than lean patients in the control group, at 17.2 and 13.3 per 100 person-years, respectively. The incidence of NIDDM was lower than in controls for each intervention strategy and within each BMI class, with the exception of a non-significant decrease in lean patients receiving only dietary intervention (Fig 2). The proportionate decrease in NIDDM incidence in patients receiving dietary and/or exercise intervention was similar for the 2 BMI classes.

Conclusions.—Lifestyle changes with respect to diet and exercise can decrease the incidence of NIDDM in patients with IGT. This is apparently the first controlled, randomized clinical trial to address this relationship and to demonstrate risk amelioration through dietary and/or exercise intervention. Further research is needed to optimize intervention strategies and to determine if these results are generalizable to the population at large.

▶ This is a massive and well-designed 6-year prospective trial from China, showing the sophistication of research that is now possible in that country, given some input from western colleagues. One tricky question of experimental design was the method of randomization, which was by clinic rather than by individual. This raised the tedious question of "units of analysis." Statistical purists would currently argue that the assessment of significance should be based on the experience of the 33 clinics, rather than that of the individual 110,660 participants. The present team of investigators were aware of this issue, and wisely used the Ryan-Einot-Gabriel-Welsch multiple F test to compare results at the various clinics. The exercise intervention was based on a table of everyday activities that were classified into 4 levels. Participants were encouraged to progress by at least 1 unit relative to this table. Based on clinic means, the proportion of patients with IGT who had diabetes develop during the 6 years dropped from 65.9% at control clinics to 44.2% at exercise clinics, and results were no better in the group that had a combination of diet plus exercise. One distinction from a western population is that initial levels of body fat were moderate, BMIs being in the range 25–26 kg/m².

R.J. Shephard, M.D., Ph.D., D.P.E.

Diabetes and Exercise: The Role of the Athletic Trainer
Jimenez CC (West Chester Univ, Pa)
J Athletic Train 32:339–343, 1997   5–7

Introduction.—Physical exercise is an important component of a healthy lifestyle, whether an individual is diabetic or not. In the management of diabetes mellitus, the role that exercise plays is defined. Guidelines for preventing and treating exercise-related complications are provided.

Methods.—A review of the literature in MEDLINE was conducted to compile the information.

Results.—Guidelines for safe exercise include wearing identification that indicates the individual is diabetic; avoiding exercise at the peak of insulin action; adjusting carbohydrate intake or insulin dosage before exercise; checking blood sugar before, after, and if possible, during exercise; preventing dehydration by consuming adequate fluids before, during, and after exercise; having access to a fast-acting carbohydrate during exercise in the event of hypoglycemia; and having blood glucose testing equipment and supplies available. Hypoglycemia is the most frequently encountered exercise risk, and the signs include shakiness, sweating, rapid heartbeat, trouble concentrating, headache, dizziness, mood changes, and tingling in the face, tongue, and lips. By giving the athlete at least 10 g of a fast-acting carbohydrate source such as half a can of nondiet soda, most cases of hypoglycemia can be reversed. Glucagon must be administered in severe cases of hypoglycemia where the athlete is unconscious or unable to swallow. Deciding how the glucose should be administered should be discussed and planned out beforehand with the athlete. Exercise should be delayed if the blood glucose level is at 250 mg/dL or higher. General guidelines for carbohydrate supplementation before different types of exercise are provided in the Table.

TABLE pg 342.—Recommended Food Intake Based on Type of Exercise and Blood Glucose Level

Exercise	Blood Glucose Level	Food Exchanges to Add*
Short-duration, low- to moderate-intensity exercise walking (½ mile) or leisurely cycling (less than 30 minute)	under 80 mg/dL over 80 mg/dL	2 fruit 1 fruit
Moderate-intensity exercise tennis, swimming, jogging, golfing, or leisurely cycling (1 hour)	under 80 mg/dL 80–180 mg/dL 180–300 mg/dL over 300 mg/dL	½ meat and 2 bread 1 fruit or 1 bread no extra food DO NOT EXERCISE
Strenuous exercise football, hockey, racquetball, basketball, strenuous cycling or swimming, or shoveling	under 80 mg/dL 80–180 mg/dL 180–300 mg/dL over 300 mg/dL	1 meat, 2 bread, 1 fruit, and 1 milk 1 meat and 2 bread 1 fruit or 1 bread DO NOT EXERCISE

*One fruit = 118 mL (4 oz) orange juice; 1 meat = 15 mL (1T) peanut butter; 1 bread = 14 g (½ oz) bagel; 1 milk = 237 mL (8 oz) 2% or skim milk.

(Adapted with permission from Lundstrom RE, Rossini AA: *A Diabetes Handbook.* Worcester, Mass, University of Massachusetts Medical Center, 1994, pp 28, 47, 81. Courtesy of Jimenez CC: Diabetes and exercise: The role of the athletic trainer. *J Athletic Train* 32:339–343, 1997.)

Conclusions.—By understanding the unique physiologic responses of diabetics to exercise, as well as the risks and benefits of exercise, the athletic trainer can help athletes with diabetes to compete safely.

▶ With guidance from the athlete's physician, the athletic trainer should be closely involved with monitoring and providing emergency care for the diabetic athlete. Each diabetic athlete may respond differently to exercise. It is important to become familiar with the individual's reactions and the appropriate responses.

F.J. George, A.T.C., P.T.

4-Hydroxycatecholestrogen Metabolism Responses to Exercise and Training: Possible Implications for Menstrual Cycle Irregularities and Breast Cancer

de Crée C, Fujimori Y, Van Kranenburg G, et al (Inst for Gyneco-Endocrinological Research, Leuven, Belgium; Univ of Maastricht, The Netherlands; Kyoto Univ, Japan)
Fertil Steril 67:505–516, 1997

5–8

Introduction.—The 4-hydroxyestrogens (4-OHE) have a strong estrogenic potency and an affinity for catechol-O-methyltransferase, an enzyme that deactivates catecholamines. The behavior of C4-substituted estrogens in response to vigorous exercise was evaluated in 6 sedentary, healthy, eumenorrheic women.

Methods.—Women were studied through 3 menstrual cycles: control cycle, moderate training cycle, and heavy training cycle. Blood samples

TABLE 3.—Absolute Changes in Follicular Phase Plasma Total Estrogen and Catecholestrogen Responses to Acute Exercise Before and After a Brief Training Period

Hormone	t_0	t_{submax}	t_{max}	t_{recov1}	t_{recov2}
			Workload		
E (pg/mL)					
Pretraining	879 ± 179	1,041 ± 170	1,267 ± 166	1,165 ± 201	1,120 ± 146
Mild training	931 ± 83	1,137 ± 118	1,191 ± 166	1,084 ± 156	1,072 ± 125
Heavy training	922 ± 198	1,152 ± 188	1,197 ± 134	1,063 ± 162	1,070 ± 129
4-OHE (pg/mL)					
Pretraining	51 ± 7	73 ± 9*	84 ± 9*	82 ± 13*	80 ± 13*
Mild training	62 ± 7	66 ± 7	64 ± 13	67 ± 13	69 ± 10
Heavy training	58 ± 11	74 ± 12	77 ± 9	87 ± 9	92 ± 12*
4-MeOE (pg/mL)					
Pretraining	<35	<35	<35	<35	<35
Mild training	<35	<35	<35	<35	<35
Heavy training	44 ± 3†	61 ± 5*‡	69 ± 5‡§	77 ± 5‡§	79 ± 6‡§
4-OHE/E					
Pretraining	0.06 ± 0.01	0.07 ± 0.01	0.07 ± 0.01	0.07 ± 0.02	0.07 ± 0.02
Mild training	0.07 ± 0.02	0.06 ± 0.01	0.05 ± 0.02	0.06 ± 0.02	0.06 ± 0.02
Heavy training	0.06 ± 0.01	0.06 ± 0.01	0.06 ± 0.01	0.06 ± 0.02	0.06 ± 0.03*
4-MeOE/4-OHE					
Pretraining	0.34	0.28	0.30	0.30	0.30
Mild training	0.50†	0.52†	0.48†	0.44†	0.46†
Heavy training	0.75 ± 0.10‡	0.82 ± 0.16‡	0.90 ± 0.23‡	0.88 ± 0.17‡	0.86 ± 0.20‡

Note: Values are means ± SEM. Conversion factors to SI units areas follow: E_1, 3.699; E_2 3.671; $4\text{-}OHE_1$, 3.492; $4\text{-}OHE_2$, 3.467; $4\text{-}MeOE_1$ 3.329; and $MEOE_2$, 3.307.

*Acute exercise-induced plasma concentration significantly different from baseline values within the same phase of training, $P < 0.05$.

†Posttraining plasma concentration significantly different from pretraining values at the same level of exercise intensity, $P < 0.05$.

‡Posttraining plasma concentration significantly different from pretraining values at the same level of exercise intensity, $P < 0.01$.

§Acute exercise-induced plasma concentration significantly different from baseline values within the same phase of training, $P < 0.01$.

Abbreviations: 4-OHE, 4-hydroxy estrogens; *4-MeOE,* 4-hydroxyestrogen-monomethylethers.

(Reprinted by permission from the American Society for Reproductive Medicine from de Crée C, Fujimori Y, Van Kranenburg G et al: 4-Hydroxycatecholestrogen metabolism responses to exercise and training: Possible implications for menstrual cycle irregularities and breast cancer. *Fertil Steril* 67:505–516, 1997.)

were collected during follicular and luteal phases on the same day as exercise tests. Serum samples were analyzed for: follicular and luteal phase plasma E_2, luteinizing hormone, catecholamines, prolactin, total unconjugated and conjugated estrogens, total hydroxyestrogens (4OHE), and 4-hydroxyestrogen-monomethylethers (4-MeOE).

Results.—At pretraining baseline, 4-OHE levels were significantly higher in the luteal phase, compared to the follicular phase, and 4-MeOE values were below minimal detection. Catecholamines, prolactin, E_2, unconjugated and conjugated estrogens, 4-OHE, and 4-MeOE all increased during incremental training. The increases in 4-OHE during exercise were more pronounced before training, compared to 4-MeOE, which was highest after training. There was a significant increase in the 4-MeOE:4-OHE ratio with progressive training (Table 3).

Conclusion.—The acute exercise-induced increase in 4-OHE with positive correlation to lactate levels may signify a key process in the pathogenesis of exercise-associated menstrual irregularities. Exercise triggered an even more important increase in baseline 4-MeOE:4-OHE in either the follicular or luteal phase. This limited circulation of the active carcinogenic-potent form, which may be important in the postulated immunoprotective effect of sports participation on reproductive cancers.

▶ Although the evidence is not entirely unanimous, there is growing support for the idea that regular vigorous physical activity protects women against breast cancer. This benefit has usually been linked to a negative energy balance and the suppression of menstrual function, and it has traditionally been suggested that vigorous exercise reduces the secretion of potentially carcinogenic estrogens—either by a direct influence of physical activity on pituitary function, or through a depletion of body fat stores. The present article notes the carcinogenic action of catecholestrogens[1, 2] and suggests that the beneficial effect of vigorous training comes from an increase in O-methylation of these dangerous compounds.

R.J. Shephard, M.D., Ph.D., D.P.E.

References

1. Ashburn SP, Han X-L, Liehr JG: Microsomal hydroxylation of 2- and 4-fluoroestradiol to catechol metabolites and their conversion to methyl ethers: Catechol estrogens as possible mediators of hormonal carcinogenesis. *Mol Pharmacol* 43:534–541, 1993.
2. Lemon HM, Heidel JW, Rodriguez-Sierra JR: Increased catechol estrogen metabolism as a risk factor for non-familial breast cancer. *Cancer* 69:457–465, 1992.

Reproductive Function in Male Endurance Athletes: Sperm Analysis and Hormonal Profile
Lucía A, Chicharro JL, Pérez M, et al (Fundación Laboral Instituto Nacional de Industria, Madrid)
J Appl Physiol 81:2627–2636, 1996   5–9

Introduction.—The effects of strenuous physical exercise on the menstrual cycle of female athletes are well documented, but less attention has been directed toward the impact of endurance training on male reproductive function. A study of 40 men, 31 who engaged in strenuous physical activity and 9 who were sedentary, examined the effects of endurance exercise on semen characteristics and sex hormones.

Methods.—Eligible participants ranged in age from 20 to 39 years, were in good health, had no history of chronic disease or depressive illness, and had not used medications that could alter the hypothalamic-pituitary-gonadal (H-P-G) axis. The study group included 12 professional cyclists, 9 elite triathletes, 10 recreational marathon runners, and 9 sedentary controls. All reported to the laboratory on 3 occasions for hormonal measurements, semen ejaculate analysis, and determination of body fat percentage. Test session times corresponded to precompetition (winter), competition (spring), and rest (fall) periods. Comparisons in measured parameters were made within groups, between groups in each of the 3

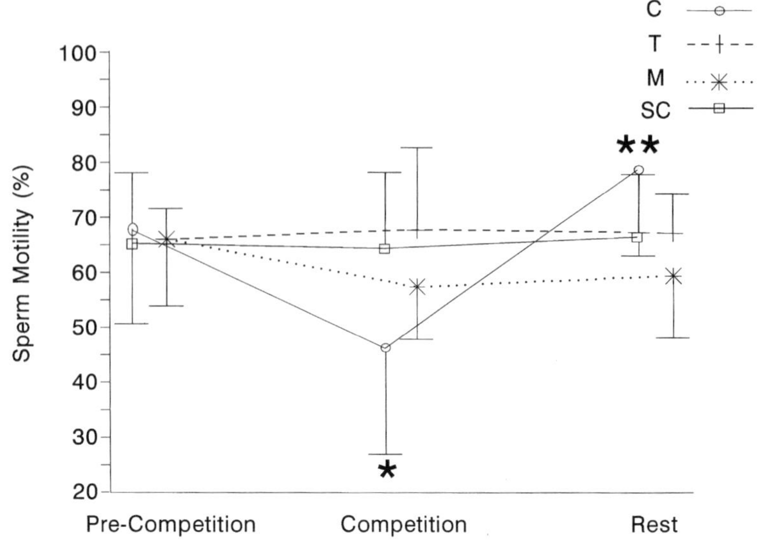

FIGURE 8.—Seminal analysis: sperm motility. Values are means ± SD. *C vs. T, M, and SC in competition period, $P < 0.05$; and C in competition period vs. other 2 periods, $P < 0.01$. **C vs. M in rest period, $P < 0.05$. *Abbreviations:* C, cyclists; T, triathletes; M, marathoners; SC, sedentary controls. (Courtesy of Lucía A, Chicharro JL, Pérez M, et al: Reproductive function in male endurance athletes: Sperm analysis and hormonal profile. *J Appl Physiol* 81:2627–2636, 1996.)

periods, and over time. Athletes also performed maximal exercise tests before the study protocol and were assessed for volume and intensity of training during the competition season.

Results.—Within-group comparisons for body fat showed no significant differences, except that marathon runners were significantly leaner during the competition period than they were during the rest period. In between-group comparisons, the percentage of body fat was higher in controls for all periods and was higher in marathoners than it was in cyclists. Average levels of all hormones evaluated were consistently within normal limits for all 4 groups throughout the study. Semen analysis yielded similar findings with few differences. One exception was a lower sperm motility (Fig 8) among cyclists during the competition period, an alteration that was transient and probably the result of friction against the saddle rather than alterations in the H-P-G axis.

Conclusion.—Men who participated in strenuous physical exercise, even at a professional level, did not exhibit any alterations in the H-P-G axis. Hormonal profiles and results of semen analysis were similar in athletes and sedentary controls.

► Feminists have long argued that there is little difference between men and women with regard to the temporary suppression of sexual function induced by repeated bouts of prolonged endurance exercise.[1] In both sexes, the anthropological reason for the phenomenon seems to be a need to avoid reproduction at times when a relative deficiency of food causes a negative energy balance. Commonly reported manifestations in men include reduced levels of total and free testosterone and alterations in the release of luteinizing hormone. There also have been suggestions that the ejaculate of high-mileage runners shows decreased sperm motility, an increased proportion of immature cells, and sperm with an abnormal morphology. In this report, the main clinical finding is a decreased sperm motility in distance cyclists at the time of peak training. The authors did not find any changes in the output of reproductive hormones (although they did not test the pulsatile secretion of luteinizing hormone or follicle-stimulating hormone). The cyclists showed an associated decrease in body fat, from a low initial value of 10.2% to 9.0%, in keeping with the anthropological hypothesis. Nevertheless, no hormonal changes were detected. Lucía et al thus advanced alternative explanations of their findings, such as testicular microtrauma or an increase of intrascrotal temperature. The main take-home message is that any exercise-induced changes in reproductive function are short-lived and, in these days of world overpopulation, should not be a major concern to competitors.

R.J. Shephard, M.D., Ph.D., D.P.E.

Reference

1. Pryor JL: Reproduction: Exercise-related adaptations and the health of women and men, in Bouchard C, Shephard RJ, Stephens T, et al (eds): *Exercise, Fitness and Health*. Champaign, Ill., Human Kinetics, 1990, pp 661–676.

Drug and Sport: Research Findings and Limitations
Clarkson PM, Thompson HS (Univ of Massachusetts, Amherst)
Sports Med 24:366–384, 1997   5–10

Introduction.—Although drug use may disqualify an athlete from competition, many types of drugs are used by athletes in an attempt to improve performance. The literature on 3 categories of drugs—stimulants, drugs used to reduce tremor or heart rate, and drugs used to alter body composition—was reviewed.

Stimulants.—Drugs used as stimulants to enhance performance include amphetamines, ephedrine, and cocaine. Amphetamines stimulate the CNS, causing release of noradrenaline from sympathetic nerves and possibly increasing the release of dopamine from the brain. Studies of the effects of amphetamines on performance, however, have yielded equivocal results. There is considerable variability among individual responses, and the drugs may actually diminish performance. Ephedrine, used in the treatment of asthma, causes an augmentation in myocardial contraction and cardiac output. The drug has also been used in an attempt to lose weight. Data on the effects of ephedrine on performance are limited. Cocaine stimulates the CNS and the sympathetic nervous system. Virtually no recent studies have examined the effects of cocaine on athletic performance, and none have proven to be beneficial.

Drugs Used to Reduce Tremor and Heart Rate.—Included in this category are β-adrenergic blockers, which can be useful in sports requiring steadiness, such as shooting and archery. Because of variations in individual responses, however, an athlete may experience a poorer performance after taking β-blockers.

Drugs to Alter Body Composition.—This category includes anabolic-androgenic steroids (AAS), human growth hormone (hGH), β-agonists, and diuretics. The use of anabolic-androgenic steroids during training does enhance strength and may provide significant psychological benefits. The effects of hGH are similar, promoting increased muscle strength or mass. Although most drug testing screens cannot detect hGH, its prohibitive cost has limited its use. When administered orally, β2-agonists such as clenbuterol and salbutamol appear to improve muscular strength. The body loss resulting from diuretics has led to their use in sports with strict body-weight classifications, but these agents may limit performance.

Conclusion.—Most drugs taken to enhance athletic performance produce a large interindividual variability in response. A particular drug may improve performance, have no effect, or have a negative effect. In highly trained athletes, the margin of improvement is often quite low. In addition, all of these drugs may have harmful health consequences.

▶ This comprehensive account of the various pharmacologic agents used to facilitate athletic performance is recommended reading for all those involved in the care of athletes. The authors emphasize many factors including the large variability in response, safety or lack thereof, and the fact that there is little research to substantiate the efficacy of many agents.

J.S. Torg, M.D.

General Practitioner Knowledge of Prohibited Substances in Sport
Greenway P, Greenway M (Langley Corner Surgery, West Sussex, England)
Br J Sports Med 31:129–131, 1997   5–11

Background.—In Britain, most sports-governing bodies subscribe to a list of prohibited substances for athletes, as published in the British National Formulary. But are general practitioners also aware of this list? Certainly these physicians are typically the first medical person an athlete seeks when he or she is not feeling well. This study evaluated the knowledge of general practitioners regarding which drugs are prohibited in athletes.

Methods.—Of 400 surveys sent to general practitioners in West Sussex, 157 were returned (39.2% response rate). The questionnaire asked 4 questions, as discussed below.

Results.—Question 1 asked whether the general practitioner knew where he or she could obtain the listing of prohibited substances; 35% gave the correct answer, 23% gave an incorrect answer, and 42% admitted they did not know. Question 2 addressed which specific drugs were prohibited; Table 2 reveals that from 15% (dihydrocodeine) to 80% (salbutamol) of practitioners gave a correct answer, and from 13% to 30% of general practitioners did not know. Question 3 asked whether anabolic steroids could be prescribed for nonmedical indications; 71% gave the correct answer of no, 12% answered yes, and 17% did not know. Finally, question 4 addressed whether the respondent had ever been asked to prescribe anabolic steroids for a nonmedical purpose; 18% had been asked, and 82% had not been asked.

Conclusions.—Controlling drug abuse among athletes requires the co-operation not only of the sports authority and the athlete, but also of the medical community at large. This study shows that general practitioners have room for improvement in understanding which substances are prohibited in athletes. Particularly as the list of prohibited drugs changes, a means of keeping the general practitioner aware of the list is sorely needed.

▶ I have long argued that the medical school and continuing education curricula for family physicians should focus less on medical curiosities that they are unlikely either to see or to treat, and more on preventive medicine, particularly appropriate management of the person who wishes to undertake vigorous physical activity. Most practitioners are likely to encounter a few people who are involved in competitive athletics, and the level of ignorance disclosed by this simple survey is disturbing, particularly since the 39% of respondents presumably comprised those who were best informed.

R.J. Shephard, M.D., Ph.D., D.P.E.

Trends in Anabolic-Androgenic Steroid Use Among Adolescents
Yesalis CE, Barsukiewicz CK, Kopstein AN, et al (Pennsylvania State Univ, University Park; Natl Inst on Drug Abuse, Rockville, Md; Human Kinetics Publishers, Champaign, Ill)
Arch Pediatr Adolesc Med 151:1197–1206, 1997   5–12

Objective.—Adolescents report using anabolic steroids to enhance athletic performance and to improve appearance. Because prolonged use may affect maturation, create psychologic dependence, and lead to other high-risk behaviors, a survey was conducted of secondary school students to examine the trends in adolescent steroid use in the United States since 1988.

Methods.—Local, state, and national cross-sectional surveys of illicit use of anabolic steroids by adolescents, aged 12 to 18 years, were identified through computer and manual searches. The surveys, using anonymous self-administered questionnaires, were conducted in the school or home by the Monitoring the Future study, the Youth Risk and Behavior Surveillance System and the National Household Survey on Drug Abuse.

Results.—Approximately 3% to 12% of adolescent boys and 0.5% to 2% of adolescent girls admitted to having used anabolic steroids. Youth Risk and Behavior Surveillance System 1995 data estimate that 375,000 boys and 175,000 girls have tried anabolic steroids at least once. Whereas the surveys show that anabolic steroid use by adolescent boys has remained the same or declined from the period 1991 to 1995, surveys reveal an increased use during this same period among adolescent girls. The latter trend is a cause for concern because some of the effects of androgenic steroids are irreversible. Although the veracity of self-reported survey results is always questionable, it is likely that any bias lies in the direction of underreporting.

Conclusion.—Traditional education and prevention programs using "scare tactics" have not been effective in stemming the use of anabolic steroids and may actually stimulate use out of curiosity. Combining traditional programs with approaches on how to combat peer and media pressure that teach resistance skills and are sex specific are recommended.

▶ We often review anabolic steroid use among adolescents.[1] This thoughtful, comprehensive article is an update by experts, worth reading in its entirety. It concludes that since 1991, steroid use by adolescent boys has remained stable but by adolescent girls has increased. Three percent to 12% of high school boys and 0.5% to 2% of high school girls admit to using steroids some time during their lives. Among other good reasons to try to deter use by adolescents, the increasing use by females is of particular concern because some of the androgenic effects in females are irreversible. These experts argue that our traditional "cognitive and affective approach" to prevention of steroid use has not worked well—and that "scare tactics" may even backfire. They think we should put more emphasis on a "social influence approach"—on teaching adolescents to recognize and resist peer and media pressures to use steroids.

E.R. Eichner, M.D.

Reference

1. 1994 Year Book of Sports Medicine, pp 345–349; pp 352–354.

Detection of Anabolic Steroid Administration: Ratio of Urinary Testosterone to Epitestosterone vs the Ratio of Urinary Testosterone to Luteinizing Hormone
Perry PJ, MacIndoe JH, Yates WR, et al (Univ of Iowa, Iowa City)
Clin Chem 43:731–735, 1997   5–13

Introduction.—The analysis of urinary steroids has been the primary method for detecting illicit anabolic steroid use. Although this method has been successful for most steroids, the detection and monitoring of anabolic compounds is not fail-safe. It is difficult, for example, to detect the illicit use of testosterone, a naturally occurring anabolic steroid. The luteinizing hormone is a potentially useful marker for detecting administration of exogenous testosterone, but it is unknown whether the testosterone to luteinizing hormone ratio is more sensitive than the testosterone to epitestosterone ratio, which was adopted by the Medical Commission of the International Olympic Committee in Los Angeles. Which laboratory test was more sensitive for the detection of the administration of exogenous testosterone was determined.

Methods.—Nineteen men were given testosterone cypionate injections of 250 or 500 mg/week for 14 weeks after 2 weekly placebo injections. They were then given 14 weeks of placebo injections. If patients had a negative test result 9 weeks after their last injection, they were considered to have ceased taking testosterone cypionate.

Results.—A false negative rate of 46% and a false positive rate of 4% were found with the detection of illicit or supraphysiologic testosterone cypionate use with the urinary testosterone to epitestosterone ratio of

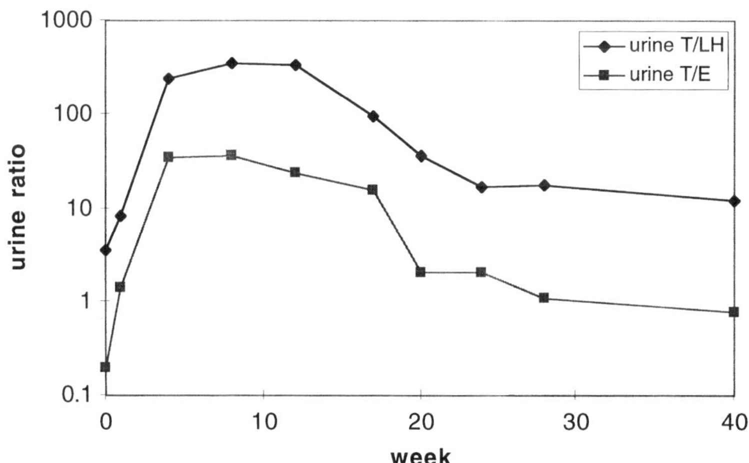

FIGURE 1.—Urine testosterone to luteinizing hormone (*T/LH*) ratios and testosterone to epitestosterone (*T/E*) ratios in 19 men receiving testosterone cypionate, 250 or 500 mg/week. (Courtesy of Perry PJ, MacIndoe JH, Yates WR, et al: Detection of anabolic steroid administration: Ratio of urinary testosterone to epitestosterone vs the ratio of urinary testosterone to luteinizing hormone. *Clin Chem* 43:731–735, 1997.)

greater than or equal to 6. A false negative rate of only 24% and a false positive rate of 13% were found with a urinary testosterone to luteinizing hormone ratio of greater than or equal to 30. One of every 2 participants using injectable testosterone cypionate will give a false negative urine drug screen during injection periods and for 9 weeks afterward with the testosterone to epitestosterone ratio cutoff of greater than or equal to 6, the traditional laboratory marker.

Conclusion.—The urinary testosterone to luteinizing hormone ratio of greater than or equal to 30 is a more sensitive marker of illicit or supraphysiologic testosterone cypionate use than is the urinary testosterone to epitestosterone ratio of greater than or equal to 30, and it is sensitive for twice as long as is the urinary testosterone to epitestosterone ratio (Fig 1).

▶ Many abusers of steroids have switched to testosterone preparations in recent years, and this has posed the need to evaluate critically the use of testosterone to epitestosterone ratios in the detection of this particular abuse. The ratio of 6:1, adopted by the Medical Commission of the International Olympic Committee in 1982, has inevitably led to some false accusations of doping, because some 0.8% of the general public who are not abusing anabolic steroids show a ratio that exceeds this arbitrary ceiling.[1] In the present study, the International Olympic Committee standard proved thoroughly unsatisfactory, with a false negative rate of 46%, and a false positive rate of 4%. Some investigators have suggested use of the testosterone to luteinizing hormone ratio as an alternative screening method; using a cut-off ratio of 30:1, this did not seem any more satisfactory than the testosterone to epitestosterone ratio, with a false negative rate of 24% and a disastrous false positive level of 13%. In assessing the proportion of false positive values, it may be noted that participants had been administering testosterone to themselves until 9 weeks before testing, although it was assumed that 97% of the effect of this treatment had abated. The actual numbers of false positive results were 2 and 4 cases for the 2 criteria. Observations are thus needed on a larger sample, including individuals who have never had anabolic hormones administered. Nevertheless, it is becoming clear that Olympic laboratories will never design a test that will detect all participants who have defied the rules of competition.

R.J. Shephard, M.D., Ph.D., D.P.E.

Reference

1. Catlin DH, Hatton CK: Use and abuse of anabolic and other drugs for athletic enhancement. *Adv Intern Med* 36:399–424, 1991.

Use of Filter Paper for Sample Collection and Transport in Steroid Pharmacology

Howe CJ, Handelsman DJ (Univ of Sydney, Australia)
Clin Chem 43:1408–1415, 1997   5–14

Purpose.—There are technical difficulties involved in performing pharmacologic studies of long-acting steroids in the field, including the need to collect, process, and store blood samples in a central facility. A simpler, less invasive method of obtaining blood samples is needed. Filter paper spots, already used in population screening programs, are investigated for use in measuring steroid concentrations.

Methods.—The study examines the feasibility of making pharmacokinetic and pharmacodynamic measurements of nandrolone and testosterone in capillary blood spots collected by fingerprick and dried on filter paper. The hormone radioimmunoassays were modified for use in extracts from capillary blood spots. Each punched spot measured 7.9 mm in diameter, and contains 14.9 µL of dried blood. The stability of the measurements was assessed under adverse conditions, such as high temperatures, in the laboratory. Field studies, with dried spots sent through the postal system, were also performed. In addition, a pilot pharmacologic study was done.

Results.—Assays in punched spots accurately measured levels of testosterone as low as 0.4 nmol/L from a single spot and of nandrolone down to 0.9 nmol/L from 2 spots. Under moderate environmental conditions of storage or postal transport, the apparent androgen concentrations were unaffected. Under extreme conditions—particularly storage at high temperatures—there was an increase in final nandrolone concentration and, to a lesser extent, testosterone (when corrected for tracer recovery). The tritiated tracer, rather than the unlabeled androgens, appeared susceptible to thermal degradation.

In the pilot pharmacologic study, subjects received IM injections of nandrolone decoanate, 100 mg, in 1 mL of arachis oil. There was good agreement between the nandrolone concentrations measured in concurrent plasma specimens and venous and capillary blood spots. Agreement was very high between testosterone concentrations measured in contemporaneous plasma specimens and venous blood spots.

Conclusion.—Dried blood spots on finger paper appear to be a useful technique for sample collection and transport in field studies of steroid pharmacology. This technique could allow subjects in the field to collect fingerprick blood samples themselves and mail them to a central laboratory for steroid measurements. The authors are conducting further studies for applying the filter paper technique.

▶ There is still a need for a simple method of sampling human steroid concentrations that could be widely applied in spot checks. Blood samples require rapid access to a specialized laboratory, and although the analysis of saliva specimens has shown some promise, steroid concentrations in saliva are low because of the absence of binding proteins, and samples are easily invalidated by minor oral abrasions that lead to contamination with blood or delays in analysis.

The results presented here suggest that some types of filter paper can be used successfully to collect, store, and analyze samples of capillary blood, at least under temperate conditions. However, the success of the analysis varies from 1 type of filter paper to another, and the accuracy of data deteriorates if samples are transported under hot conditions. The published figures show a surprisingly close correlation of reported concentrations between plasma samples and venous spots, and it will be interesting to see whether the technique can be refined sufficiently to allow an extension from its present pharmacologic and anthropologic applications to issues of athletic doping.

R.J. Shephard, M.D., Ph.D., D.P.E.

Exposure to Anabolic-Androgenic Steroids Shortens Life Span of Male Mice

Bronson FH, Matherne CM (Univ of Texas, Austin; Bayer Corp, West Haven, Conn)
Med Sci Sports Exerc 29:615–619, 1997   5–15

Introduction.—Some athletes and body builders take a variety of steroids at doses up to 40 times normal androgenic maintenance levels, often in combination with growth hormone and IGF-1. A pattern of steroid use and washout periods can continue for years. The potential pathologic consequences of exposure to anabolic-androgenic steroids were examined in male mice.

Methods.—The animals were assigned to 3 experimental groups that were matched for average and range of body mass. For a 6-month period, 2 groups were exposed to a combination of 4 anabolic-androgenic steroids at doses either 5 or 20 times greater than required to maintain normal-sized seminal vesicles in castrated CF-1 male mice. The third group served as a control. The kinds of steroids and their relative levels were intended to be similar to the usage of human athletes and body builders. Mice were followed up for age at death and cause of death; those not found dead but appearing moribund were killed.

Results.—By age 20 months, 26 of 50 (52%) male mice treated with the high dose of steroids had died or been killed. In contrast, 33% of those given the low dose and 12% of controls had died or been killed (Fig 1). In the steroid-treated groups, most of the mice dying before 1 year of age were found to have glomerulonephropathy; most of those dying after 1 year of age had tumors, usually in the liver and/or kidney. Other findings in steroid-treated animals included heart damage and pulmonary adenomas.

Discussion.—The number, kinds, and relative doses of steroids to which mice were exposed were comparable to those taken by athletes and body

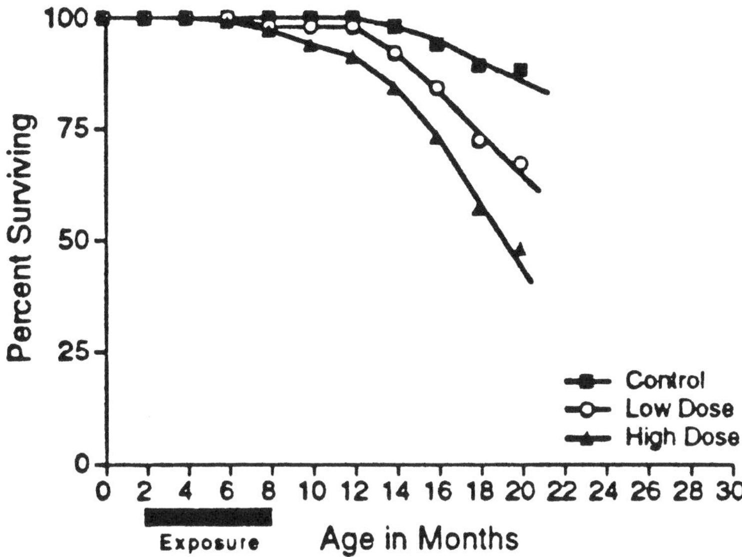

FIGURE 1.—Survival curves for male mice treated for 6 months with 1 or 2 doses of anabolic steroids vs. control males given no exogenous hormones. The experiment was terminated 1 year after exposure to steroids ceased when the survivors were 20 months old. At that time, 52% of the high dose males and 33% of the low dose males had died, compared with only 12% of the control males. (Courtesy of Bronson FH, Matherne CM: Exposure to anabolic-androgenic steroids shortens life span of male mice. *Med Sci Sports Exerc* 29:615–619, 1997.)

builders. Duration of exposure in male mice, however, amounted to about one fifth of their life expectancy. This extreme exposure to steroids reduced the animals' life span and produced a broad array of pathologic effects.

▶ There are many anecdotal reports that the abuse of androgenic steroids can lead to hepatic carcinoma, but there seem to be only 13 or 14 cases actually detailed in the medical literature. It is plainly unethical to conduct deliberate experiments to induce such tumors in human subjects, and there is, thus, some interest in what happens when small mammals are given androgenic steroids over long periods. Bronson and Matherne were careful to match the dose given to their mice with that used by unscrupulous athletes (5 to 20 times normal maintenance levels), but the duration of exposure (6 months) was equal to a fifth of the mice's life span, much longer than would be likely for most athletes. The pattern of exposure (continuous administration, without "time out") was also atypical of human doping schedules. Nevertheless, the types of liver damage observed (peliosis hepatis and hepatocytic carcinoma) seem typical of what has been described in human cases. It is particularly disturbing that many of the more serious pathologies did not appear until long after the steroid administration had ceased, raising the disquieting possibility that an undetected "iceberg" of adverse effects may yet develop in athletes that have abused androgens in large doses over the past 10–20 years.

R.J. Shephard, M.D., Ph.D., DPE

6 Medical Conditions

High Incidence of Scintigraphic Myocardial Uptake Defects at Rest and During Exercise in Male Elite Runners
Bouvier F, Nejat M, Berglund B, et al (South Hosp, Stockholm; Karolinska Hosp, Stockholm; Huddinge Univ, Sweden)
Heart 77:252–255, 1997   6–1

Introduction.—The prevalence of ischemic heart disease is increasing in younger patients, particularly males. Ischemic heart disease is of concern, even among athletes younger than 30 years. Single photon emission tomography (SPECT) is a valuable tool for diagnosis of ischemic disease. Normal values for SPECT are based mostly on data from older and relatively untrained men and women. Norms for these values may be different for young athletes. Maximum exercise stress and rest scintigraphy were performed in healthy male elite runners and compared with semiquantitative scintigraphic data from 2 reference groups.

Methods.—Sixteen healthy male elite runners, a reference group of 11 sedentary or moderately physically active men (Swedish group), and a commonly used reference group from Emory University Hospital underwent stress-rest myocardial scintigraphy (MIBI-SPECT), polar map reconstruction with and without uniform attenuation correction.

Results.—Compared to the 2 reference groups, most runners had uptake defects on polar maps. When compared to the Swedish group, 13 of 16 runners had defects during stress and 11 of 16 had defects during rest. Defects during stress and rest were detected in 10 of 16 runners, when compared to the American reference group. Ninety-one percent of defects were fixed and were located in the anterior, lateral, and posterior regions of the left ventricle. Use of a uniform attenuation correlation algorithm enhanced rather than decreased perfusion defect size.

Conclusion.—If myocardial perfusion scintigraphy is used with SPECT to assess elite athletic males, the existing normal reference files for semiquantitative evaluation may be inadequate.

▶ The number of diagnostic errors that arise from the performance of laboratory tests on symptom-free individuals is rapidly approaching crisis proportions. In consequence, patients and insuring agencies face much unnecessary expense, there is unwarranted limitation of physical activity, and often iatrogenic "disease." The present study demonstrates once more how widely test results differ between well-trained athletes and the general public, and how fallacious it can be to use norms based on sedentary individuals when advising well-trained subjects. There is much to commend the practice of my mentor, the late Dr. Maurice Campbell, founding editor of the *British Heart Journal*. He would never allow any special investigation until the physician under his supervision had reached a diagnosis on the basis of a careful history and clinical examination.

R.J. Shephard, M.D., Ph.D., D.P.E.

An Echocardiographic Study Comparing Male Swedish Elite Orienteers With Older Elite Endurance Athletes

Henriksen E, Landelius J, Wesslén L, et al (Central Hosp, Västerås, Sweden; Univ Hosp, Uppsala, Sweden; Karolinska Inst, Stockholm; et al)
Am J Cardiol 79:521–524, 1997   6–2

Background.—In orienteering, a popular sport in Sweden, athletes find (with map and compass) and traverse on foot the fastest path through rough terrain. The sport is intensely physical, and some elite orienteers have participated despite symptoms of respiratory tract infection. From 1979 to 1992, 16 young (mean age 25 years) Swedish orienteers (15 male) had sudden unexpected cardiac death; 5 had reported heart symptoms. Myocarditis was common at autopsy, suggesting electric instability and ventricular arrhythmias as the cause of death.

Methods.—The study group was 96 young (mean age 22 years) elite male orienteers age-matched with 47 control elite male endurance athletes similar in height, body mass, body surface area, and heart rate. Echocardiography with color-flow mapping and continuous and pulsed spectral Doppler recording were performed with ECG.

Results.—Most left and right cavities and left ventricular wall measurements were slightly larger in controls than orienteers. Left ventricular wall motion abnormalities (mild hypokinesia and 2 cases of severe hypokinesia or akinesia) were found in 9 orienteers (9%) and 2 control subjects (4%), with samples too small for statistical significance. Mean number of abnormal segments was 2.8 in orienteers and 2 in controls. There were no abnormalities in the right ventricular wall. Five orienteers had abnormalities on ECGs, but abnormal wall motion and abnormalities on ECG were concurrent in only 1 case.

Conclusions.—Similar unexpected deaths have not been seen in other Swedish endurance sports, and no cardiac deaths in orienteers have been reported since November 1992. This may be because of advice to reduce training and competition for 6 months and also not to train or compete when infectious symptoms are present.

▶ Scandinavian sports physicians were concerned by a rash of unexpected deaths among orienteers during the period 1979 to 1992.[1] Uncharitable individuals speculated that this might reflect some form of doping, such as

the administration of hemopoietin. Autopsy suggested myocarditis in 12 of 16 cases, raising a second possibility of immunosuppression by sustained endurance effort, with localization of unrestrained viruses to the heart. None of the group met recent criteria for hypertrophic cardiomyopathy,[2] and it is unlikely that the incidents could have been avoided by a preliminary clinical examination. There remain 2 puzzling features of the episode: an absence of similar deaths in other types of endurance sports, and a disappearance of the problem since 1992. Possibly, the string of deaths prompted sports physicians to issue stronger warnings against competing when symptoms of infection were apparent.[1]

R.J. Shephard, M.D., Ph.D., D.P.E.

References

1. Wesslén L, Pählson C, Lindqvist O, et al: An increase in sudden unexpected cardiac deaths among young Swedish orienteers during 1979–1992. *Eur Heart J* 17:902–910, 1996.
2. Maron BJ, Pellicia A, Spirito P: Cardiac disease in young trained athletes: Insights into methods for distinguishing athlete's heart from structural heart disease, with particular emphasis on hypertrophic cardiomyopathy. *Circulation* 91:1596–1601, 1995.

Basic Fibroblast Growth Factor as a Biochemical Marker of Exercise-induced Ischemia

Gu J-W, Santiago D, Olowe Y, et al (Columbia-Presbyterian Med Ctr, New York)
Circulation 95:1165–1168, 1997
6–3

Background.—Several biochemical markers may be used in the diagnosis of myocardial infarction. However, there are currently no reliable biochemical tests available to complement the clinical, imaging, and ECG techniques used in the diagnosis of myocardial ischemia. Basic fibroblast growth factor (bFGF) is a mitogenic polypeptide secreted in response to ischemia or hypoxia that is more intensely expressed during myocardial ischemia in animal models. Concentrations of bFGF are elevated in patients with 1 of several types of tumors and are detectable in the urine of these patients. The usefulness of urinary bFGF as a marker of exercise-induced ischemia was evaluated.

Methods.—Eighty-six patients completed an exercise thallium study for evaluation of chest pain during 4 months at a single hospital. Each patient was tested for myocardial ischemia by ECG and/or scan guidelines during the procedure. Urine bFGF concentration was determined for each patient by enzyme-linked immunosorbent assay 2–4 hours after exercise. Concentrations of bFGF were corrected for glomerular filtration rate by comparison with urine creatinine concentrations and were expressed as the ratio of bFGF to creatinine (pg/g).

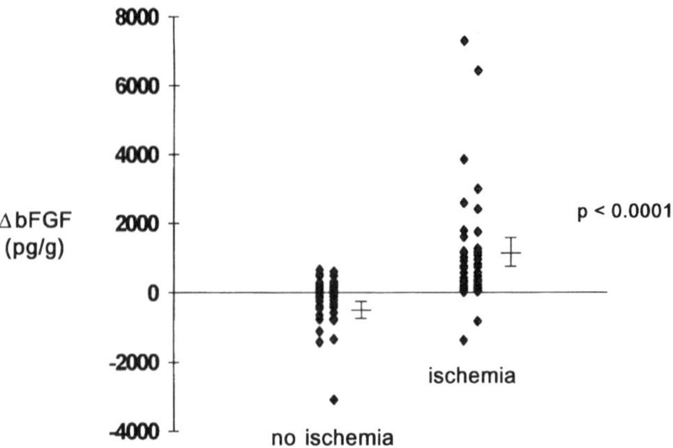

FIGURE.—Scatterplot showing the change in urine basic fibroblast growth factor (*bFGF*) after exercise for patients with and without exercise-induced ischemia. Error bars represent mean ± standard error of the mean. (Courtesy of Gu J-W, Santiago D, Olowe Y, et al: Basic fibroblast growth factor as a biochemical marker of exercise-induced ischemia. *Circulation* 95:1165–1168, 1997. Reproduced with permission of *Circulation*. Copyright 1997, American Heart Association.)

Results.—Exercise-induced myocardial ischemia occurred in 43 (50%) of the 86 patients. Increased urine bFGF concentrations were strongly associated with occurrence of myocardial ischemia during exercise, changing by 1,052 or −278 pg/g in patients with or without myocardial ischemia, respectively ($P < 0.0001$) (Figure). Urine bFGF concentrations of greater than 700 pg/g were indicative of myocardial ischemia in each of the 21 patients with values in this range.

Conclusions.—Exercise-induced myocardial ischemia, defined by thallium scintigraphy and ECG, is associated with an increased urinary excretion of bFGF. Additional research is needed to define more fully the utility of this biochemical marker in clinical diagnosis of myocardial ischemia.

▶ Despite advances in our understanding of enzyme markers of myocardial infarction, it takes several days to get a clear picture of creatine kinase and serum glutamic oxalacetic transaminase changes. It is thus of considerable interest that bFGF can be detected a few hours after myocardial ischemia that has been documented by ECG and thallium scintigraphy. However, there remains a need for substantially more research before these observations can be used to form a clinical test. There is no isoform to distinguish skeletal from cardiac muscle ischemia, and there is some evidence that exercise can cause a release of bFGF even in the absence of clinically significant ischemia. Further, urinary concentrations of this substance will be influenced by the volume of urine production and the timing of urine samples relative to a putative ischemic incident.

R.J. Shephard, M.D., Ph.D., D.P.E.

Significance of Slow Upsloping ST-Segment Depression on Exercise Stress Testing
Sansoy V, Watson DD, Beller GA (Univ of Virginia, Charlottesville)
Am J Cardiol 79:709–712, 1997
6–4

Introduction.—Demonstration of at least 1.0 mm of horizontal or downsloping ST-segment depression is the standard indication of an abnormal exercise test. This study examined the supplementary value of varying degrees of upsloping ST-segment depression recorded during treadmill exercise testing to the accuracy of the exercise ST-segment response for detection of ischemia.

Methods.—Patients included in the study were undergoing testing in conjunction with ^{201}Tl imaging over a 1-year period. Of 456 found to have ^{201}Tl redistribution, 199 met the study criteria, 168 men (mean age 58 years) and 31 women (mean age 61 years). The normal population consisted of 336 patients with a normal ^{201}Tl scintigram, 168 men (mean age 51 years) and 31 women (mean age 54 years). Upsloping ST-segment depression during a symptom-limited or submaximal exercise test was considered positive if the ST segment was still depressed $\geq$1.0, $\geq$1.5, or $\geq$2.0 mm below the baseline at 0.08 seconds after the J point. Patients were encouraged to exercise for an additional 60 seconds after 2.0 mCi of ^{201}Tl was injected intravenously at peak exercise. Planar images were acquired 5 minutes after exercise and 2.5–3 hours later. Exercise ECG results were reviewed without knowledge of thallium-201 imaging results.

Results.—The exercise ECG was normal in 61% of the normal patients; 55 had $\geq$1.0 mm horizontal or downsloping ST-segment depression, 24 had $\geq$1.5 mm, and 9 had $\geq$2.0 mm upsloping ST-segment depression. In the coronary artery disease group, 98 had $\geq$1.0 mm horizontal ST-segment depression; 25 had $\geq$1.0 mm, 13 had $\geq$1.5 mm, and 6 had $\geq$2.0 mm upsloping ST-segment depression. The addition of upsloping ST-segment depression to the criteria for a positive exercise test result increased sensitivity for detection of ischemia (Table 1), but specificity decreased, and the positive predictive value of the test was significantly lower.

Discussion.—Findings confirm that ^{201}Tl redistribution is more prevalent than horizontal or downsloping ST-segment depression for detection of ischemia. Only 49% of patients in this series with reversible ^{201}Tl defects had at least 1.0 mm horizontal or downsloping ST segment. No matter what criterion is used with respect to upsloping ST-segment depression, there is a significant reduction in the positive predictive value of the ST-segment response.

▶ It is easy to recognize and interpret a horizontal or downsloping ST segment that develops during exercise. However, a larger proportion of records shows an upsloping ST segment, and the question arises whether such observations can be used to increase the information yield from an exercise ECG. A recent trial found that even if only massive upward ST slopes (beginning from a depression of less than 20 mm at the J point) are

TABLE 1.—Sensitivity, Specificity, and Accuracy of Varying Degrees of Upsloping ST-Segment Depression When Added to Horizontal or Downsloping ST-Segment Depression for Detection of Ischemia

ST-Segment Depression	Sensitivity (%)	Specificity (%)	Positive Predictive Value (%)	Negative Predictive Value (%)	Accuracy (%)
≥ 1.0 mm of horizontal or downsloping	49	84	64	74	71
Addition of:					
1) ≥2.0 mm upsloping	52, p = 0.31 (NS)	81, p = 0.21 (NS)	62	74	70, p = 0.89 (NS)
2) ≥1.5 mm upsloping	59, p = 0.035	74, p = 0.001	57	75	68, p = 039 (NS)
3) ≥1.0 mm upsloping	71, p <0.0001	56, p <0.0001	49	77	61, p = 0.0015

(Courtesy of Sansoy V, Watson DD, Beller GA: Significance of slow upsloping ST-segment depression on exercise stress testing. *Am J Cardiol* 79:709–712, 1997. Reprinted by permission of the publisher. Copyright 1997 by Excerpta Medica, Inc.)

considered, the accuracy of ECG interpretation is less than an assessment based on the traditional criteria of horizontal or downsloping ST segments.

R.J. Shephard, M.D., Ph.D., D.P.E.

Simple Clinical Data Are Useful In Predicting Effect of Exercise Training After Myocardial Infarction

Heldal M, Sire S, Sandvik L, et al (Aker Univ Hosp, Oslo, Norway; State Rehabilitation Inst, Oslo, Norway; Med Stat Research, Lillestrom, Norway)
Eur Heart J 17:1821–1827, 1996　　　　　　　　　　　　　　　　6–5

Introduction.—A study of patients who entered a cardiac rehabilitation program after myocardial infarction sought to identify variables that might predict increase in exercise capacity. Because most participants in such programs have been middle-aged men, physicians may be less likely to direct older patients and women to exercise training.

Methods.—During a 2.5 year period, 309 patients ages 68 or younger were discharged alive from the study institution after myocardial infarction; 170 met entry criteria, and 142 were eventually included in the training program. Of these patients, 37 dropped out or were excluded from analysis, leaving 105 in the final evaluation. Patients exercised for 2 hours daily, 5 days a week for 4 weeks. The aim was to achieve a heart rate 85% of the maximum achieved at the first exercise test. Training effect was defined as an absolute increase in cumulative work from pretraining to posttraining exercise tests. Twenty-eight variables were selected as possible predictors of a training effect.

Results.—Patients who completed the training program demonstrated a 49% increase in mean cumulative work, from 46.7 to 69.5 kJ. The following 3 discrete variables were significantly related to the training effect in univariate analysis: (1) male sex, (2) angina pectoris at the start of training, and (3) the ability to exercise to exhaustion at the baseline exercise test (Table 2). The following 5 variables were identified in multi-

TABLE 2.—Discrete Variables Significantly Associated With the Training Effect in Univariate Analysis

	n	CW baseline	CW incease	
Gender				
Males	83	51·2 ± 22·6	24·9 ± 18·5	*P*<0.001
Females	22	29·7 ± 12·6	14·9 ± 9·6	
Angina pectoris at start of training				
+	30	40·3 ± 17·2	18·5 ± 19·3	*P*=0.037
−	75	49·2 ± 24·1	24·5 ± 16·5	
Ability to exercise to exhaustion at baseline exercise test				
+	82	48·8 ± 24·.0	25·1 ± 18·1	*P*=0.0013
−	23	41·4 ± 16·3	14·4 ± 11·7	

Abbreviation: CW, cumulative work (kJ). The study population (n = 105) is divided according to parameter label. *P* values are for between-group differences in the training effect.

(Courtesy of Heldal M, Sire S, Sandvik L, et al: Simple clinical data are useful in predicting effect of exercise training. *Eur Heart J* 17:1821–1827, 1996. Copyright 1996. Reprinted by permission of the publisher, W B Saunders Company Limited London.)

variate analysis as having a significant independent relationship to the training effect: (1) peak aspartate aminotransferase, (2) higher age, (3) male sex, (4) β-blocker treatment, and (5) the ability to exercise to exhaustion at baseline. These 5 variables explained one third of the variations in effect from training.

Discussion.—Exercise training is beneficial after myocardial infarction, but not all patients will increase their exercise capacity. Five simple clinical parameters can be used to predict improvement in exercise capacity. Older age and treatment with β-blockers were associated with a lower effect from training. Myocardial infarct size, male sex, and ability to exercise to exhaustion at baseline predicted a better training effect.

▶ It has long been realized that not all postcoronary patients respond to a training program. Some, possibly because of old age or more extensive cardiac damage, show little increase of aerobic function with training.[1] The present study confirms the importance of age and infarct size to exercise response. It also notes a better response in men than in women and in those who are able to exercise to exhaustion, along with an adverse response in those receiving β-blocker treatment. The issue that has received the greatest discussion in recent years is the poor response of women. There seem a number of reasons for this. Women generally sustain a myocardial infarction at an older age than men. Doctors are less likely to refer women to a formal cardiac rehabilitation program, and, in part because of family responsibilities, women are more likely than men to drop out or to have a sporadic attendance at exercise classes. Where women complete a full rehabilitation program, their response does not seem to differ from that of the men.

R.J. Shephard, M.D., Ph.D., D.P.E.

Reference

1. Kavanagh T, Shephard RJ, Doney H, et al: Intensive exercise in coronary rehabilitation. *Med Sci Sports* 5:34–39, 1973.

Non-invasive Measurement of Cardiac Output and Ventricular Ejection Fractions in Chronic Cardiac Failure: Relationship to Impaired Exercise Tolerance
Steele IC, Moore A, Nugent A-M, et al (Royal Victoria Hosp, Belfast, Northern Ireland)
Clin Sci (Colch) 93:195–203, 1997 6–6

Introduction.—There are continued questions regarding how cardiac output limitation affects exercise pathophysiology in patients with chronic cardiac failure (CCF). Patients with CCF and controls show comparable oxygen intake during steady-state exercise; the possible differences in cardiac output are unknown. This study compares cardiac output re-

sponses to steady-state submaximal exercise between patients with CCF and controls.

Methods.—The study included 10 men with stable CCF and 10 age-matched controls. All patients performed a 3-day series of exercise tests, consisting of a familiarization exercise test, a symptom-limited maximal exercise test, and 2 submaximal exercise tests. The carbon dioxide rebreathing method was used to measure cardiac output. Other measurements included oxygen consumption, ventilation, Borg-perceived level of exertion, venous lactate concentration, and ejection fraction. The data were analyzed to see whether the reduced exercise tolerance of the CCF group was related to reduced cardiac output or to peripheral factors.

Results.—Median peak oxygen consumption was 1.18 L/min in the CCF group vs. 1.935 L/min in the control group. The CCF group also had a lower peak venous lactate concentration, although there was no difference in overall level of perceived exertion. During submaximal exercise at a similar absolute work-rate, oxygen consumption was 0.67 L/min in the CCF group and 0.62 L/min in the control group; cardiac outputs were 6.92 and 7.3 L/min, respectively. However, the CCF group had a higher level of perceived exertion, (4 vs. 3), higher venous lactate concentration (1.6 vs. 1.14 mmol/L), and faster heart rate (106 vs. 87 beats/min).

Conclusion.—In response to submaximal exercise, patients with cardiac failure have lower exercise tolerance but similar maximal oxygen intake and cardiac output compared with controls. Heart rate is increased in patients with CCF to maintain cardiac output in the presence of reduced stroke volume. The findings suggest that peripheral factors—as opposed to abnormalities of central cardiac function—play a key role in the abnormal exercise response of patients with CCF.

▶ The last few years have seen a remarkable transition in the treatment of patients with stable congestive heart failure. It is now recognized that substantial improvements in both functional capacity and the quality of life result from participation in a program of progressive exercise rehabilitation. However, there is little relationship between initial disability and the cardiac ejection fraction, and many authors find little change in cardiac output after patient participation in a program that leads to substantial functional gains.

The study of Steele et al. sits a little uneasily on the fence between a central and a peripheral limitation of function. A normal relationship of cardiac output to oxygen consumption is suggested for a given intensity of submaximal exercise, but the authors rightly warn that this conclusion may be compromised by difficulties in applying the CO_2 rebreathing method to patients with congestive heart failure. Further, the greater increase in blood lactate, respiratory gas exchange ratio, and rating of perceived exertion relative to healthy individuals points to some peripheral limitation of function, perhaps as a consequence of the deconditioning of muscles.

R.J. Shephard, M.D., Ph.D., D.P.E.

Exercise-related Ventilatory Abnormalities and Survival in Congestive Heart Failure

MacGowan GA, Janosko K, Cecchetti A, et al (Univ of Pittsburgh, Pa)
Am J Cardiol 79:1264–1266, 1997   6–7

Purpose.—With a shortage of available hearts for transplantation, it is important to identify those patients with congestive heart failure who are at greatest short-term risk. Although peak exercise oxygen consumption and right ventricular function provide useful information, other variables are needed to help identify patients for priority transplantation. Ventilatory equivalent for carbon dioxide was studied for its ability to provide additional prognostic information beyond that provided by peak oxygen consumption.

Methods.—Exercise tests with gas exchange analyses were performed in 104 patients with chronic heart failure who were being considered for cardiac transplantation. Most patients had idiopathic dilated cardiomyopathy or ischemic cardiomyopathy and were in New York Heart Association class 2 or 3. The tests included ventilation studies. The ratio of minute ventilation to carbon dioxide production at anaerobic threshold was the definition of the ventilatory equivalent for carbon dioxide.

Results.—The patients were followed up for a mean of 1.5 years after exercise testing. Seventy-four patients were still alive, 18 were dead, and 12 had undergone cardiac transplantation. Mean ventilatory equivalent for carbon dioxide was 35 in survivors vs. 47 in nonsurvivors (Fig 1). Peak oxygen consumption was 17 vs. 13, respectively. In that order, these were the 2 variables most significantly different between survivors and nonsur-

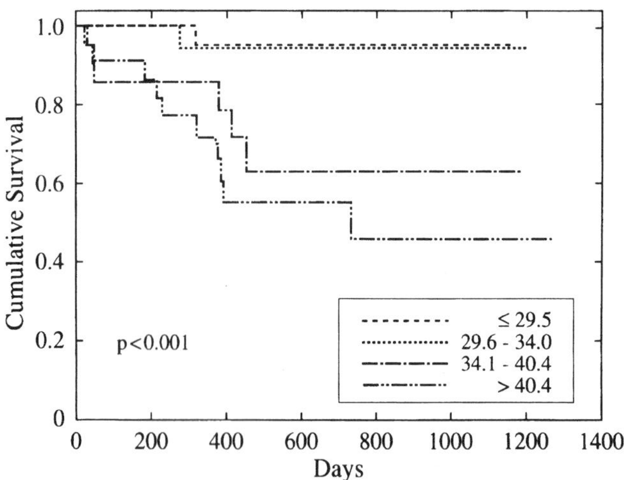

FIGURE 1.—Survival curves for the ventilatory equivalent for carbon dioxide at anaerobic threshold divided into 4 groups based on the range of values in each quartile. (Reprinted by permission of the publisher, from MacGowan GA, Janosko K, Cecchetti A, et al: Exercise-related ventilatory abnormalities and survival in congestive heart failure. *Am J Cardiol* 79:1264–1266, Copyright 1997 by Excerpta Medica, Inc.)

vivors on univariate analysis. On Cox proportional hazards modeling, survival tended to be related to the ventilatory equivalent for carbon dioxide and was unrelated to peak exercise oxygen consumption. Eighty-nine percent of patients who died had a peak oxygen consumption of 15 mL/[kg·min}. Among patients at this level of peak oxygen consumption, ventilatory equivalent for carbon dioxide differentiated between survivors and nonsurvivors, whereas peak oxygen consumption did not. These 2 values were used to construct an index for predicting survival; the index had a specificity of 93%, sensitivity of 56%, and accuracy of 79%.

Conclusions.—In patients with chronic heart failure, the ventilatory equivalent for carbon dioxide, measured at anaerobic threshold, provides prognostic information in addition to that provided by peak oxygen consumption. The index described in this study, consisting of peak oxygen consumption and ventilatory equivalent for carbon dioxide, may be useful in identifying which patients should be considered high priority for cardiac transplantation. The index has high sensitivity, though only modest specificity.

▶ An increase in patient demands for cardiac transplantation, coupled with a laudable decrease in the number of fatalities from drunk driving, has caused a rapid lengthening of waiting lists for this type of surgery. It is thus important to screen waiting lists carefully to determine who really needs such treatment. MacGowan and associates here suggest that ventilatory abnormalities including the ventilatory equivalent for carbon dioxide provide a valuable indication of patients who have poor survival prospects. When a ventilatory equivalent for carbon dioxide in excess of 50 is combined with a peak oxygen intake of less than 15 mL/kg/min, there is a strong probability of early death (specificity 93%, sensitivity 56%). For the intended screening purpose, the authors suggest that a high specificity is more important than a high sensitivity.

R.J. Shephard, M.D., Ph.D., D.P.E.

Physical Training Improves Exercise Capacity in Patients With Mitral Stenosis After Balloon Valvuloplasty
Douard H, Chevalier L, Labbe L, et al (Hôpital Cardiologique du Haut Lévèque, Pessac, France)
Eur Heart J 18:464–469, 1997   6–8

Introduction.—Percutaneous mitral valvuloplasty is an effective curative treatment for patients with severe mitral valve stenosis. The excellent hemodynamic results are often in contrast with the disappointing functional results. However, training can increase exercise capacity, even in patients with severe cardiac failure. Twenty-six patients with mitral stenosis were evaluated to determine the potential of physical training to improve physical capacity after balloon valvuloplasty.

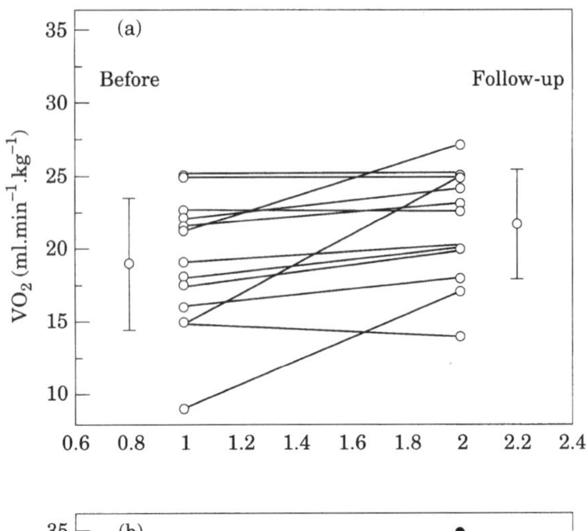

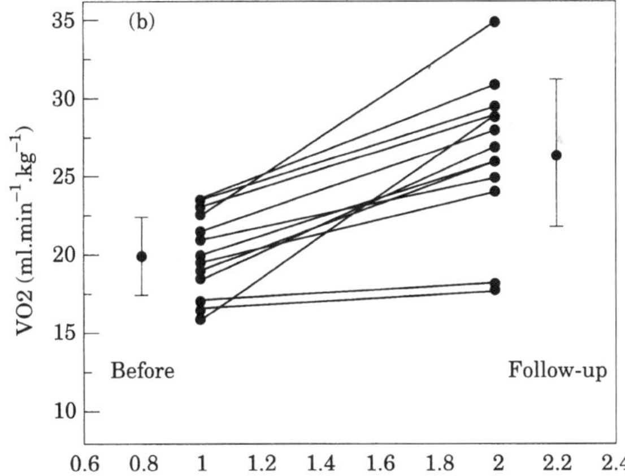

FIGURE 1.—Peak $\dot{V}O_2$ before and after percutaneous transvenous mitral commissurotomy in control (**A**) and trained (**B**) patients. (Reprinted from Douard H, Chevalier L, Labbe L, et al: Physical training improves exercise capacity in patients with mitral stenosis after balloon valvuloplasty. *Eur Heart J* 18:464–469, 1997, by permission of the publisher WB Saunders Company Limited London.)

Methods.—After balloon valvuloplasty, 13 patients participated in a 3-month rehabilitation program and the 13 patients who did not acted as controls. Respiratory gas analysis was performed during exercise tests performed 24 hours before and 3 months after valvuloplasty.

Results.—Patients in the training and control groups had similar increases in the mitral valve orifice area. Between-group cardiopulmonary parameters were similar before valvuloplasty. Patients in the training group had significant increases in peak workrate, peak oxygen uptake, $\dot{V}O_2$, and $\dot{V}O_2$ at anaerobic threshold (Figure 1).

Conclusion.—Patients with mitral stenosis who undergo balloon valvuloplasty can benefit considerably from regular exercise.

▶ The benefits of an exercise rehabilitation program subsequent to surgery have been demonstrated for many types of cardiac patients. The present report shows a striking 3-month advantage of exercised patients vs. some well-matched controls after mitral valvuloplasty. There remains a need for a longer-term follow-up, to see if the exercise program merely speeds the rehabilitation process, or whether it confers a permanent advantage relative to controls who receive standard treatment.

R.J. Shephard, M.D., Ph.D., D.P.E.

The Asthmatic Athlete: Metabolic and Ventilatory Responses to Exercise With and Without Pre-exercise Medication
Ienna TM, McKenzie DC (Univ of British Columbia, Vancouver, Canada)
Int J Sports Med 18:142–148, 1997   6–9

Introduction.—The severity of bronchoconstriction in athletes with exercise-induced asthma (EIA) is influenced by the type, duration, and intensity of exercise and by environmental conditions. Inhaled salbutamol, often used as a preventive measure, can virtually abolish bronchoconstriction when taken 10 to 15 minutes before exercise. A group of athletes with asthma was studied to determine whether they would have normal physiological responses to exercise without pre-exercise medication.

Methods.—The study group included highly trained athletes (5 women and 4 men with a mean age of 26) and moderately trained athletes (7 men and 1 woman, mean age 24 years). All had EIA and all but 3 had a history of asthma. A methacholine challenge test was used to assess bronchial reactivity of each participant, and each performed a maximal oxygen uptake test. Both groups of athletes were studied under 2 conditions: salbutamol, 200 µg taken via inhaler 15 minutes before exercise or placebo. Two exercise tests were completed about 1 week apart.

Results.—Highly trained and moderately trained athletes differed in maximal oxygen consumption, but men and women did not differ in this measure. Placebo or salbutamol pretreatments did not differ in their effects on oxygen consumption, minute ventilation, heart rate, respiratory exchange ratio, % saturation, and blood lactate. Among highly trained athletes, however, mean heart rate averaged over the 4 exercise conditions was significantly higher under the placebo condition. Pre-exercise peak expiratory flow rates (PEFR) were significantly higher when salbutamol was the pretreatment (Fig 1).

Discussion.—Both highly trained and moderately trained athletes with EIA had normal physiological responses during submaximal and maximal exercise, and no differences were found in measured responses with salbutamol or placebo pretreatment. Salbutamol was confirmed to be an effective bronchodilator; mean PEFR measures during exercise and recovery conditions were significantly higher with this medication than with placebo.

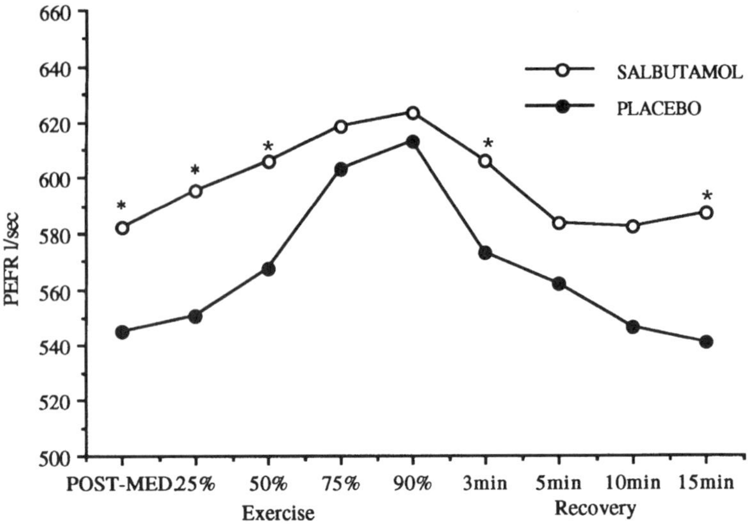

FIGURE 1.—PEFR ($1 \cdot sec^{-1}$) measures during exercise and recovery, all subjects data (n = 17). Mean (*p >0.05). *Abbreviation: PEFR,* peak expiratory flow rate. (Courtesy of Ienna TM, McKenzie DC: The asthmatic athlete: Metabolic and ventilatory responses to exercise with and without pre-exercise medication. *Int J Sports Med* 18:142–148, 1997. Georg Thieme Verlag.)

▶ As many as 11% of athletes competing in the Olympic Games claim to suffer from some form of asthma, although in some individuals this may be a pretext for the use of drugs that they hope will enhance their performance. There has been much discussion as to whether drugs used for the relief of asthma do indeed enhance endurance performance. The article by Ienna and McKenzie shows that a standard dose of inhaled salbutamol (the permitted route of administration for international competitors) had no influence on systemic metabolic parameters.

The authors note the well-accepted finding that some top level athletes develop arterial unsaturation during intensive effort. The probable reason for this arterial unsaturation is a dispersion of ventilation/perfusion ratios, so that there is inadequate time for equilibration of gas pressures between the alveoli and the capillaries in those alveoli that have rapidly perfused capillaries. Thus, the present authors had anticipated that such problems might be made worse by asthma. In fact, they were not, in part because the asthma was not very severe, even at rest, and in part because enough catecholamines were secreted during maximal exercise to overcome bronchoconstriction in both salbutamol-treated and placebo groups.

R.J. Shephard, M.D., Ph.D., D.P.E.

Qualitative Aspects of Exertional Breathlessness in Chronic Airflow Limitation
O'Donnell DE, Bertley JC, Chau LKL, et al (Queen's Univ, Kingston, Ont, Canada)
Am J Respir Crit Care Med 155:109–115, 1997   6–10

Background.—For most patients with severe chronic airflow limitation (CAL), breathlessness is the major symptom limiting exercise tolerance. In normal subjects, breathing discomfort known as dyspnea limits exercise capacity. It is unknown whether the symptoms experienced by patients with CAL and normal subjects are qualitatively different or different only in magnitude. The qualitative nature of exercise-induced breathlessness was compared for patients with CAL vs. normal controls, with attention to the physiologic rationale for any differences observed.

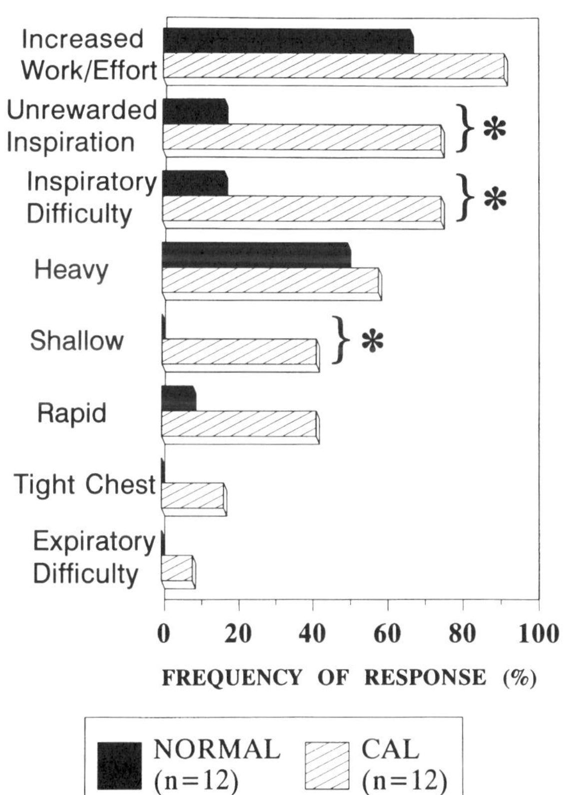

FIGURE 1.—Selection frequency of descriptor clusters for exertional breathlessness in normal subjects and in patients with chronic airflow limitation (CAL). *Asterisk* indicates *P* less than 0.05; significant difference between groups using Fisher's exact test. (Courtesy of O'Donnell DE, Bertley JC, Chau LKL, et al: Qualitative aspects of exertional breathlessness in chronic airflow limitation. *Am J Respir Crit Care Med* 155:109–115, 1997. Official Journal of the American Thoracic Society. Copyright American Lung Association.)

Methods.—The study included 12 patients with severe CAL; they had a mean age of 66 years and a mean forced expiratory volume in 1 sec of 37% predicted. Both groups performed a symptom-limited incremental cycle ergometer exercise test, during which several variables were measured: perceived inspiratory difficulty (Borg$_{IN}$); inspiratory effort, expressed as esophageal pressure as a fraction of maximal esophageal pressure at isovolume (Pes/PImax); breathing patterns; and operational lung volumes, expressed as end-expiratory/inspiratory lung volumes (EELV/EILV). In both groups, these parameters were compared at a standard oxygen consumption per unit time of 50% predicted maximum. Immediately after the exercise session, the subjects were asked to select qualitative terms describing their experience of breathlessness.

Results.—In choosing descriptors, both groups selected terms expressing increased "work/effort" and "heaviness" of breathing. In addition, patients in the CAL group endorsed terms such as "increased inspiratory difficulty," "unsatisfied inspiratory effort," and "shallow breathing" (Fig 1). The factor most strongly correlated with standardized Borg$_{IN}$ on stepwise regression analysis was the ratio of Pes/PImax to tidal volume/predicted VC. There was also a strong correlation between Borg$_{IN}$—as an indicator of the relationship between effort and ventilatory output—and dynamic EELV/total lung capacity at isotime.

Conclusion.—The sensation of exercise-induced breathlessness is qualitatively different for patients with CAL vs. normal subjects. The nature of these differing sensations may involve thoracic hyperinflation leading to a mismatch between inspiratory effort and ventilatory output. As patients with CAL continue to exercise, the disparity between effort and ventilatory output increases; much greater effort than normal is needed to achieve a given change in volume.

► Is dyspnea always perceived in the same manner? Sports physicians have long argued that the dyspnea of disease differs substantially from that associated with vigorous exercise in an athlete. It is less clear whether the explanation resides in the mechanics of breathing or in differences of cognitive appraisal between the anxiety of disease and the mind-set of a person who is bent on achieving a tangible goal of athletic performance. O'Donnell and associates here point to hyperinflation of the lungs as an important biomechanical feature of lung mechanics in patients with chronic chest disease. The hyperinflation causes a mismatch between inspiratory effort and ventilatory output. Using a questionnaire with 16 predetermined descriptors of dyspnea, the authors found that relative to normal exercising subjects, the patients had a strong clustering of responses relating to inspiratory difficulty and unsatisfied inspiration.

R.J. Shephard, M.D., Ph.D., D.P.E.

Exercise-induced Anaphylaxis: Useful Screening of Food Sensitization
Guinnepain M-T, Eloit C, Raffard M, et al (Unité d'Allergologie-Hôpital de l'Institut Pasteur, Paris)
Ann Allergy 77:491–496, 1996   6–11

Background.—Exercise-induced anaphylaxis was once an unusual occurrence but is now more frequently reported. In 19 severe cases, previously latent food sensitization was found. Avoidance of specific foods for 5 hours before exercise averted symptoms, suggesting a role of food allergy.

Methods.—In 19 patients with severe systemic anaphylaxis during or right after exercise, causal relationships with foods were investigated systematically.

Results.—No patients had a food allergy history, but skin tests showed food sensitization in 17. Results were positive for several antigens, most commonly wheat flour. Antigen avoidance 5 hours before exercise averted anaphylaxis in 17 cases, even if the previously provocative exercise was performed as often as 4 times weekly. Two had recurrences despite elimination diets, but repeated evaluation allowed successful avoidance of additional foods.

Conclusions.—Although the pathophysiology of exercise-induced anaphylaxis is not yet clear, subjects can exercise strenuously without symptoms after avoiding specific foods for 5 hours. Food allergens play an important role, so skin tests should be done in all cases.

▶ The present report is encouraging in suggesting that exercise-induced anaphylaxis is largely a dietary phenomenon. It seems that with due attention to diet, the affected individuals can undertake vigorous exercise safely. Reasons why exercise precipitates severe spasm are as yet unclear. Probably, many of the factors associated with exercise-induced asthma may be at work. Some authors have hypothesized that triggering is a result of a decrease in pH,[1] and there have been suggestions that the administration of 3 g of sodium bicarbonate can prevent the disorder.

R.J. Shephard, M.D., Ph.D., D.P.E.

Reference

1. Katsunuma T, Iiikura Y, Asakawa A, et al: Wheat-dependent exercise-induced anaphylaxis: Inhibition by sodium bicarbonate. *Ann Allergy* 68:184–188, 1992.

Blocking Effect of Vitamin C in Exercise-induced Asthma
Cohen HA, Neuman I, Nahum H (Pediatric Ambulatory Clinic, Petach, Tiqva, Israel; Tel Aviv Univ, Israel)
Arch Pediatr Adolesc Med 151:367–370, 1997   6–12

Objective.—Some studies have shown that vitamin C has a beneficial effect on individuals with exercise-induced asthma (EIA). Results of a study comparing the effects of ascorbic acid on hyperactive airways at rest and after the physical provocation of exercise are presented.

Methods.—Pulmonary function tests were performed at rest and 1 hour after administering oral ascorbic acid (2g) to 20 patients (7 females and 13 males, aged 7 to 28 years), with EIA. Patients were then given either placebo or ascorbic acid (2g) in a randomized, double-blind fashion 1 hour before a 7-minute exercise program, and pulmonary function tests were repeated after exercise and again after an 8-minute rest. Patients were crossed-over to the opposite study arm 1 week later, and the procedure was repeated.

Results.—Pulmonary function test results decreased significantly in 9 patients and somewhat in 2 patients 1 hour after ingesting ascorbic acid compared with results after ingesting placebo. Four of 5 patients who benefited from administration of ascorbic acid continued to take it and benefited from it for an additional 2 weeks.

Conclusion.—Vitamin C may have a protective effect on airway hyper-reactivity in some patients with EIA.

▶ Linus Pauling is smiling down from above: Vitamin C even prevents asthma! In this study, a single dose of 2 g of ascorbic acid prevented exercise-induced asthma in 9 of 20 individuals during a 7-minute treadmill exercise bout. In 2 other individuals, vitamin C reduced EIA. These 2 latter patients were 22 and 28 years of age, whereas all 9 of the former were no older than 15, and most were younger than 13 years. Maybe vitamin C works better in children; I haven't had much luck with it yet in collegiate athletes with EIA. The 2-week follow-up trial, in which 5 individuals took 0.5 g/day of vitamin C and were retested, is too small and uncontrolled to matter. I doubt this study will hold up.

E.R. Eichner, M.D.

Association Between Type of Training and Risk of Asthma in Elite Athletes
Helenius IJ, Tikkanen HO, Haahtela T (Helsinki Univ; Research Inst for Olympic Sports, Jyväskylä, Finland)
Thorax 52:157–160, 1997   6–13

Introduction.—There is a high prevalence of asthma in endurance athletes. Whether there is an association between type of training and risk of asthma is not known. The prevalence of asthma in 2 different athlete groups whose training and competition are very different was compared with that of a control group.

Methods.—A respiratory questionnaire was completed by 106 speed and power athletes, 107 long distance runners, and 124 medical students. Answers concerning physician-diagnosed asthma were confirmed. Differences in prevalence rates and trends in prevalence rates of asthma were examined statistically.

Results.—The prevalence of physician-diagnosed asthma was not significantly related to age, sex, or family history. Speed and power athletes had a higher prevalence of exercise-induced asthma (8%) and long-distance runners had a significantly higher prevalence of exercise-induced asthma than did controls (17% vs. 3%).

Conclusion.—The risk of developing asthma is increased in elite athletes, with long-distance runners having a significantly higher prevalence of exercise-induced asthma than controls.

▶ Recent studies suggest that asthma is uniquely prevalent in distance runners and cross-country skiers, the hypothesis being that such athletes necessarily breathe more cold air and pollen than do other athletes.[1] This study tends to support the hypothesis, with questionnaire results suggesting that the type of training matters: distance runners have the most asthma, followed by speed and power athletes, followed by nonathletes. But these authors have shown that the expression of exercise-induced asthma depends in part on how and where athletes exercise. Fully one quarter of 32 top "nonasthmatic" runners had bronchospasm when they exercised hard for 7 minutes in the cold.[2] A likely flaw in this hypothesis is that even if you have a propensity to get exercise-induced asthma, you won't get it if you don't exercise (nonathlete) or if you exercise only briefly (sprinter).

E.R. Eichner, M.D.

References

1. 1994 Year Book of Sports Medicine, pp 400–401.
2. Helenius IJ, Tikkanen HO, Haahtela T: Exercise-induced bronchospasm at low temperature in elite runners. *Thorax* 51:628–629, 1996.

Gene Therapy in Sports Medicine
Lamsam C, Fu FH, Robbins PD, et al (Univ of Pittsburgh, Pa)
Sports Med 25:73–77, 1998   6–14

Introduction.—A great deal of basic science and clinical research has been conducted with the aim of enhancing the healing potential of tissues with limited healing capability—including articular cartilage, menisci, the anterior cruciate ligament, and sheathed tendons—that are commonly involved in athletic injuries. Various growth factors have been identified that stimulate events related to the healing process, but these factors may be lacking in tissues with limited power to heal themselves. In this situation, it might be possible to enhance healing through exogenous application or increased endogenous synthesis of growth factors. The problem has been the lack of a suitable delivery system. The current state of gene therapy to help heal sports injuries was reviewed.

Gene Therapy for Athletic Injury.—Problems with delivering growth factors to injured tissues may be overcome by the use of gene transfer techniques, in which gene therapy works as a local growth factor delivery system. This approach could be useful in initiating and accelerating the processes of cartilage, meniscus, tendon, and ligament repair. Gene transfer may be done ex vivo, in which target cells are isolated, cultivated, genetically modified, and reintroduced to the patient; or in vivo, in which gene vectors are introduced directly into the body. Either approach would require information on the appropriate growth factors and the molecular and the relevant cellular repair mechanisms. Previous studies have demonstrated the transfer of marker genes to synovium, chondrocytes, meniscal fibrochondrocytes, tenocytes, and ligamental fibroblasts. Studies suggest that retroviruses may be the most effective approach for ex vivo gene transfer, whereas adenoviruses could be used for in vivo gene transfer.

Discussion.—Preliminary research suggests that gene therapy may offer new approaches to promoting healing of athletic injuries. It will be a long time before these techniques are ready for clinical application. However, the results so far warrant further development of gene transfer approaches to promote healing of joint tissues with limited healing capability.

▶ This is an interesting report dealing with the basic concepts of gene therapy. The authors admit, however, that although they believe gene therapy will be particularly useful in initiating and accelerating the repair of cartilage, meniscus, tendon, and ligaments, today "it is in its infancy." Specifically, at this time, there is no clinically useful way to effect gene transfer for the treatment of athletic injuries.

J.S. Torg, M.D.

Randomised Controlled Trial of Graded Exercise in Patients With the Chronic Fatigue Syndrome
Fulcher KY, White PD (Royal London Med School)
BMJ 314:1647–1652, 1997   6–15

Background.—In chronic fatigue syndrome (CFS), patients fatigue more from exercise than do healthy subjects. Consequent reduced physical activity may have adverse physical and psychological effects; exercise offers countervailing benefits. Programs of graded aerobic exercise have reduced symptoms in similar chronic conditions.

Methods.—In a controlled, randomized, control-treatment crossover trial at a CFS clinic, 66 patients with CFS but not psychiatric disorder or sleep disturbance were randomly assigned to 12 weeks of graded aerobic exercise or flexibility and relaxation. Patients rated their own progress,

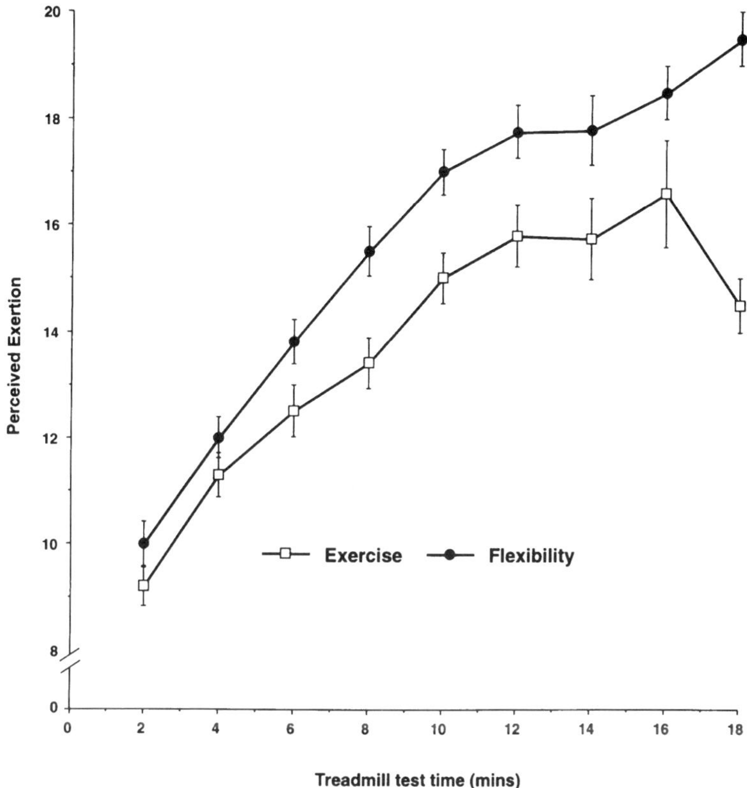

FIGURE 2.—Mean perceived exertion scores during treadmill testing after treatment. *Bars* are SEM. (This figure was first published in Fulcher KY, White PD: Randomised controlled trial of graded exercise in patients with the chronic fatigue syndrome. *BMJ* 314:1647–1652, 1997, and is reproduced by permission of the BMJ.)

with "very much better" or "much better" considered significant improvements.

Results.—Of 29 subjects who completed the exercise program, 16 reported significant improvement, vs. 8 of 30 in the flexibility group ($P = 0.05$). In 2 patients (1 per group), major depression was concurrent with perceived worsening of CFS. Of 7 who dropped out (4 exercise and 3 flexibility), 2 (1 per group) claimed that treatment made CFS worse. By intent to treat, 17 of 33 benefited from exercise and 9 of 33 from flexibility ($P = 0.04$). Mean submaximal perceived exertion scored 14.5 with exercise and 16.2 with flexibility ($P = 0.04$; Fig 2). Twenty-three patients crossed over to exercise; of 22 who completed that program, 12 noted improvement. Physiologic gains were maintained or better 3 months after program completion. At 1 year, 35 of 47 responding patients in the exercise group (74%) noted improvement.

Conclusions.—Only a few patients with CFS declined or dropped out of the graded exercise program, and only 1 who completed it reported worsened CFS, with benefit sustained at 1 year. For patients with CFS but not psychiatric disorder or sleep disturbance, graded exercise is more effective than relaxation and flexibility treatment.

▶ The CFS is notoriously difficult to treat, and some older texts have recommended the avoidance of physical activity until the condition has been resolved. The present controlled trial compared 12 weeks of graded aerobic exercise with flexibility exercises and relaxation therapy, showing the advantage of the more active treatment. However, it is important to note that before randomization, the authors excluded all patients with a psychiatric disorder or an appreciable sleep disturbance. They were thus treating only milder examples of the syndrome, a little over half of their total sample. It may be of importance that the 2 patients who felt worse after exercise treatment had depressive illnesses.

R.J. Shephard, M.D., Ph.D., D.P.E.

Recreational Physical Activity and Breast Cancer Risk Among Women Under Age 45 Years
Gammon MD, Schoenberg JB, Britton JA, et al (Columbia School of Public Health, New York; New Jersey Dept of Health and Senior Services, Trenton; Stanford Univ, Calif; et al)
Am J Epidemiol 147:273–280, 1998   6–16

Objective.—Data from a population-based case-control study were analyzed to examine the relationship between recreational physical activity and risk of breast cancer and to determine whether risk reduction applies to both pre- and postmenopausal women, whether there is an optimal period for exercise, and whether intensity, frequency, or duration of activity is important.

Methods.—Women (n=1,668) aged less than 45 in whom breast cancer was diagnosed between 1990 and 1992 in 3 U.S. geographic areas were frequency-matched to 1,505 control women by 5-year age group and geographic area. All were interviewed about contraceptive and reproductive histories, exogenous hormone use, medical history, family history of cancer, lifetime alcohol use, adolescent diet, smoking, and demographic characteristics and completed 100-item food frequency questionnnaire. Anthropometric measurements were made, and frequency of vigorous and moderate physical activity was determined. Level of physical activity was stratified into quartiles and examined over 3 time periods, ages 12–13, age 20, and the past year.

Results.—Breast cancer was unrelated to recreational physical activity at ages 12–13 (OR=0.94), age 20 (OR=1.08), or the past year (OR=1.18), level of physical activity at any time period, climbing versus never climbing 2 or more flights of stairs without stopping during the past year, age at menarche, age at diagnosis, menopausal status, body mass index, or caloric intake during the past year.

Conclusion.—Recreational physical activity is not associated with a lower risk of breast cancer.

▶ The conflicting results from the many studies attempting to find a relationship between physical activity and breast cancer has left us in limbo. At present, the evidence of a protective effect is not sufficiently convincing to add breast cancer to the list of diseases that may be prevented by exercise. A reference in this article to changes in menstrual characteristics as having a potentially positive effect on risk of breast cancer suggests that those involved in the effort to link exercise to breast cancer would be well advised to become familiar with the negative consequences of delayed menarche or oligomenorrhea and amenorrhea to bone.

B.L. Drinkwater, Ph.D.

Physical Activity and the Risk of Breast Cancer
Thune I, Brenn T, Lund E, et al (Univ of Tromsø, Norway; Cancer Registry of Norway, Oslo)
N Engl J Med 336:1269–1275, 1997   6–17

Introduction.—The menstrual cycle can be interrupted by vigorous exercise, perhaps by suppressing gonadotropin-releasing hormone. A woman's exposure to estrogen may be lowered by this effect. The risk of breast cancer may also be influenced by energy balance, but this has not been thoroughly examined in humans. In premenopausal and postmenopausal women, the influence of physical activity at work and during leisure time on the risk of breast cancer was examined.

Methods.—There were 25,624 women, aged 20–54 years, who enrolled in health surveys and answered questionnaires about activity at work and during leisure time. An assessment of their physical activity was made and categorized from grade 1–4, with grade 1 assigned to those whose leisure time was spent reading, watching television, or doing other sedentary activities, and grade 4 assigned to those who had regular, vigorous training or participated in competitive sports several times a week.

Results.—Among the 25,624 women, 351 women had invasive breast cancer during a median follow-up of 13.7 years. After adjustments for age, body-mass index, height, parity, and county residence had been made, greater leisure-time activity was associated with a reduced risk of breast cancer among women who exercised compared with those who did not (Table 5). The reduction in risk was greater in premenopausal women than in postmenopausal women and greater in women younger than 45 years than in older women, of those who exercised regularly. In lean women who exercised at least 4 hours per week, the risk of breast cancer was lowest. Women who had higher levels of activity at work also had a reduced risk, and this effect was more noticeable among women who were premenopausal than those who were postmenopausal.

TABLE 5.—Adjusted Relative Risk of Breast Cancer According to Body-Mass Index and Overall Level of Physical Activity During Leisure Time in the 1974–1978 and 1977–1983 Surveys*

OVERALL LEVEL OF PHYSICAL ACTIVITY†	ALL WOMEN		BODY-MASS INDEX, <22.8		BODY-MASS INDEX, 22.8–25.7		BODY-MASS INDEX, >25.7	
	CASES OF BREAST CANCER	RELATIVE RISK (95% CI)‡	CASES OF BREAST CANCER	RELATIVE RISK (95% CI)§	CASES OF BREAST CANCER	RELATIVE RISK (95% CI)§	CASES OF BREAST CANCER	RELATIVE RISK (95% CI)§
Consistently sedentary	29	1.00	13	1.00	7	1.00	9	1.00
Moderately active	283	0.90 (0.61–1.32)	112	0.76 (0.43–1.35)	81	0.87 (0.40–1.88)	90	1.14 (0.57–2.27)
Consistently active	34	0.67 (0.40–1.10)	6	0.23 (0.09–0.60)	13	0.83 (0.33–2.09)	15	1.38 (0.60–3.17)
P for trend		0.09		0.002		0.73		0.42

*The sedentary group is the reference group.

†Participants with a consistently sedentary level of activity were classified as sedentary in both surveys (grade 1). Participants who remained active, reporting moderate (grade 2) or regular (grade 3 or 4) exercise in the first survey and regular exercise (grade 3 or 4) in the second survey, were classified as being consistently active. Participants were classified as moderately active if they did not meet the criteria for the other 2 categories.

‡Variables were adjusted for age at entry, body-mass index, height, county of residence, and number of children.

§Variables were adjusted for age at entry, height, county of residence, and number of children.

Abbreviation: CI, confidence interval.

(Reprinted by permission of *The New England Journal of Medicine*. Courtesy of Thune I, Brenn T, Lund E, et al: Physical activity and the risk of breast cancer. *N Engl J Med* 336:1269–1275, copyright 1997, Massachusetts Medical Society.)

Conclusion.—A reduced risk of breast cancer is associated with physical activity during leisure time and at work. In inactive women, exposure to estrogen may be greater, which underscores the importance of avoiding obesity.

▶ There has been considerable debate about the issue of whether regular leisure activity reduces the risk of breast cancer. This large prospective study goes some way to answer the controversy. Some benefit is apparently shown from both leisure activity and physical activity at work. The dilemma is that few of a prospective sample have breast cancer develop (351 of 25,624 women); the average benefit from leisure activity is substantial (risk ratio, 0.67), but because few women get regular leisure exercise (36 of the 351 who had breast cancer develop), the 95% confidence limits of the leisure effect (0.44–1.00) are such that traditional statistical significance is not reached ($P < 0.08$).

R.J. Shephard, M.D., Ph.D., D.P.E.

Exercise, Occupational Activity, and Risk of Endometrial Cancer
Olson SH, Vena JE, Dorn JP, et al (State Univ of New York, Buffalo; Mem Sloan-Kettering Cancer Ctr, New York)
Ann Epidemiol 7:46–53, 1997   6–18

Background.—The risk of some cancers may be decreased by regular physical activity. Endometrial cancer has been linked to body mass and exogenous estrogen, which in turn may be related to physical activity.

Methods.—Interviews assessed vigorous physical activity and walking in a case-control study of 232 postmenopausal women with adenomatous carcinoma of the endometrium and 631 control women. Also included was occupational history for physical activity. Response rates were 50% for case-patients and 51% for controls.

Results.—Case-patients were more likely than age-adjusted controls to have high body mass index, to have diabetes, not to smoke, not to have as many children, to have earlier menarche and later menopause, and to have used unopposed estrogens. Enough exercise to produce sweat was associated with some reduction in risk. Moderate physical activity at age 16 and 20 years before the interview was associated with lower risk than no activity, but higher activity did not reduce risk further. At 2 and 10 years before the interview, the highest category of physical activity carried the lowest risk, but risk was not statistically significantly lower than for women who did not exercise at all. Walking varied considerably among the periods studied; Table 3 shows that walking at least 24 km (15 miles) per week at age 16 years was associated with slightly (but nonsignificantly) reduced risk. Among women who walked 20 and 10 years before the interview, however, the risk was actually slightly higher. Excluding body mass index did not substantially change the results. Job-related physical activity was unrelated to risk.

TABLE 3.—Risk of Endometrial Cancer According to Miles per Week Walked for Exercise, Pleasure, or Transportation at Various Time Periods, Western New York, 1986–1991

Exercise characteristic		Cases	Controls	Adjusted OR*	95% CI
Age 16					
None		31	83	1.00	...
< 8 miles		54	146	.96	(0.53–1.75)
8–14 miles		49	151	.69	(0.38–1.27)
≥ 15 miles		72	189	.64	(0.36–1.16)
P (trend test)	0.09				
20 years ago					
None		99	304	1.00	...
< 4 miles		45	133	1.28	(0.80–2.04)
≥ 4 miles		62	156	1.35	(0.89–2.09)
P (trend test)	0.48				
10 years ago					
None		104	313	1.00	...
< 4 miles		52	137	1.21	(0.78–1.88)
≥ 4 miles		53	152	1.17	(0.75–1.81)
P (trend test)	0.81				
2 years ago					
None		96	244	1.00	...
< 4 miles		64	189	1.00	(0.65–1.53)
≥ 4 miles		55	177	1.04	(0.66–1.63)
P (trend test)	.31				

*Adjusted for age, education, body mass index, diabetes, smoking, parity, age at menarche, menopausal status, and use of unopposed estrogens.

Abbreviations: OR, odds ratio; *CI*, confidence interval.

(Reprinted by permission of the publisher from Olson SH, Vena JE, Dorn JP, et al: Exercise, occupational activity, and risk of endometrial cancer. *Ann Epidemiol* 7:46–53, copyright 1997 by Elsevier Science Inc.)

Conclusions.—Endometrial cancer risk may be reduced by walking at age 16 and by vigorous exercise at some but not all times during life. Occupational activity did not reduce risk. Very high physical activity may reduce risk, but sample size is insufficient for statistical confidence.

▶ A number of studies have suggested the possibility that regular physical activity reduces the risk of endometrial cancer. Unfortunately, most of the available data are similar to the study of Olson and associates—an effect that is clinically of considerable importance (a risk ratio of 0.67–0.72) but a sample size that is inadequate to reach statistical significance. Possibly, the time will soon be ripe to attempt a meta-analysis of available information.

R.J. Shephard, M.D., Ph.D., D.P.E.

Leisure-Time Physical Activity, Body Size, and Colon Cancer in Women
Martínez ME, Giovannucci E, Spiegelman D, et al (Harvard Med School, Boston)
J Natl Cancer Inst 89:948–955, 1997   6–19

Background.—Although physical inactivity carries a higher risk of colon cancer in women, whether leisure-time activities are associated with colon cancer risk is not known. These authors analyzed data from a large group of women to determine any relationship between leisure-time activities and the risk for colon cancer.

Methods.—Female nurses 30–55 years old who were free of cancer, ulcerative colitis, or Crohn's disease were enrolled in 1976. Participants completed a biennial questionnaire to indicate medical events and risk factors. The 1986 questionnaire included questions on leisure-time physical activity during the past year, including walking or hiking outdoors; jogging; running; bicycling; lap swimming; playing tennis, squash, or racquet ball; calisthenics, aerobics, aerobic dance, or the use of a rowing machine; the number of flights of stairs climbed each day; and the subject's usual walking pace. The energy expended was calculated as metabolic equivalent (MET)—hours per week; this value was calculated by multiplying the hours per week spent participating in an activity by the activity's typical energy expenditure, then summing activities over the week to arrive at a total score. Also, in 1986 subjects reported the size of their waist at the umbilicus and of their hips at the largest circumference. Regression analysis was adjusted for confounding variables including age, family history of colorectal cancer, smoking, aspirin use, red meat consumption, alcohol use, and postmenopausal hormone use.

Findings.—Data were available on 67,802 subjects, representing 385,819 person-years of follow up. Colon cancer occurred in 212 subjects (97 distal, 88 proximal, and 27 unknown site). The risk of colon cancer was significantly associated with leisure-time physical activity (Table 2). Compared with subjects who had < 2 MET-hours/week of activity, those who expended > 21 MET-hours/week had a relative risk of colon cancer of 0.54. This significant association was based mainly on cancer of the distal colon, whereas cancer of the proximal colon had no significant association with leisure-time physical activity. Participating in high-intensity activities for $\geq$ 30 min/day or in moderate-intensity activities for $\geq$ 1 hr/day dramatically reduced the risk for colon cancer (range 0.61 to 0.69). However, the relative risk was not reduced with low-intensity activities at any frequency. A higher BMI was also significantly associated with an increased risk of distal colon cancer: Subjects with a BMI $\geq$ 29 kg/m^2 had a relative risk of 1.96 compared with subjects whose BMI was < 21 kg/m^2. Finally, the risk for distal colon cancer increased as the waist-to-hip ratio increased (trend not statistically significant).

Conclusions.—As leisure-time activity increased, the risk of cancer of the distal colon decreased significantly. Even activities of moderate intensity performed for an hour a day significantly reduced colon cancer risk.

TABLE 2.—Relative Risk (*RR*) of Colon Cancer According to Level of Leisure-time Physical Activity (in MET-hours*) in 1986†, Nurses' Health Study, 1986–1992

	MET-hours per week					
	<2	2–4	5–10	11–21	>21	Two-sided
Person-years	63,734	51,413	66,435	60,769	58,817	*P* for trend‡
Colon cancer§						
No. of cases	47	26	36	29	23	
Age-adjusted RR	1.00 (referent)	0.69	0.74	0.65	0.52	
Multivariate RR‖	1.00 (referent)	0.71	0.78	0.67	0.54	.03
95% CI¶	—	0.44–1.15	0.50–1.20	0.42–1.07	0.33–0.90	
Distal colon cancer						
No. of cases	21	15	17	14	6	
Age-adjusted RR	1.00 (referent)	0.89	0.78	0.70	0.31	
Multivariate RR‖	1.00 (referent)	0.92	0.81	0.71	0.31	.01
95% CI¶	—	0.48–1.79	0.43–1.55	0.36–1.41	0.12–0.77	
Proximal colon cancer						
No. of cases	19	8	15	11	13	
Age-adjusted RR	1.00 (referent)	0.53	0.76	0.61	0.73	
Multivariate RR‖	1.00 (referent)	0.54	0.79	0.62	0.77	.67
95% CI¶	—	0.23–1.22	0.40–1.56	0.30–1.32	0.38–1.58	

*Metabolic equivalent (MET)-hours = sum of the average time per week spent in each leisure-time physical activity multiplied by the MET value for each activity; MET value = (caloric need/kilogram body weight per hour activity)/(caloric need/kilogram body weight per hour at rest).

†Data were based on 67,802 respondents. Data on leisure-time physical activity were missing for 51 case patients and 84, 651 person-years.

‡Test for trend was calculated by use of the median of each MET-hours per week category as a continuous variable in the multiple regression model.

§Includes 22 cases lacking data on anatomic site.

‖Adjusted for age, cigarette smoking, family history of colorectal cancer, body mass index, postmenopausal hormone use, aspirin use, intake of red meat, and alcohol consumption.

¶*CI*, Confidence interval.

(Courtesy of Martínez ME, Giovannucci E, Spiegelman D, et al. Leisure-time physical activity, body size, and colon cancer in women. *J Natl Cancer Inst* 89:948–955, 1997, by permission of Oxford University Press.)

These findings are yet another good argument for increasing levels of physical activity.

▶ Once again, it appears that moderate activity is effective in reducin the risk of a serious disease. However, although the authors attempted to control for the overall healthier lifestyle of the active women, they apparently did not adjust the data for the higher intake of dietary fiber among the more active women. Since intake of dietary fiber has been linked to a lower risk of colon cancer, this seems a strange omission. This may have been addressed in another report from the Nurses' Health Study Research Group, but it is a "missing piece" in the analysis of data from this study.

B.L. Drinkwater, Ph.D.

Sport and Delinquency: an Examination of the Deterrence Hypothesis in a Longitudinal Study
Begg DJ, Langley JD, Moffitt T, et al (Univ of Otago, Dunedin, New Zealand; Univ of Wisconsin, Madison; Univ of North Carolina, Chapel Hill)
Br J Sports Med 30:335–341, 1996   6–20

Background.—Some authorities believe that participating in sports will moderate delinquent behavior. This notion is called the "deterrence hypothesis." Whether mid-adolescent sports involvement would deter delinquent behavior in late adolescence was investigated.

Methods.—Data were obtained from 1,037 participants in a longitudinal study of the health, development, attitudes, and behavior of a cohort born in Dunedin, New Zealand. Interviews conducted at 15 and 18 years of age included questions on physical activity and delinquent behavior. Data were analyzed by logistic regression models.

Findings.—After controlling for delinquent behavior and psychosocial variables at 15 years of age, delinquency at 18 years of age was significantly more likely to be found among girls with moderate or high levels of sports activity and among boys with high levels of sports activity than in those with low levels of sports activity. Sports activity was not significantly related to aggressive behavior. Team sports participation was unassociated with delinquency and aggressive behavior.

Conclusions.—These findings do not suppot the deterrence hypothesis. High involvement in sports, though not in team sports, was correlated with an increase in delinquent behavior later in adolescence.

▶ Most coaches claim that sports build character. Surely, most coaches—and many parents—would believe that playing team sports would likely decrease delinquency among juveniles. This longitudinal study of a cohort of about 800 kids born in Dunedin, New Zealand, finds no influence of team sports on delinquency. Its more surprising finding is that sports activity in general is tied to delinquency. Among the boys, those who had a high level of sports activity at age 15 were almost twice as apt to report delinquent behavior by age 18 as boys with a low level of sports activity. This trend was even more pronounced among the girls. So sports is no panacea for juvenile delinquency. In fact, the role of sports one way or the other was small; the best predictor of delinquency at age 18 was delinquency at age 15. Maybe sports activity just happens to track with delinquency, each peaking at age 18 or so. Maybe that's why they call delinquency juvenile.

E.R. Eichner, M.D.

Psychological Effects of Chronic Injury in Elite Athletes
Shuer ML, Dietrich MS (Vanderbilt Univ, Nashville, Tenn)
West J Med 166:104–109, 1997   6–21

Introduction.—Athletes who compete in National Collegiate Athletic Association Division I programs often train in a state of pain or injury. Those with chronic-overuse injuries may enter a rehabilitative netherworld, with inadequate care for their psychological recovery. In this self-report study, researchers examined the level of emotional distress in athletes who engage in active training while suffering from a musculoskeletal injury.

Methods.—Study participants were 280 elite National Collegiate Athletic Association Division I athletes with an average age of 19.5; 49% were men and 51% women. Sports represented included tennis, swimming, volleyball, track and field, water polo, softball, and gymnastics. Athletes completed the Impact of Event Scale (IES), a 15-question instrument. Various symptoms of the injury were quantified using the 2 subscales of the IES: Intrusion ("an involuntary entry into awareness") and Avoidance ("a conscious attempt to divert thoughts"). A reference group consisted of earthquake and fire victims and orthopedic patients.

Results.—Of the athletes sampled, 48% were classified as injured; 87% of these were considered to have chronic injuries. Most injured athletes were actively training and present at practice. Common sites of injury were the shoulder (29%), knee (20%), and ankle (11%). Athletes with chronic injuries and victims of natural disasters had similar IES Intrusion scores, but scores on the Avoidance/Denial subscale were higher for the athletes. The injured athletes' scores on the Avoidance subscale were comparable to those of a group of orthopedic patients who required hospital admission with surgical fixation. Intrusion scores were similar for male and female athletes, but female athletes had significantly higher Avoidance scores. Increased duration of injury did not result in a statistically significant decline in subscale scores.

Conclusion.—Chronic injuries, even when considered "minor," are associated with both physical and psychological problems, particularly when athletes continue to train just below the pain threshold. There is a need for educational programs directed toward athletes, coaches, physicians, and parents so that these elite athletes can be assisted in all aspects of their recovery.

▶ Recognizing that "you can't make the club while sitting in the tub" and "hurt is temporary, pride is forever," the authors point out that "emotional rehabilitation of elite athletes, most specifically those with chronic-overused injuries, has not been adequately addressed by medical or athletic establishments." However, I am not convinced that it has been established that it need be. Injury was defined by the authors as a musculoskeletal injury that rendered the athlete "less than 100%" on the day of the study. To be noted, although the article presumably deals with chronic injury, this term is not really defined. The authors believe that athletes with chronic-overuse injuries appear to be suffering from stress-response syndrome and, on the basis of the study instrument, equate these athletes with victims of the Oakland-Berkeley fire and the Loma Prieta earthquake. On the basis of this presumed analogy, it is suggested that perhaps psychiatrists should become members of the "multi-disciplinary sports medicine team." What is needed, however, is a clear clinical and real-life demonstration that this is necessary.

J.S. Torg, M.D.

Coagulation and Fibrinolysis After Moderate and Very Heavy Exercise in Healthy Male Subjects

Weiss C, Seitel G, Bärtsch P (Universität Heidelberg, Germany)
Med Sci Sports Exerc 30:246–251, 1998   6–22

Background.—Previous research suggests that moderate exercise may predominantly activate the fibrinolytic system and that very heavy exercise along with plasmin formation may give rise to thrombin and fibrin formation. The relationship between exercise intensity and activation of coagulation and fibrinolysis has not been studied systematically using neoantigens that indicate in vivo activity. Molecular markers of platelet activation, thrombin, fibrin, and plasmin formation, as well as markers of the fibrinolytic activity, were determined in healthy trained young men before, during, and after 1 hour of moderate and very heavy exercise.

Methods and Findings.—Twelve men ran on a treadmill at different exercise intensities. During moderate exercise, plasma levels of tissue plasminogen activator (t–PA) antigen increased from a mean 3.7 to 14.6 ng·mL^{-1} and of plasminogen-α-antiplasmin (PAP) complexes from 2.1 to 4.2 nmol·L^{-1}. Prothrombin fragment 1+2 (PTF1+2), thrombin-antithrombin III (TAT) complexes and fibrinopeptide A (FPA) did not change significantly during moderate exercise. During very heavy exercise, mean plasma levels of t-PA antigen and PAP complexes exceeded normal values by 2.5– and 2–fold, respectively. Plasma levels of PTF1+2, TAT, and FPA increased significantly within the normal range (Figs 1 and 2).

Conclusions.—Exercise-induced activation of coagulation appears to be well balanced by fibrinolytic system activation in healthy young men. Moderate exercise results in increased plasmin formation only, whereas plasmin production during very heavy exercise seems to exceed that of thrombin and fibrin.

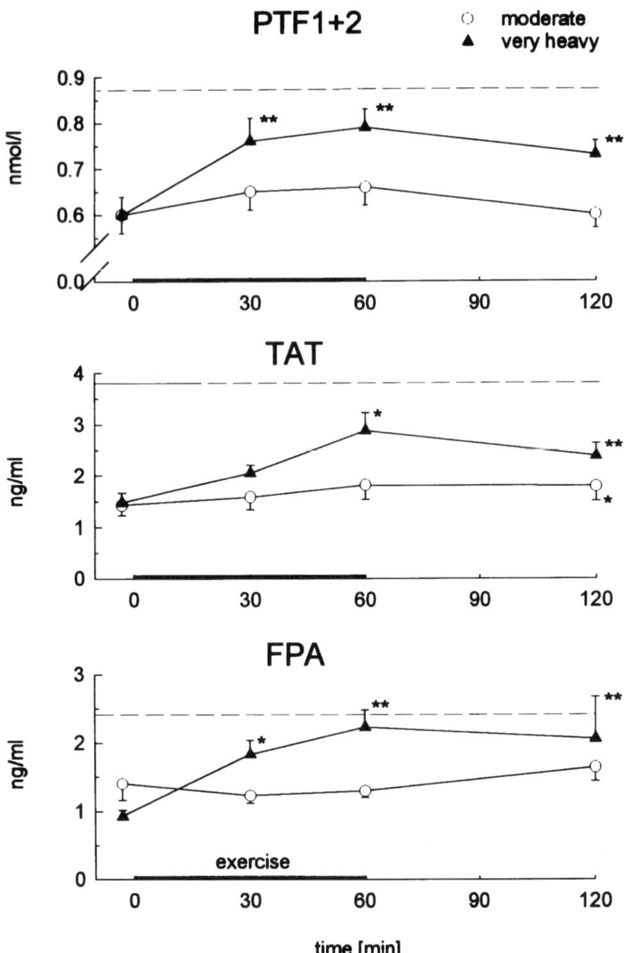

FIGURE 1.—Exercise-induced changes of PTF1+2, thrombin-antithrombin III complexes TAT, and FPA in 12 healthy male subjects. Data were obtained before (0), during (30), immediately after (60), and 1 hour after (120) running on a treadmill for 1 hour at 2 different intensities corresponding to moderate and very heavy exercise. Results are given as means ± SE, and dashed lines denote the upper limit of normal values (mean + 2 SD). *$P < 0.05$, **$P < 0.01$ compared with baseline values. (Courtesy of Weiss C, Seitel G, Bärtsch P: Coagulation and fibrinolysis after moderate and very heavy exercise in healthy male subjects. *Med Sci Sports Exerc* 30:246–251, 1998.)

▶ It is well known that running a marathon, for example, evokes a sharp increase in fibrinolysis. We have also reviewed articles showing that a single, brief bout of exercise increases fibrinolysis in proportion to effort and that active men have more brisk baseline fibrinolysis than do inactive men.[1, 2] However, strenuous exercise can, in theory, also be "prothrombotic" in that it can increase platelet count and activate coagulation. In a previous study of "both edges of the sword," this group found balanced activation of coagulation and fibrinolysis after a 2-hour triathlon; if anything, the increase in

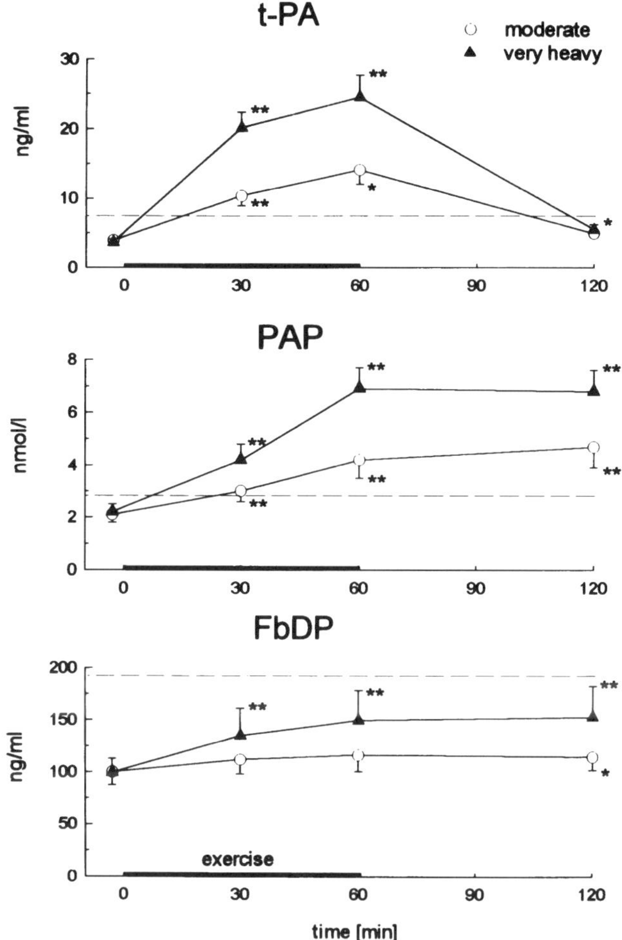

FIGURE 2.—Exercise-induced changes of t-PA, PAP, and FbDP in 12 healthy male subjects. Further explanations are given in the legend to Fig 1. (Courtesy of Weiss C, Seitel G, Bärtsch P: Coagulation and fibrinolysis after moderate and very heavy exercise in healthy male subjects. *Med Sci Sports Exerc* 30:246–251, 1998.)

fibrinolysis overrode the activation of coagulation, suggesting the net effect was antithrombotic.[3] This same reassuring note appears here: Moderate exercise resulted in increased plasmin formation only, and during very heavy exercise, the generation of plasmin seemed to exceed that of thrombin and fibrin. In summary, young healthy trained men are at no risk of thrombosis during exercise.

E.R. Eichner, M.D.

References

1. 1995 YEAR BOOK of SPORTS MEDICINE, pp 451–453.
2. 1995 YEAR BOOK of SPORTS MEDICINE, pp 468–470.
3. 1996 YEAR BOOK of SPORTS MEDICINE, pp 243–244.

Effects of Chronic Exercise and Deconditioning on Platelet Function in Women

Wang J-S, Jen CJ, Chen H-I (Natl Cheng-Kung Univ, Tainan, Republic of China)
J Appl Physiol 83:2080–2085, 1997   6–23

Background.—A previous study of men suggests that moderate-intensity acute exercise and exercise training suppress platelet adhesiveness and aggregability. The current study determined the effects of chronic exercise and deconditioning on platelet function in women.

Methods.—Sixteen healthy sedentary women were assigned to an exercise or control group. Women in the exercise group cycled on an ergometer at 50% maximal oxygen consumption for 30 min/day, 5 days/week, for 2 consecutive menstrual cycles. These women were then deconditioned for 3 menstrual cycles. Measures were obtained during this period before and immediately after a progressive exercise test in the midfollicular phase.

Findings.—After exercise testing, resting heart rates and blood pressures were decreased, and exercise performance was improved. In addition, resting platelet function was reduced, whereas plasma nitrite and nitrate levels and platelet cGMP contents were increased. Platelet function potentiation by acute strenuous exercise was reduced, whereas plasma nitrite and nitrate levels and platelet cGMP content were increased by acute exercise. Deconditioning reversed these effects.

Conclusions.—Nitric oxide may mediate training-induced platelet functional changes in women in the midfollicular phase. These findings provide new insight into the possible protective effects of exercise training against the risk of cardiovascular disease in women.

▶ Several lines of epidemiological evidence suggest that hyperreactive platelets are a risk factor for coronary heart disease.[1] In a pioneering randomized trial in overweight, middle-aged men, a 12-week program of brisk walking and slow jogging seemed to reduce platelet hyperreactivity.[2] The same trend—a reduction in platelet adhesiveness and aggregability—occurs in young sedentary women after 2 months of moderate aerobic training. The platelet benefits may be mediated by release of nitric oxide. Deconditioning reverses the benefits. This same group showed similar trends in an earlier study of healthy young men.[3]

E.R. Eichner, M.D.

References

1. Thaulow E, Erikssen J, Sandvik L, et al: Blood platelet count and function are related to total and cardiovascular death in apparently healthy men. *Circulation* 84:613–617, 1991.
2. Rauramaa R, Salonen JT, Seppanen K, et al: Inhibition of platelet aggregability by moderate-intensity physical exercise: a randomized clinical trial in overweight men. *Circulation* 74:939–944, 1986.
3. Wang J-S, Jen CJ, Chen H–I: Effects of exercise training and deconditioning on platelet function in men. *Arterioscler Thromb Vasc Biol* 15:1668–1674, 1995.

Red Cell Membrane Skeletal Changes in Marathon Runners

Jordan J, Kiernan W, Merker HJ, et al (Free Univ, Berlin; Humboldt Univ, Berlin)
Int J Sports Med 19:16–19, 1998   6–24

Background.—Hemolysis during endurance exercise may be associated with structural changes in red blood cell (RBC) membrane skeletal proteins. This possibility was investigated in marathon runners.

Methods.—Thirteen men were assessed before and after participating in a marathon race. Scanning electron microscopy (SEM) and transmission electron microscopy (TEM) were used to observe RBC membrane skeletons.

Findings.—No changes in RBC were seen with TEM. However, SEM showed disrupted RBC membrane skeletons. Compared with RBC before the race, RBC after the race appeared to have lost membrane material. A 30% increase in RBC membrane skeletal areas was noted. A 57% decline in plasma haptoglobin values indicated hemolysis (Figs 1 and 2).

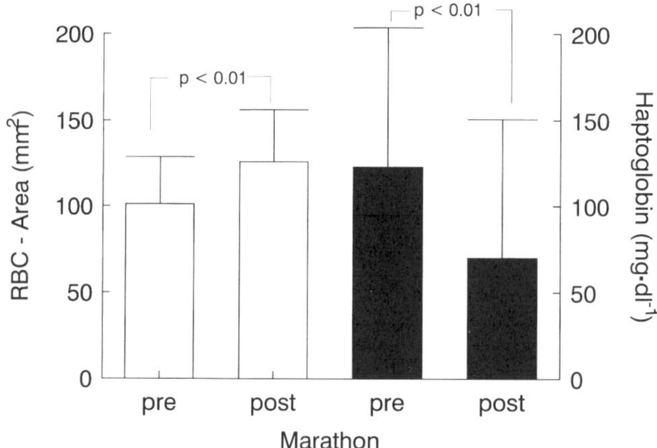

FIGURE 1.—RBC membrane skeleton area (RBC area) and plasma haptoglobin concentration pre- and post-marathon. (Courtesy of Jordan J, Kiernan W, Merker HJ, et al: Red cell membrane skeletal changes in marathon runners. *Int J Sports Med* 19:16–19, 1998 Georg Thieme Verlag.)

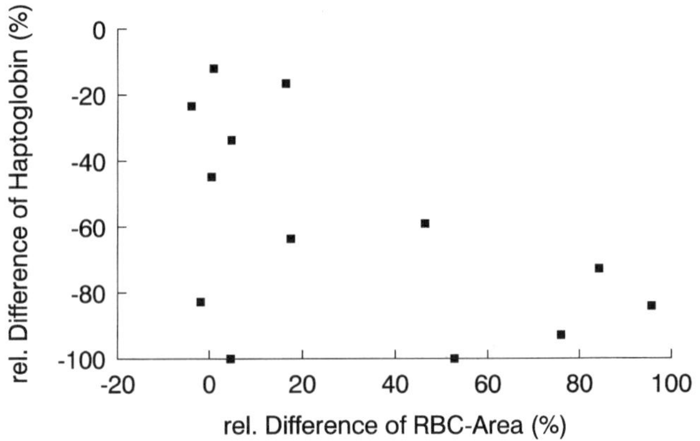

FIGURE 2.—Relationship between membrane skeletal area increase and change in plasma haptoglobin concentration. The relationship (r = 0.53, p = 0.06) is borderline significant. (Courtesy of Jordan J, Kiernan W, Merker HJ, et al: Red cell membrane skeletal changes in marathon runners. *Int J Sports Med* 19:16–19, 1998 Georg Thieme Verlag.)

Conclusions.—In this study of marathon runners, structural changes in RBC membrane skeletons occured after the race. These changes may be associated with increased susceptibility to chemical and physical stress and contribute to hemolysis during endurance exercise.

▶ Interest continues in footstrike or exertional hemolysis, which occurs in runners, aerobic dancers, rowers, weight lifters, even distance swimmers. This study using SEM shows disrupted RBC membrane skeletons in concert with intravascular hemolysis (as shown by the decline in haptoglobin concentration) after a marathon race. But this modest decline in haptoglobin here reflects the main message about exertional hemolysis: It rarely is important clinically. Because exertional hemolysis rarely exhausts the supply of plasma haptoglobin, it does not drain iron stores. Similarly, because exertional hemolysis is generally mild, it can easily be offset by mild reticulocytosis.

E.R. Eichner, M.D.

Effects of Hydroxyurea Adminstration on the Body Weight, Body Composition and Exercise Performance of Patients With Sickle-cell Anaemia
Hackney AC, Hezier W, Gulledge TP, et al (Univ of North Carolina, Chapel Hill)
Clin Sci 92:481–486, 1997   6–25

Introduction.—Sickle cell anemia is a common genetic illness, with a gene frequency of approximately 8%. Hydroxyurea is an inhibitor of the enzyme ribonucleotide reductase and has beneficial hematologic effects on patients with sickle cell anemia. The effect of body mass, body composition, and exercise performance on patients with sickle cell anemia taking hydroxyurea was defined.

Methods.—Six men and 4 women received hydroxyurea while 8 men and 6 women received placebo. During 4 separate 24-hour admissions at baseline, 6 months, 12 months, and 18 months, data for each patient were collected. A dual x-ray absorptiometer was used to measure body composition. Cycle ergometry was used to measure exercise testing. A Wingate protocol was used to assess anaerobic performance. A steady-state submaximal exercise protocol was used to examine aerobic performance.

Results.—The hydroxyurea- and placebo-treated groups had no significant differences in any of the parameters at baseline. An average body mass gain of 3.16 kg was seen at 18 months in the hydroxyurea-treated patients. The placebo-treated participants had an average gain in mass of 1.82 kg. Both lean and fat components accounted for the additional mass in both groups. An increase in peak muscle power of 104.9 W was seen in anaerobic performance in the patients given hydroxyurea. The placebo group had a more modest increase of 57.7 W. The hydroxyurea-treated men had the most marked improvement in anaerobic performance. A decrease in peak heart rate response to a standardized workrate of 15.2 beats/min was seen in the aerobic performance of the hydroxyurea-treated patients. The placebo-treated participants had a decrease of only 4.3 beats/min.

Conclusion.—Hydroxyurea administration produced an improvement in physical capacity of patients with sickle cell anemia when the data combined the overall gain in body mass with increases in anaerobic muscular performance and aerobic cardiovascular efficiency.

▶ Sickle cell disease reflects the presence of an abnormal variant of the hemoglobin molecule, which has difficulty in unfolding during gas exchange. A surprisingly large proportion of African Americans are affected by this condition (up to 8%). In 1987, Charache and associates reported clinical benefit from administration of an inhibitor of the enzyme ribonucleotide reductase, hydroxyurea.[1] The present controlled trial showed increased weight gain, improvements in anaerobic muscle performance, and a lower heart rate during submaximal aerobic work in patients receiving hydroxyurea than in those receiving a placebo. The authors speculate that part of the benefit from the drug results from a reduction in hemolysis following administration of hydroxyurea. Less energy is then needed for synthesis of erythrocytes, and more is available for synthesis of lean tissue. However, the gain in hemoglobin during 18 months of treatment (4 vs. 3 g/L) was only marginally greater than in control subjects, and the final value (90 g/L) remained well below normal limits.

R.J. Shephard, M.D., Ph.D., D.P.E

Reference

1. Charache S, Dover GL, Moyer MA, et al: Hydroxyurea-induced augmentation of fetal hemoglobin production in patients with sickle-cell anemia. *Blood* 69:109, 1987.

Hormonal, Immunological, and Hematological Responses to Intensified Training in Elite Swimmers

Mackinnon LT, Hooper SL, Jones S, et al (Univ of Queensland, Brisbane, Australia)

Med Sci Sports Exerc 29:1637–1645, 1997　　　　　　　　　　　6–26

Background.—Overtraining syndrome is characterized by excessive fatigue, mood state changes, and performance decrements usually refractory to short-term rest or recovery training. The term *overreaching* refers to similar but more transitory symptoms. Hormonal, immunologic, and hematologic variables in athletes with overreaching symptoms were compared with those in well-trained athletes during intensified training.

Methods.—Training volume was increased progressively during 4 weeks in 24 elite swimmers (16 women and 8 men). Overreaching symptoms were identified in 8 swimmers based on decrements in swimming performance, persistent high fatigue ratings, and log book comments indicating poor adaptation to increased training.

Findings.—Urinary excretion of norepinephrine was significantly decreased in overreached compared to well-trained swimmers during the 4 weeks. The 2 groups did not differ significantly in levels of plasma norepinephrine, cortisol, and testosterone; testosterone-to-cortisol ratio; peripheral blood leukocyte and differential counts; neutrophil-to-lymphocyte ratio; CD4-to-CD8 cell ratio; serum ferritin and blood hemoglobin concentrations; erythrocyte number; hemotocrit; or mean red cell volume. Both groups showed significant increases in mean red cell volume during the 4-week period, suggesting increased red blood cell turnover.

Conclusions.—Urinary norepinephrine excretion appears to be the only variable measured that distinguishes overreached from well-trained swimmers during short-term intensified training. Low urinary norepinephrine excretion was seen 2–4 weeks before overreaching symptoms appeared, indicating that neuroendocrine changes may precede and possibly contribute to the development of overreaching and overtraining syndromes.

▶ The hunt continues for the elusive laboratory marker of "overtraining." Followed here were 16 hormonal, immunologic, or hematologic variables in 24 elite swimmers who "overtrained" by increasing their swim volume 10% a week for 4 weeks. Among these 16 variables, few changed much, even though 8 swimmers had performance or subjective signs of overreaching. Testosterone/cortisol ratio, proposed by others as a marker of overtraining,[1] was no help here. Urinary norepinephrine excretion was the strongest "discriminator" of those who overreached, but it was low in these swimmers at the *start* of the study, and did not fall during the study. Still, the authors conclude that overreaching/overtraining may be a neuroendocrine disorder. Time will tell. The swimmers as a group (those who overreached and those who did not) did have dilutional pseudoanemia (likely from an expanded plasma volume) and the increase in erythrocyte mean cell volume that likely reflects exertional hemolysis, described before in runners and swimmers.[2, 3]

E.R. Eichner, M.D.

References

1. 1994 YEAR BOOK OF SPORTS MEDICINE, pp 342–343.
2. Eichner ER: Runner's macrocytosis: A clue to footstrike hemolysis. *Am J Med* 78:321–325, 1985.
3. Selby GB, Eichner ER: Endurance swimming, intravascular hemolysis, anemia and iron depletion: A new perspective on athlete's anemia. *Am J Med* 81:791–794, 1986.

Prolonged Submaximal Eccentric Exercise Is Associated With Increased Levels of Plasma IL–6
Rohde T, MacLean DA, Richter EA, et al (Univ of Copenhagen)
Am J Physiol 273:E85–E91, 1997
6–27

Background.—Severe eccentric exercise results in muscle damage and plasma cytokine increases. The cause of muscle damage, increased protein breakdown, and the role of cytokines are not clear, though several mechanisms have been proposed, including mechanical overload and Ca^{2+}–mediated proteolysis. Supplementing branched–chain amino acids (BCAA) before and during exercise can decrease the amount of net muscle protein degradation and the release of essential amino acids from muscle that normally occurs during prolonged exercise. The relationship among a continuous submaximal eccentric bout, plasma cytokine response, and the cellular immune system was investigated.

Methods.—Six men performed 2 trials of prolonged eccentric exercise of one leg. The first was a BCAA supplementation trial, and the second was a control trial.

Findings.—In the BCAA trial, the release of amino acids from muscle during and after eccentric exercise was reduced, suggesting that the net muscle protein degradation was suppressed. Mean plasma interleukin (IL)–6 levels rose from 0.75 to 5.02 pg/mL in the control trial and from 1.07 to 4.15 pg/mL in the BCAA supplementation trial. Eccentric exercise did not affect concentrations of neutrophils, lymphocytes, CD16+/CD56+, CD4+, CD8+, CD114+/CD38+, lymphocyte proliferative response, or cytotoxic activities. However, BCAA supplementation decreased the concentration of CD14+/CD38+ cells.

Conclusions.—The concentration of IL-6 in plasma is increased after prolonged eccentric exercise. The cytokine response appears to be independent of the muscle proteolysis seen during exercise.

▶ This group has long explored how exercise influences immunity. Exercise may alter immune function by releasing stress hormones or cytokines. Strenuous eccentric exercise tends to damage muscles and release cytokines; this study explores whether submaximal eccentric exercise alters immune markers and whether release of cytokines (IL–6) correlates with muscle damage. Earlier research suggests exercise releases (into the serum) IL–6 more than other cytokines.[1] IL-6 causes fever and stimulates ACTH release, and is the main inducer of the acute-phase reaction of the liver. So IL-6 is a likely "immunomodulator of exercise." This study shows that supplementation with branched chain amino acids (leucine, valine, and isoleucine) reduces muscle damage and proteolysis from eccentric exercise but does not reduce the release of IL–6. But other researchers have correlated muscle damage to release of IL–6.[1] In any case, in this exercise model (one-leg, submaximal, prolonged, eccentric exercise), very little immunomodulation was seen, so very little can be concluded.

E.R. Eichner, M.D.

Reference

1. Weinstock C, et al: Effect of exhaustive exercise stress on the cytokine response. *Med Sci Sports Exerc* 29:345–354, 1997.

In Vivo Cell-mediated Immunity and Vaccination Response Following Prolonged, Intense Exercise

Bruunsgaard H, Hartkopp A, Mohr T, et al (Univ of Copenhagen; Rigshospitalet, Copenhagen; Panum Inst, Copenhagen; et al)
Med Sci Sports Exerc 29:1176–1181, 1997   6–28

Introduction.—Prolonged, intense exercise results in a depression of the number of lymphocytes in the blood and impairment in the function of natural killer and B cells. This period of immunological suppression may increase an individual's susceptibility to micro-organisms. A study was designed to determine whether an in vivo impairment of cell-mediated immunity and antibody production exists after intense, long-term exercise.

Methods.—Study participants, all men, were 33 triathletes (group A) who performed a training competition, 11 healthy non-exercising triathletes (controls; group B), and 22 healthy moderately trained individuals (controls; group C). All underwent a skin test (7 different antigens applied on the forearm) and vaccinations with tetanus and diphtheritis toxoid and pneumonococcal polysaccharide. Immunizations were performed in group A after the period of intense exercise. Antibody titers were measured before and 2 weeks after the exercise; the skin test was read 48 hours after application.

Results.—Compared with control groups B and C, the athletes who had completed one half of an ironman competition exhibited a significantly lower skin test response to the tetanus antigen. The group A triathletes also demonstrated a smaller cumulative response, consisting of the sum of the diameters of indurations and number of positive skin-test spots (responses were similar in groups B and C). Assessment of the vaccination response showed levels of specific antibodies to be similar among the 3 groups.

Conclusion.—In the early days after prolonged, high-intensity exercise, in vivo cell-mediated immunity was impaired in these athletes. Two weeks after the vaccination, however, no impairment of the in vivo antibody production was observed. Thus transient, early suppression of immunity after exercise may increase the risk of acute infection but does not affect the subsequent establishment and generation of specific immunity.

▶ As we frequently review, exercise-related immune changes tend to be mild, mixed, and brief, making their clinical import moot.[1, 2] Most studies rely on in vitro tests of immunity. Even from the same research group, results are mixed, depending in part on study populations. One group, for example, finds baseline natural killer cell activity to be increased in marathoners but not in endurance athletes compared to controls.[3, 4] This article summarizes results of in vivo tests to gauge exercise-related changes in immunity. But as in prior studies using in vitro tests, any changes are small and of dubious clinical import. Here the skin tests (not read blindly) after the triathlon suggest a decrease in cellular immunity. But the antibody response to vaccinations after the marathon was normal, as in an early study with tetanus toxoid.[5] Exercise-related immune changes remain a phenomenon in search of a clinical role.

E.R. Eichner M.D.

References

1. 1997 YEAR BOOK OF SPORTS MEDICINE, pp 415–416.
2. 1996 YEAR BOOK OF SPORTS MEDICINE, pp 373–376.
3. Nieman DC, Buckley KS, Henson DA, et al: Immune function in marathon runners versus sedentary controls. *Med Sci Sports Exerc* 27:986–992, 1995.
4. Nieman DC, Brendle D, Henson DA, et al: Immune function in athletes versus nonathletes. *Int J Sports Med* 16:329–333, 1995.
5. Eskola J, Ruuskanen O, Soppi E, et al: Effect of sport stress on lymphocyte transformation and antibody formation. *Clin Exp Immunol* 32:339–345, 1978.

Effects of Bovine Colostrum Supplementation on Serum IGF-I, IgG, Hormone, and Saliva IgA During Training

Mero A, Miikkulainen H, Riski J, et al (Univ of Jyväskylä, Finland; Turku Technology Ctr, Finland)
J Appl Physiol 83:1144–1151, 1997   6–29

Objective.—Bovine colostrum is known to be very important to the health of calves. It contains growth factors and antimicrobial factors in addition to nutrients. The most abundant growth factors present are insulin-like growth factors (IGF) I and II, which stimulate cell growth and may act as endocrine hormones and as paracrine and autocrine growth factors. Drinking colostrum or colostrum supplements might increase IGF-I concentration in human blood. Bovine colostrum supplement is commercially available in Europe as Bioenervi and is not banned in Olympic competition. This article studies the effects of serum IGF-I on physiologic responses in human athletes.

Methods.—The randomized, crossover study included 9 drug-free male sprinters and jumpers. The athletes took part in 3 experimental training treatment periods, each separated by 13 days. In each period, the subjects consumed a drink of 125 mL/day. Two of the drinks contained Bioenervi, 25 or 125 mL/day, and a third was a placebo. During each treatment, the subjects took part in an identical strength and speed training program. The effects of Bioenervi supplementation on serum IGF-I, IgG, hormone, and amino acid levels and on saliva IgA concentrations were assessed.

Results.—Serum IGF-I increased with Bioenervi treatments relative to placebo—especially at the higher dose—with both Bioenervi treatments, the 8-day change in IGF-I was significantly and positively correlated with the change in insulin concentration during the same period. There were no significant differences in serum IgG, hormone, and amino acid levels or saliva IgA response between the 3 treatments.

Conclusion.—For athletes in strength and speed training, Bioenervi bovine colostrum supplement significantly increases serum IGF-I concentrations. This could result from direct absorption of IGF-I from Bioenervi or from stimulation of endogenous IGF-I synthesis. No significant effects on saliva IgA, serum IgG or amino acid concentrations are apparent.

▶ Bovine colostrum whey is not yet approved for sale in North America, but its use is permitted in some European countries. Although the product contains large quantities of various immunoglobulins relative to normal milk, it does not appear to boost salivary IgA levels, at least in normal, healthy subjects. Of equal interest to the sports physician, it increases concentrations of serum IGF-I, and may, thus, enhance muscle hypertrophy during strength training. To date, the substance is not banned by the International Olympic Committee, but it would seem time for the Medical Committee to make a ruling on the use of this substance by competitors.

R.J. Shephard, M.D., Ph.D., D.P.E.

Effect of Exercise on Milk Immunoglobulin A

Gregory RL, Wallace JP, Gfell LE, et al (Indiana Univ, Indianapolis; Indiana Univ, Bloomington)
Med Sci Sports Exerc 29:1596–1601, 1997   6–30

Background.—The immunologic effects of maximal exercise on breast milk have not been well documented. Because immunoglobulin A (IgA) is the main Ig in human secretions, the influence of exercise on breast milk IgA and IgA subclasses was studied.

Methods.—Seventeen lactating women were studied. Breast milk was collected before and after randomly ordered periods of exercise and non-exercise. Exercise consisted of a maximal graded treadmill test. After milk

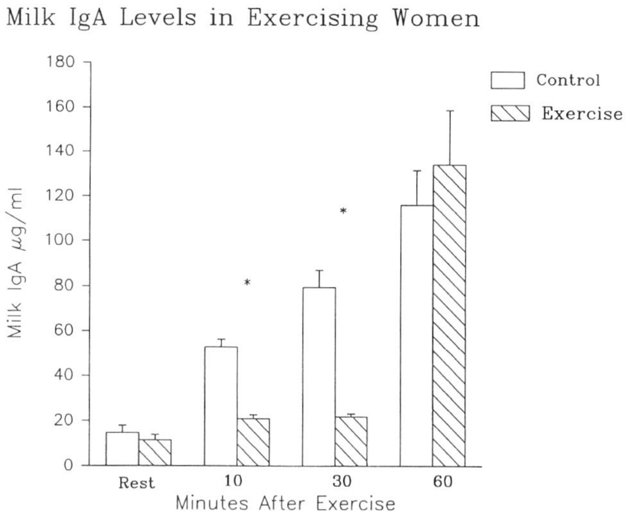

Milk IgA Levels in Exercising Women

FIGURE 1.—Concentrations of breast milk IgA from 17 postpartum exercising and control women during rest and 10, 30, and 60 minutes after exercise. Samples were collected during rest, the breasts were emptied, and the subjects either exercised or rested, and samples were collected 10, 30, and 60 minutes after exercise or control rest periods. Values are means (μg·mL^{-1}) ± SEM. Every woman served as both an exercising volunteer and control subject on different days. Significant differences ($P \leq 0.05$) between control and exercise milk IgA values are marked with an asterisk above the bars. (Courtesy of Gregory RL, Wallace JP, Gfell LE, at al: Effect of exercise on milk immunoglobulin A. *Med Sci Sports Exerc* 29:1596–1601, 1997.)

was collected at rest, additional samples were obtained 10, 30, and 60 minutes after exercise or after 30-minute rest periods.

Findings.—Milk obtained 10 and 30 minutes after exercise showed significantly lower IgA concentrations than milk obtained after the control period. Exercise and control samples were similar at 1 hour, indicating that milk IgA production had recovered by this time. A similar significant reduction in IgA1 was seen 10 minutes after exercise, which normalized by 30 and 60 minutes. No significant changes occurred in milk IgA2 levels at any of the times studied. In both exercise and control groups, milk IgA concentrations rose significantly after the breasts were emptied, suggesting that breast emptying stimulated milk IgA synthesis (Fig 1).

Conclusions.—Exercise appears to change milk IgA and IgA1 concentrations for 10–30 minutes after exhaustive exercise, but recovery occurs within 1 hour. The current data also provide more evidence of the effects of exercise on the mucosal immune system.

▶ This study augments earlier research from one of the investigators to offer practical guidelines for young, athletic mothers who breast-feed. The profiles of IgA (vs. its subclasses) in breast milk over time show a puzzling lack of concordance, which the authors attribute to different tests and reagents. But the trend seems clear: women have a "transient milk IgA deficiency" following maximal exercise compared with when they rest (see Figure 1). This fits with most (but not all) prior research on salivary IgA, which tends to fall after maximal exercise in skiers, cyclists, swimmers, and runners.[1] Earlier work from one of these investigators showed that, at the same times postexercise that IgA level is low (10 minutes and 30 minutes), lactic acid levels are high and make milk taste sour and unappealing.[2] So the practical guidelines are: (1) exercise moderately to avoid accumulating lactic acid; (2) nurse before exercise or collect preexercise milk to feed later; or (3) discard milk produced during the first 30 minutes after maximal exercise.

E.R. Eichner, M.D.

References

1. 1994 YEAR BOOK OF SPORTS MEDICINE, pp 394–395.
2. Wallace JP, Rabin J: The concentration of lactic acid in breast milk following maximal exercise. *Int J Sports Med* 12:328–331, 1991.

Carbohydrate Affects Natural Killer Cell Redistribution but Not Activity After Running

Nieman DC, Henson DA, Garner EB, et al (Appalachian State Univ, Boone, NC; Univ of South Carolina, Columbia; Loma Linda Univ, Calif)
Med Sci Sports Exerc 29:1318–1324, 1997   6–31

Introduction.—In previous studies of marathon runners, the authors demonstrated that natural cell cytotoxic activity (NKCA) is strongly depressed during recovery from running. A cortisol-induced redistribution of blood natural killer (NK) lymphocytes from the blood compartment to other tissues appears to account for the decrease in NKCA. This randomized study examined the influence of carbohydrate supplementation on the NK cell response to 2.5 hours of high-intensity running.

Methods.—Study participants, 24 men and 6 women aged 25 to 29, were marathon runners with 4 years or more of running experience. All had completed at least 2 marathon events during the previous year. Seventeen were randomized to carbohydrate and 13 to placebo supplement groups. The runners and sedentary controls were both tested during the months of May and June. After a 12-hour fast and resting condition, runners had a blood sample taken, then consumed 0.75 L of a 6% carbohydrate (Gatorade) or placebo beverage. The marathoners ran on treadmills for 2.5 hours at a pace adjusted to elicit a workload approximating 75% to 80% of VO_{2max}. Every 15 minutes they ingested 0.25 L of carbohydrate or placebo fluid. Blood samples were obtained immediately after the run and at 3 periods in the next 5 hours.

Results.—The carbohydrate and placebo groups were comparable in training and fitness parameters and in energy intake during the 3 days before testing. Runners lost an average of 0.35 kg of body weight during the exercise protocol. The pattern of change in glucose, cortisol, and the blood concentration of NK cells (Fig 1) differed significantly between carbohydrate and placebo groups, but the 2 groups did not significantly differ in NKCA after 2.5 hours of intensive running (Fig 2). Changes in

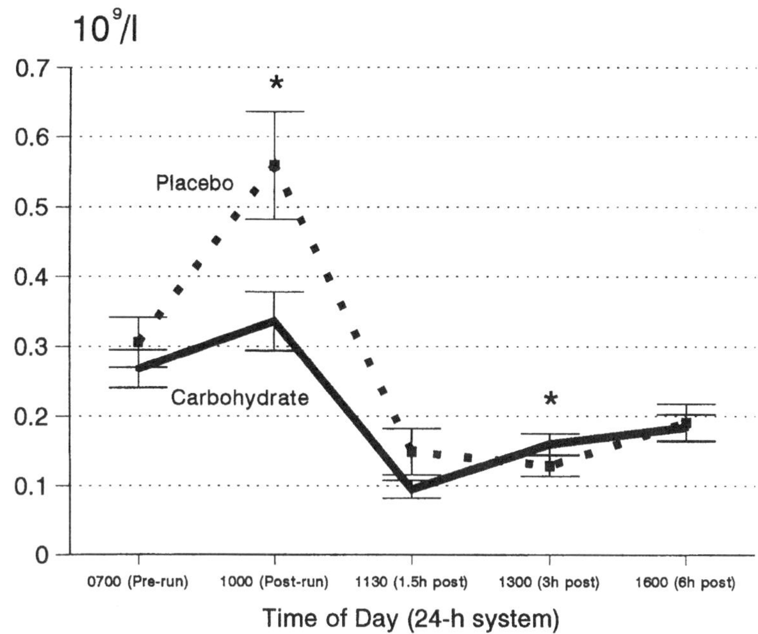

FIGURE 1.—A significant difference in the pattern of change between groups over time was found for blood natural killer cell counts, highlighted by a greater increase in the placebo group immediately postrun and a greater decrease 3 hours postrun [$F_{(4,25)}$ = 3.79]. *P less than 0.05 = significant difference from baseline (pre-exercise) between groups. (Courtesy of Nieman DC, Henson DA, Garner EB, et al: Carbohydrate affects natural killer cell redistribution but not activity after running. *Med Sci Sports Exerc* 29:1318–1324, 1997.)

plasma epinephrine and norepinephrine from pre- to immediate postrun tended to be higher in runners given the placebo drink.

Conclusion.—Post-2.5-hour-run plasma glucose concentrations, stress hormone concentrations, and leukocyte subset and NK cell trafficking are affected by carbohydrate vs. placebo supplementation. This finding confirms the need to control for carbohydrate ingestion during exercise immunology experiments.

▶ Can sports drinks bolster your immunity on the run? Well, maybe. In theory, by curbing falls in blood volume and blood glucose, sports drinks like Gatorade can minimize surges in stress hormones and so minimize wide swings in NK cell counts during and after the race. That's what happened here. After the long run, placebo drinkers had lower glucose, higher norepinephrine, and higher cortisol levels than did Gatorade drinkers. And sure enough, during the run placebo drinkers had wider swings (sharper rise, sharper fall) in NK cell counts. But NK cell activity was not affected. We need more research on whether these modest changes have clinical import. Meanwhile, I'll keep quaffing Gatorade.

E.R. Eichner, M.D.

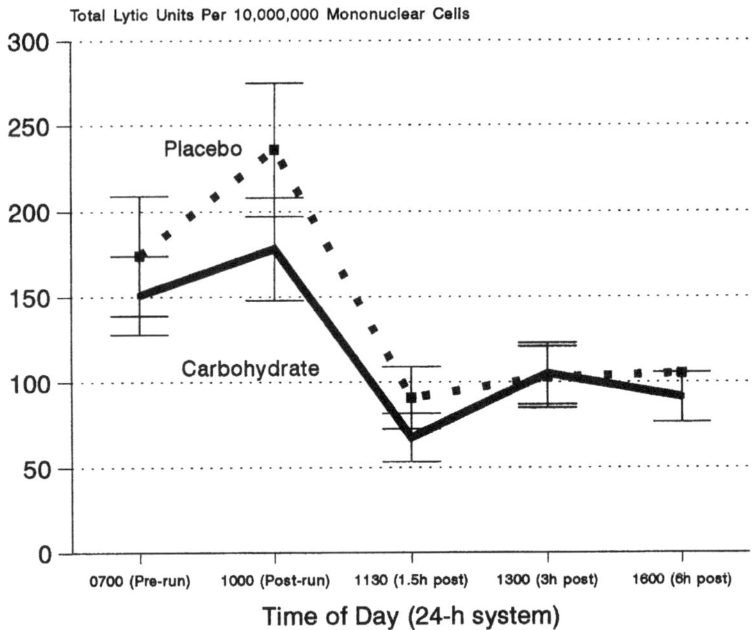

FIGURE 2.—The pattern of change over time between groups was not significantly different for natural killer cell cytotoxic activity when expressed as total lytic U [$F(4,112) = 0.80$, P = 0.530]. For all subjects combined, a significant time effect was observed [$F(4,112) = 18.6$, P less than 0.001], with NKCA decreasing below prerun levels during 6 hours of recovery. *Abbreviation: NKCA,* natural killer cell cytotoxic activity. (Courtesy of Nieman DC, Henson DA, Garner EB, et al: Carbohydrate affects natural killer cell redistribution but not activity after running. *Med Sci Sports Exerc* 29:1318–1324, 1997.)

Effects of Exercise Intensity on Natural Killer Cell Activity in Women

Strasner A, Davis JM, Kohut ML, et al (Univ of South Carolina, Columbia)
Int J Sports Med 18:56–62, 1997
6–32

Introduction.—The natural killer cell may be one potential biologic explanation for the relationship between exercise and altered risk of infection and cancer. Natural killer cells can initiate spontaneous cytolytic activity against virally infected and malignant cells without requiring antibodies or antigens, earning them the reputation as a first and extended line of defense against foreign pathogens and cancer. Acute exercise includes a transient increase in natural killer cytolytic activity just after exercise followed by a drop to below baseline levels within 2 hours of recovery, and the magnitude of these phases correlates with exercise intensity. The effects of high-intensity vs. moderate-intensity cycle ergometer exercise on natural killer cell activity in women using oral contraceptives was investigated. The potential role of epinephrine, norepinephrine, and cortisol as mediators of these effects was investigated.

Methods.—Eight women participated in 3 conditions of 25 minutes of cycle ergometer exercise at high intensity (80% VO_2 max), at moderate

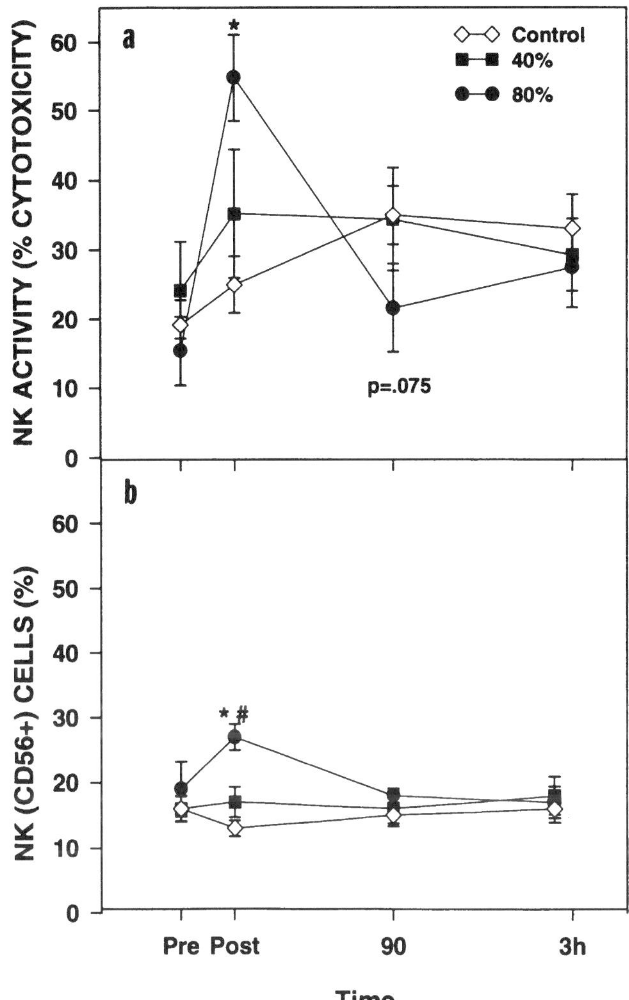

FIGURE 1.—a, natural killer cell cytolytic activity in response to high-intensity exercise, moderate-intensity exercise, and resting control sessions in 8 active females. *P ≤0.05 vs. control. These data represent natural killer cell activity at the 80:1 ratio. Similar results were obtained at the other effector: target cell ratios. b, percentage of natural killer cells (CD56$^+$) relative to peripheral blood mononuclear cells in response to high-intensity exercise, moderate-intensity exercise, and resting control sessions. *P ≤0.05 vs. control. # = P ≤0.05 vs. moderate-intensity exercise (n=8). (Courtesy of Strasner A, Davis JM, Kohut ML, et al: Effects of exercise intensity on natural killer cell activity in women. *Int J Sports Med* 18:56–62, 1997 Georg Thieme Verlag.)

intensity (40% VO$_2$ max), and a control session in which they remained seated on the cycle but did not exercise. Blood was obtained just before, immediately after, and 90 minutes and 3 hours after exercise.

Results.—Natural killer cell activity gradually increased during the control session, and cortisol concentration gradually decreased during the approximately 3½-hour experimental periods. High intensity increased natural killer cell activity, %CD56[+] natural killer cells, and plasma nor-epinephrine immediately after exercise, as compared with controls (Fig 1). At 90 minutes after exercise, there was a trend for decreased natural killer activity. At 3 hours after exercise, there were no differences among the treatment groups. There were no differences from the control in any variable at any time in the moderate-intensity group.

Conclusion.—A brief increase of natural killer cell response followed by a more prolonged suppression occurs in women using oral contraceptives in response to intense exercise as it does in men.

▶ As the authors point out in their discussion, the conclusions drawn from this study would be quite different had they relied on each subject serving as her own control rather than incorporating a resting control session into the experimental design. Time and money saved by using preexercise values as a baseline against which exercise effects are compared are time and money wasted if the variable of interest does not remain constant over time under resting conditions.

B.L. Drinkwater, Ph.D.

Carbohydrate Supplementation Affects Blood Granulocyte and Monocyte Trafficking but not Function After 2.5 h of Running
Nieman DC, Fagoaga OR, Butterworth DE, et al (Appalachian State Univ, Boone, NC; Loma Linda Univ, Calif; Univ of South Carolina, Columbia)
Am J Clin Nutr 66:153–159, 1997   6–33

Introduction.—Various measures of immune function, including natural killer cell cytotoxic activity and mitogen-induced lymphocyte proliferation, are depressed in marathon runners during intensive running. Sustained neutrophilia, monocytosis, and lymphopenia are also associated with endurance running. The interaction between exercise and immune function may be modulated by nutritional status. Higher blood glucose and lower cortisol and epinephrine responses have been associated with carbohydrate ingestion during prolonged endurance exercise. The immune response may also be altered by ingestion of carbohydrate during intensive running. The influence of supplemental carbohydrate on the immune response was investigated during 2.5 hours of intensive running.

Methods.—Of 30 experienced marathon runners, 17 were assigned to carbohydrate supplement and 13 received placebo. Before a blood sample was taken at 7:15 AM, the individuals rested for 10–15 minutes, then ingested 0.75 L of carbohydrate beverage or placebo. Fifteen minutes later, they began running at 75% to 80% of VO_{2max} for 2.5 hours. Every 15 minutes, they drank 0.25 L carbohydrate or placebo fluid. Another blood sample was taken immediately after the 2.5-hour run. Samples were then taken at 1.5 hours, 3 hours, and 6 hours.

Results.—The pattern in plasma glucose and cortisol and the blood concentration of neutrophils and monocytes were significantly changed in

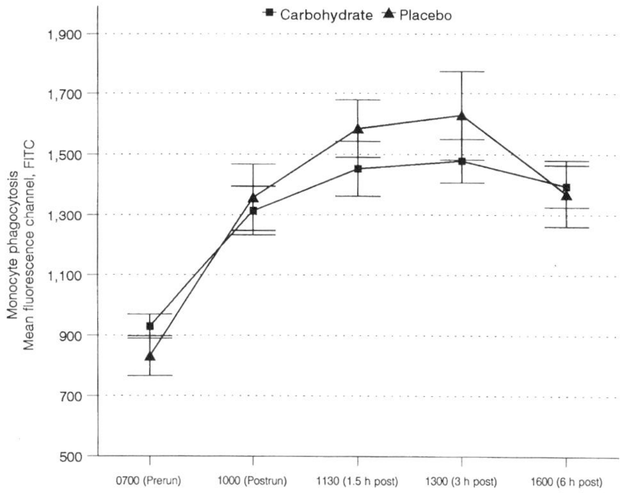

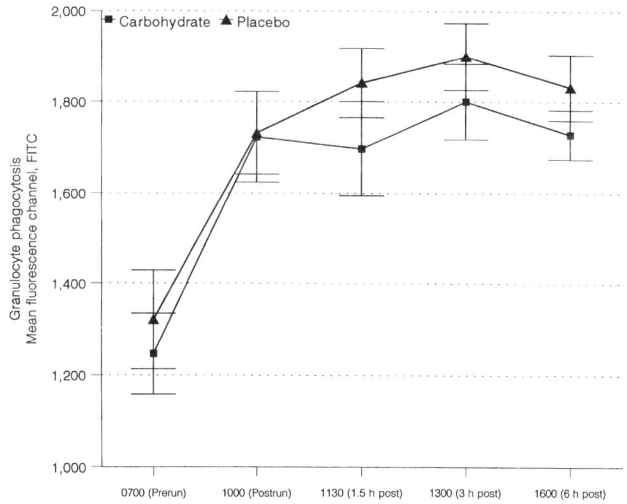

FIGURE 1.—Pattern of change in blood monocyte or granulocyte phagocytosis for the carbohydrate and placebo groups over time. No significant differences were found. *Abbreviation: FITC,* fluorescein isothiocyanate. (Courtesy of Nieman DC, Fagoaga OR, Butterworth DE, et al: Carbohydrate supplementation affects granulocyte and monocyte trafficking but not function after 2.5 h of running. *Am J Clin Nutr* 66:153–159, 1997, copyright *Am J Clin Nutr*, American Society for Clinical Nutrition.)

the carbohydrate-drinking group when compared with those of the placebo-drinking group. However, the blood granulocyte and monocyte phagocytosis or oxidative burst activity after 2.5 hours of intensive running were not changed by carbohydrate intake (Fig 1).

Conclusion.—A significant effect in raising plasma glucose concentrations, decreasing plasma cortisol, and attenuating changes in circulating leukocyte subsets resulted from carbohydrate supplementation before, during, and after 2.5 hours of intensive running. However, blood granulocyte and monocyte function were not affected.

▶ A recent review drew attention to the possible modulation of immune responses by changes in nutritional status.[1] In particular, prolonged exercise might deplete glycogen reserves, thus reducing the availability of key amino acids needed for lymphocyte proliferation, or a decrease in overall metabolism might avert the adverse effects associated with the generation of reactive species during metabolism. Nieman and associates carried out a nice controlled experiment to test the effect of administering glucose supplements over a 2.5-hour run. They pointed out that the experimental manipulation not only increased blood glucose levels, but also modified many key hormone concentrations, including epinephrine and cortisol, and they suggest that it was probably the manipulation of these hormones that modified neutrophil and monocyte response to the bout of exercise. The changes in leukocyte count, although statistically significant, were relatively small, and probably had no great clinical significance.

R.J. Shephard, M.D., Ph.D., D.P.E.

Reference

1. Shephard RJ, Shek PN: Heavy exercise, nutrition and immune function: Is there a connection? *Int J Sports Med* 16:491–497, 1995.

7 Environmental Factors

Interactions of Physical Training and Heat Acclimation: The Thermo-physiology of Exercising in a Hot Climate
Aoyagi Y, McLellan TM, Shephard RJ (Univ of Toronto; Defence and Civil Inst of Environmental Medicine, North York, Ont, Canada; Brock Univ, St Catherines, Ont, Canada)
Sports Med 23:173–210, 1997
7–1

Background.—Competing in hot climates may pose a threat to not only the performance but also the health of athletes, particularly athletes from more temperate zones. In this situation, physical training and heat acclimation can help to improve performance and/or tolerance times. The mechanisms of achieving heat balance, the effects of protective clothing, physical training, and heat acclimation on responses to exercise in the heat, and the potential interactions between physical training and heat acclimation were reviewed.

Physical Training and Heat Acclimation.—For athletes competing at high temperatures, physical training can lead to improved aerobic fitness and thus to greater cardiovascular reserve. By lowering resting body temperature, heat acclimation permits greater heat storage. These tactics can also reduce the energy cost of exercise at a given intensity, increase the sweating response at a given percentage of maximal effort, and slow the associated increases in body temperature. Cardiovascular stress may be reduced by changes in the autonomic nervous system, expansion of blood volume, and decreased peripheral blood pooling. Decreased relative intensity of exercise, reduced physiologic strain, and habituation to heat-exercise stress may lead to improved subjective tolerance of exercise in hot conditions.

Many different factors may affect the athlete's improvement in physiologic and psychological responses, including baseline level of fitness and acclimation to heat. Age, sex, hydration, sleep status, circadian rhythms, and the menstrual cycle may also have an effect. Other relevant conditions may include the use of various ergogenic aids, mode of exercise and other event conditions, and various treatment conditions.

Recommendations.—Although physical training and heat acclimation can produce similar gains in exercise tolerance at hot temperatures, there are important differences between the 2 tactics. Whereas physical training increases aerobic fitness and decreases relative work intensity, heat acclimation lowers the thermoregulatory set point and the energy cost for a given task. Good training and heat acclimation are necessary to maximize adjustment to performing in a hot environment. For a lightly clothed athlete, significant improvements can be realized with just 1–2 weeks of physical training and heat acclimation. The gains produced by either tactic will be relatively small if the athlete wears protective clothing with limited vapor permeability.

▶ This comprehensive review is exceedingly technical and, for the most part, of practical value for the exercise physiologist. However, its bibliography of 311 citations certainly provides what is probably a comprehensive list of the articles dealing with the subject matter. It is unquestionably an impressive document.

J.S. Torg, M.D.

▶ The authors present an in-depth review of current studies regarding exercising in a hot climate. They state, "maximal adjustment to work in a hot environment requires that competitors be both well trained and fully heat acclimated." They recommend fluid replacement, beginning with 400–600 mL, 20–30 minutes prior to the event and 150–250 mL every 15 minutes during the event.

F.J. George, A.T.C., P.T.

Hyperhydration: Thermoregulatory Effects During Compensable Exercise-Heat Stress
Latzka WA, Sawka MN, Montain SJ, et al (United States Army Research Inst, Boston; Boston Univ)
J Appl Physiol 83:860–866, 1997   7–2

Introduction.—It has been suggested that hyperhydration improves thermoregulation during exercise in heat above euhydration levels; reports conflict regarding the value of hyperhydration relative to euhydration. The effects of hyperhydration on thermoregulatory responses during compensable exercise-heat stress were evaluated.

Methods.—Eight heat-acclimated men with an average age of 23 years, underwent 1-hour preexercise hyperhydration [29.1 mL/kg lean body mass; with and without glycerol (1.2 g/kg lean body mass)] to determine if sweating responses could be improved and core temperature could be reduced during exercise. Each research subject completed the following exercise trials: euhydration; glycerol hyperhydration, with and without rehydration; and water hyperhydration, with and without rehydration.

Results.—The evaporative heat loss required (E_{req} = 293 W/m²) to preserve steady state core temperature was less than the maximum capacity (E_{max} = 462 W/m²) of the climate for evaporative heat loss (E_{req}/E_{max} = 63%). When research subjects exercised in the heat (35°C, 45% relative humidity), there was no difference between hyperhydration methods for

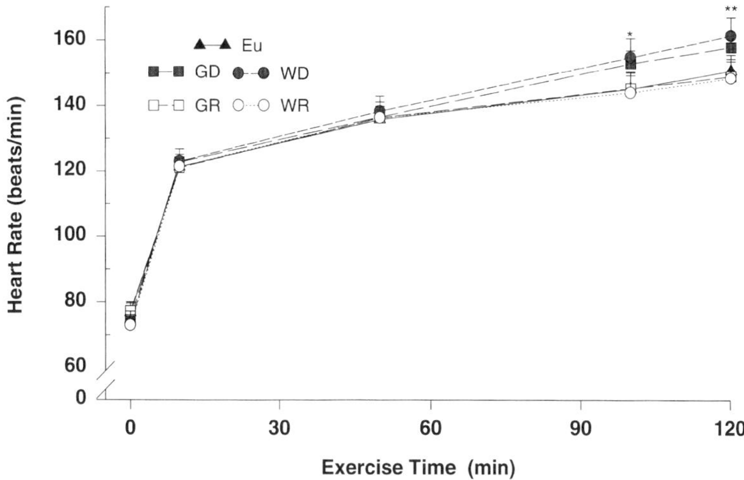

FIGURE 2.—Heart rate response during exercise-heat stress trials. Values are means ± SE; n = 8 subjects. *GD and WD values greater than WR values, $P < 0.05$. † GD and WD values greater than GR, WR, and Eu values, $P < 0.05$. *Symbols*: ▲, Euhydration (Eu); ■, glycerol hydration with no rehydration (GD); □, glycerol hyperhydration with rehydration (GR); ●, water hyperhydration with no rehydration (WD); ○, water hyperhydration with rehydration (WR). (Courtesy of Latzka WA, Sawke MN, Montain SJ: Hyperhydration: Thermoregulatory effects during compensation exercise-heat stress. *J Appl Physiol* 83:860–866, 1997.)

increasing total body water (~1.5 liters). When compared with euhydration, hyperhydration did not affect core temperature, skin temperature, whole body sweating rate, local sweating rate, sweating threshold temperature, sweating sensitivity, or heart rate (Fig 2) responses. Water and glycerol did not differ for these physiologic responses.

Conclusion.—Hyperhydration offered no thermoregulatory advantages over the maintenance of euhydration during compensable exercise-heat stress.

▶ Although adequate hydration is important to the safety of athletic competition under warm conditions, this study cuts through earlier controversy and shows clearly that there is no advantage to be gained from hyperhydration of competitors. The question has more than academic importance because in some ultra-long distance events, collapse has arisen from hyperhydration and resulting hyponatremia.

R.J. Shephard, M.D., Ph.D., D.P.E.

Dehydration Markedly Impairs Cardiovascular Function in Hyperthermic Endurance Athletes During Exercise

González-Alonso J; Mora-Rodríguez R, Below PR, et al (Univ of Texas, Austin)
J Appl Physiol 82:1229–1236, 1997   7–3

Objective.—Dehydration can stress the cardiovascular systems of endurance athletes during competition in hot environments. The resulting hyperthermia produces a decline in cardiac output and blood pressure. Whether the combination of hyperthermia and dehydration significantly increases the strain on the circulatory system resulting in inability to maintain cardiac output and blood perssure was investigated.

Methods.—The effects of dehydration were studied in 15 endurance cyclists who exercised in the heat for 100 to 120 minutes and either became dehydrated (lost 4% of body weight) or drank fluids and continued exercising for 30 minutes at 71% VO_{2max}. The cardiovascular effects of dehydration were isolated by having volunteers exercise in the cold. The vascular effects of dehydration were studied in volunteers who received an intravenous infusion of a dextran solution to replace the reduction in blood volume lost during whole body dehydration. Hyperthermia was defined as an increase in esophageal temperature of 1°C. During the 30-minute exercise period, VO_2, heart rate, esophageal temperature, mean skin temperature, cardiac output, and systolic and diastolic blood pressure were continuously monitored. Blood and plasma volumes were calculated.

Results.—Esophageal temperature and skin temperature were unchanged from baseline during the dehydration and dehydration plus blood volume restoration study but increased during the hyperthermia and hyperthermia/dehydration studies. Blood and plasma volumes, significantly lower than control levels during the dehydration and dehydration/hyperthermia studies, were reversed with dextran infusion. Serum osmolality and sodium concentration were signficantly increased during the dehydration arms. Hyperthermia significantly reduced stroke volume and increased heart rate. The combined effects of dehydration and hyperthermia significantly altered cardiovascular responses (Fig 4). Dehydration reduced stroke volume and increased heart rate.

Conclusion.—A significant increase in skin temperature can increase skin blood flow and reduce stroke volume during exercise through mechanisms other than increasing core temperature. Both hyperthermia and dehydration decrease stroke volume primarily.

▶ Prior research by this group shows that dehydration in competitive cyclists during 2 hours of exercise induces hyperthermia. The result is a fall in cardiac output and blood pressure plus vasoconstriction of skin blood vessels and a rise in systemic vascular resistance.[1] Another group finds that when subjects are hypohydrated before exercise, they become exhausted much sooner during treadmill exercise in the heat, even though they have a lower core temperature at exhaustion compared with when euhydrated.[2]

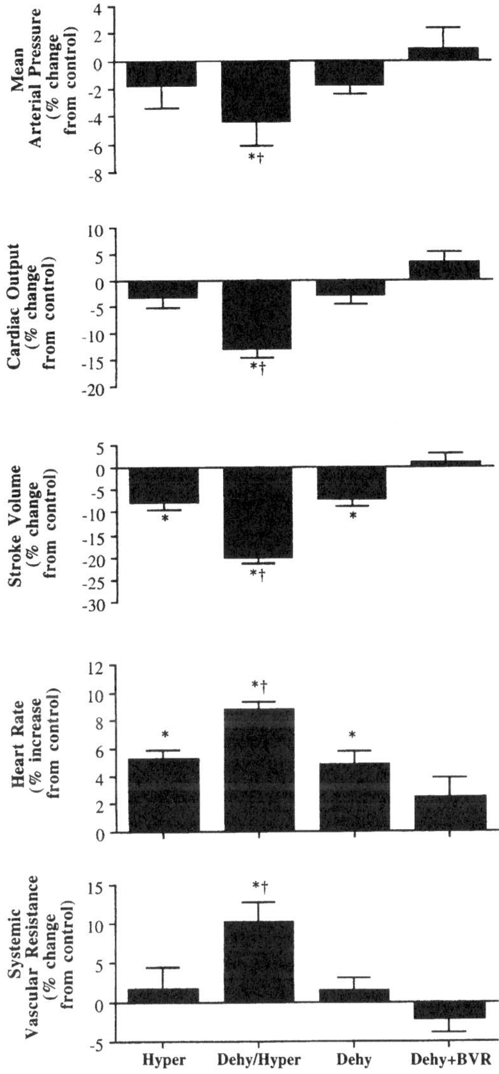

FIGURE 4.—Percent change in cardiovascular responses from control (ie, euhydrated and normothermic within a given environment) with Hyper alone (ie, without Dehy), with Dehy/Hyper, with Dehy (ie, without Hyper), and with Dehy+BVR (blood volume restoration). Values are means±SE; n = 7 and 8 subjects. *Signficantly different from control, $P < 0.05$. †Significantly different from Hyper and Dehy alone, $P < 0.05$. (Courtesy of González-Alonso J, Mora-Rodríguez R, Below PR, et al: Dehydration markedly impairs cardiovascular function in hyperthermic endurance athletes during exercise. *J Appl Physiol* 82:1229–1236, 1997.)

This study probes which limiting factor is key for athletes in the heat: hyperthermia or dehydration. The answer: both. By creative protocols, the exercise effects of hyperthermia and dehydration were separated. Either hyperthermia alone or dehydration alone lowers cardiac stroke volume 7% to

8% and increases heart rate sufficiently to prevent a decline in cardiac output. But when dehydration causes hyperthermia during exercise in the heat, the fall in stroke volume is greater (20%) and cardiac output declines (13%). Dehydration contributes to hyperthermia by evoking a sharp rise in plasma norepinephrine that constricts skin blood vessels.[3] Clinical lesson for sports medicine physicians: The dehydrated athlete is much less able to cope with hyperthermia.

E.R. Eichner, M.D.

References

1. González-Alonso J, Mora-Rodríguez R, Below PR, Coyle EF: Dehydration reduces cardiac output and increases systemic and cutaneous vascular resistance during exercise. *J Appl Physiol* 79:1487–1496, 1995.
2. Sawka MN, Young AJ, Latzka WA, et al: Human tolerance to heat strain during exercise: Influence of hydration. *J Appl Physiol* 73:368–375, 1992.
3. Mora-Rodríguez R, González-Alonso J, Below PR, et al: Plasma catecholamines and hyperglycemia influence thermoregulation during prolonged exercise in the heat. *J Physiol (London)* 491:529–540, 1996.

Hyperthermia During Olympic Triathlon: Influence of Body Heat Storage During the Swimming Stage
Kerr CG, Trappe TA, Starling RD, et al (Ball State Univ, Muncie, Ind)
Med Sci Sports Exerc 30:99–104, 1998   7–4

Introduction.—Research has indicated that wet suits decrease drag and oxygen consumption and increase buoyancy and speed of swimming. To gain this advantage, many triathletes wear wet suits regardless of environmental conditions. Wet suits are thermal insulators and may cause hyperthermia in warm conditions. This may be detrimental to subsequent cycling and running performance. The effect of the mild heat stress induced by wearing a wet suit in warm conditions on subsequent triathlon performance was analyzed.

Methods.—Five male triathletes completed 2 simulated triathlons in the laboratory using a swimming flume, cycle ergometer, and treadmill. All conditions were identical except for the swimming event, in which either a swim suit or a neoprene wet suit was worn. The environment was maintained at 32°C and 65% relative humidity. The swimming portion was standardized to 30 minutes with identical oxygen consumption, whereas the running and biking portions were completed as fast as possible.

Results.—Core temperature was not significantly different between wet suit and swim suit trials at any point. Mean skin temperature and mean body temperature were higher in the wet suit trial at 15 and 30 minutes of the swim. These differences disappeared within 15 minutes of cycling. There were no significant differences in oxygen consumption, heart rate, perceived exertion, or thermal sensation between the 2 triathlons. There were no significant differences in cycling, running, or total triathlon times between these 2 conditions.

Conclusion.—Wearing a wet suit while swimming under warm conditions in the first section of a triathlon does not alter the thermoregulatory response or adversely affect performance during subsequent cycling and running.

▶ Triathletes have found that, in general, wet suits decrease drag and increase swimming speed. It has been estimated that, depending on the skill of the swimmer, a wet suit can decrease the time of a 1,500-m swim by 1.5–3 minutes.[1] But, because wet suits are thermal insulators, they increase body temperature when worn for swimming in warm water. So in theory, the heat stress from wearing the wet suit could impair performance during the later stages of an Olympic distance triathlon in a hot and humid environment. This practical study, in time for the Sydney Olympics, is reassuring in that wearing a wet suit (vs. a swim suit) during the swimming stage of an Olympic distance triathlon in relatively warm water did not impair the thermoregulatory responses of these triathletes during the subsequent cycling and running stages.

E.R. Eichner, M.D.

Reference

1. Trappe TA, Starling RD, Jozsi AC, et al: Thermal responses to swimming in three water temperatures: Influence of a wet suit. *Med Sci Sport Exerc* 27:1014–1021, 1995.

Restoration of Fluid Balance After Exercise-induced Dehydration: Effects of Alcohol Consumption

Shirreffs SM, Maughan RJ (Univ Med School, Foresterhill, UK)
J Appl Physiol 83:1152–1158, 1997   7–5

Introduction.—Alcohol has a diuretic effect, and it is thought that alcohol-containing drinks should be avoided after exercise-induced dehydration. Because there appears to be little evidence to support this belief, a study was designed to establish whether alcohol does exert a diuretic action when consumed in a water- and electrolyte-depleted state induced by sweat loss.

Methods.—Six healthy men volunteered for the study. All were physically active and consumed alcoholic beverages on an occasional basis. Each participant undertook 4 experimental trials with 3 phases: exercise-induced dehydration, beverage ingestion, and monitoring of fluid balance for 6 hours. A different beverage was ingested in each trial: alcohol-free beer and an alcohol-free base to which was added 1%, 2%, or 4% alcohol. All drinks had a sodium concentration of 2 mmol/L and a potassium concentration of 10 mmol/L. Participants were immersed to the neck in warm water, and then they exercised in a warm and humid climatic

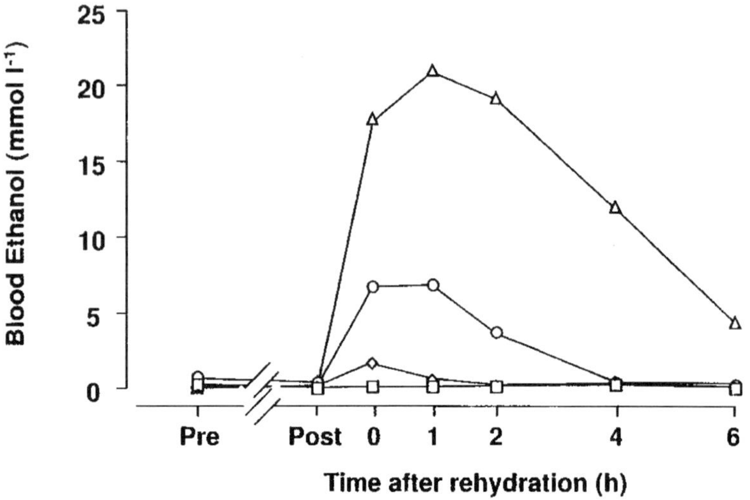

FIGURE 1.—Blood ethanol concentration over time. *Abbreviations: Pre,* pre-exercise; *Post,* postexercise. Points are median values. *Open square,* trial 0%; *open diamond,* trial 1%; *open circle,* trial 2%; *open triangle,* trial 4%. (Courtesy of Shirreffs SM, Maughan RJ: Restoration of fluid balance after exercise-induced dehydration: Effects of alcohol consumption. *J Appl Physiol* 83:1152–1158, 1997.)

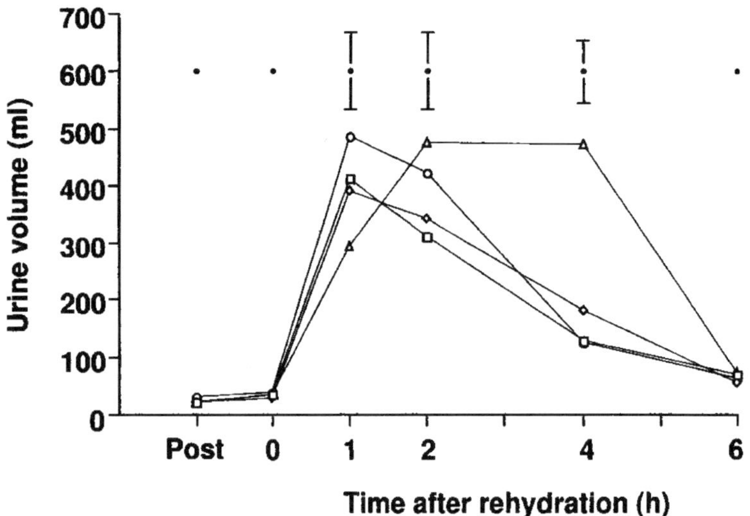

FIGURE 2.—Urine output over time. Pre-exercise sample is not shown. *Abbreviation: SE,* standard error. Points are median values. **Top,** pooled SE bars at each time point; this is SE calculated by using each subject's data from each trial at each time point. *Open square,* trial 0%; *open diamond,* trial 1%; *open circle,* trial 2%; *open triangle,* trial 4%. (Courtesy of Shirreffs SM, Maughan RJ: Restoration of fluid balance after exercise-induced dehydration: Effects of alcohol consumption. *J Appl Physiol* 83:1152–1158, 1997.)

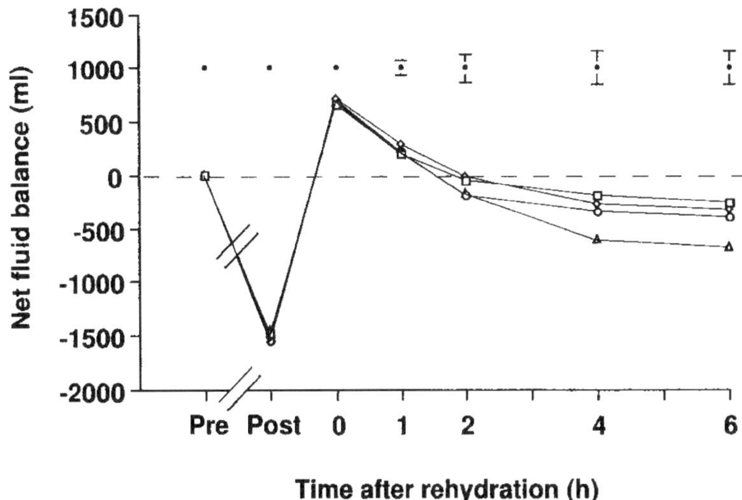

FIGURE 3.—Whole body net fluid balance calculated from estimated sweat loss, volume of fluid ingested, and urine output over course of experiment. Pre-exercise urine sample is not included in these calculations. *Abbreviation: SE,* standard error. Points are median values. **Top,** pooled SE bars at each time point; this is SE calculated by using each subject's data from each trial at each time point. *Open square,* trial 0%; *open diamond,* trial 1%; *open circle,* trial 2%; *open triangle,* trial 4%. (Courtesy of Shirreffs SM, Maughan RJ: Restoration of fluid balance after exercise-induced dehydration: Effects of alcohol consumption. *J Appl Physiol* 83:1152–1158, 1997.)

chamber. Exercise continued until body mass had fallen by almost 2%. The rehydration drinks, with a volume of 150% of estimated sweat loss, were consumed over the next hour.

Results.—The mean amount of ethanol ingested in the 4 trials was 0, 17.7, 35.9, and 68.0 g, respectively. Measured peak blood ethanol concentrations in each trial were 0, 2, 7, and 21 mmol/L, respectively (Fig 1). Although the total volume of urine produced during the 6 hours after rehydration did not differ between trials, there was a tendency for urine volume to increase with increasing quantity of ingested alcohol. Peak urine flow (Fig 2) occurred during the first hour after the rehydration period in the first 3 trials but was delayed with the 4% beverage. The 4% alcohol drink also led to a slower increase in blood and plasma volume with rehydration. There were no differences in whole body net fluid balance between trials at any time (Fig 3). Participants were positively hydrated to the same extent at the end of the rehydration period.

Conclusion.—Alcohol has a negligible diuretic effect when consumed in dilute solution after a moderate level of hypohydration induced by exercise in the heat. There seems to be no difference in recovery from dehydration whether the rehydration beverage is alcohol free or contains up to 2% alcohol, but drinks containing 4% alcohol delay recovery.

▶ This group has a solid record for practical research on rehydrating athletes, and has recently shown that drink volume and sodium content interact;[1] that a meal plus water can work better than a sports drink alone in restoring whole-body water balance;[2] and that menstrual-cycle phase does not affect rehydration.[3] But here's my favorite: Dilute beer is a sports drink! They suggest beer is more fun to quaff than other rehydration beverages. They say the beer-quaffing record is 9 liters in 20 minutes. They show that dilute beer (up to 2% alcohol) has a negligible diuretic effect after moderate hypohydration (2% of body mass) from exercising in the heat. So for "sports rehydration," provided you drink more fluid than you lose in sweat (subjects drank 150% of what they lost in sweat), dilute beer works fine. Beer in Oklahoma is 3.2% alcohol, so I figure a 50–50 mix of beer and Gatorade is ideal.

E.R. Eichner, M.D.

References

1. Shirreffs S, Taylor AJ, Leiper JB, et al: Post-exercise rehydration in man: Effects of volume consumed and drink sodium content. *Med Sci Sports Exerc* 28:1260–1271, 1996.
2. Maughan RJ, Leiper JB, Shirreffs SM: Restoration of fluid balance after exercise-induced dehydration: Effects of food and fluid balance. *Eur J Appl Physiol* 73:317–325, 1996.
3. 1997 YEAR BOOK OF SPORTS MEDICINE, pp 350–351.

Blood Lactate Threshold and Type II Fibre Predominance in Patients With Exertional Heatstroke

Hsu Y-D, Lee W-H, Chang M-K, et al (Natl Defense Med Ctr, Taipei, Taiwan, Republic of China)
J Neurol Neurosurg Psychiatry 62:182–187, 1997

7–6

Background.—The ability to sustain heat stress and prolonged exercise varies greatly among individuals. In addition to poor physical fitness, the muscle itself is an important variable in exertional heatstroke. Blood lactate threshold and type II fiber predominance were investigated in patients with exertional heatstroke.

Methods.—Thirty-seven Taiwanese military recruits with exertional heatstroke were studied. All were men, aged 19–23 years. Biopsy specimens of the vastus lateralis were obtained within 10 days of initial evaluation. Fifteen age-matched men comprised a comparison group. Twenty-nine patients also participated in a constant work load test on the treadmill 90–150 days after exertional heatstroke to determine blood lactate threshold. A second biopsy sample was taken from these subjects.

Findings.—Rhabdomyolysis developed in 24 of the 37 men with exertional heatstroke. Eighteen of these had type II fiber predominance. The patients with type II fiber predominance had a significantly shorter time to blood lactate threshold during the treadmill assessment. The highest value of blood lactate was positively correlated with the percentage of type II fibers in all subjects tested.

Conclusions.—Rhabdomyolysis is a serious complication of exertional heatstroke. Subjects with type II fiber predominance or underlying myopathy are susceptible to exertional heatstroke and rhabdomyolysis. Blood lactate threshold appears to be a good indicator of endurance capacity before training and in recovering patients.

▶ The novel suggestion—one that may apply to sports like football—is that men with type II muscle fiber predominance are more prone to exertional heatstroke. Type II fibers are "fast-twitch"—with fast contractile speed, high motor unit strength, and high glycolytic capacity; but low oxidative capacity and low fatigue resistance. Normally, about 2/3 of fibers in the vastus lateralis are fast-twitch; the rest are slow-twitch. And in the controls, 2/3 of those fibers were fast-twitch. But in the male military recruits with exertional heatstroke and the most severe rhabdomyolysis, ≥4/5 of those fibers were fast-twitch. After recovery from their illnesses, the group that had experienced exertional heatstroke and had type II predominance reached their lactate thresholds faster during a constant treadmill test meant to mimic the "medium-to-long endurance work" of army training. The novel clinical implication is that military recruits (and athletes) with type II predominance—in some exercise or sport settings—may have impaired endurance and/or generate more muscle heat, predisposing them to exertional heatstroke. Last year, we reviewed a relevant article that tied exertional heat illness in U.S. Marine recruits to fatness and lack of fitness.[1]

E.R. Eichner, M.D.

Reference

1. 1997 YEAR BOOK OF SPORTS MEDICINE, pp 301–302.

Physiological Responses to a Cold, Wet, and Windy Environment During Prolonged Intermittent Walking
Weller AS, Millard CE, Stroud MA, et al (Univ of Nottingham, England; Centre for Human Sciences, Farnborough, UK)
Am J Physiol 272:R226–R233, 1997   7–7

Background.—Adverse effects of exercise in a cold environment have been reported. However, previous studies addressing the impact of cold air on exercise physiology have either failed to assess perturbations in metabolic responses fully or have used only limited degrees of cold stress in the experimental protocol. The effects of a cold, wet, and windy environment on physiologic and thermoregulatory endpoints during prolonged exercise were examined.

Methods.—Ten men completed a 6-hour intermittent (45 minutes of exercise, 15 minutes of rest) exercise regimen in a thermoneutral environ-

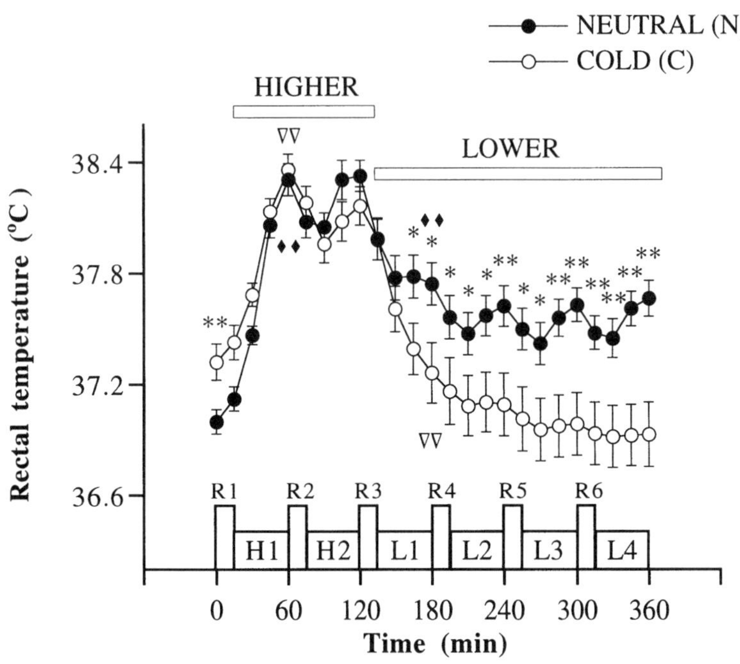

FIGURE 1.—Rectal temperature plotted against time during higher (*Higher*)- and lower (*Lower*)-intensity phases of the intermittent exercise protocol in thermoneutral (+15°C) (*Neutral*) and cold (+5°C), wet, and windy (*Cold*) conditions. Values are means ± standard error of the mean (n = 10). Significant differences between *Neutral* and *Cold*: asterisk, $P \leq 0.05$, *double asterisk*, $P \leq 0.01$. Significant differences within *Neutral* and *Cold* (from value obtained 60 minutes previously): *Neutral, double diamond, P $\leq$ 0.01; Cold, double triangle P $\leq$ 0.01*). *Abbreviations: R1–R6*, rest periods 1–6; *H1* and *H2*, work periods during *Higher*; *L1–L4*, work periods during *Lower*. (Courtesy of Weller AS, Millard CE, Stroud MA, et al: Physiological responses to a cold, wet, and windy environment during prolonged intermittent walking. *Am J Physiol* 272:R226–R233, 1997, copyright by the American Physiological Society.)

ment (15°C), and again in a cold (5°C), wet, and windy environment. Exercise was performed on a treadmill inclined at 10 degrees at 6 km/hr for the first 2 45-minute periods at each temperature (higher intensity) and on a horizontal treadmill at 5 km/hr (lower intensity) for the remaining periods. Rectal and skin temperatures, heart rate, ventilation rate, expired air composition, and plasma concentrations of free fatty acid, catecholamine, glucose, glycerol, lactate, and β-hydroxybutyrate were monitored.

Results.—Mean rectal temperature did not differ between participants in the cold and thermoneutral environments during higher intensity exercise, but was significantly lower, by 0.59°C, in the cold than the thermoneutral environment during lower intensity exercise (Fig 1). Heart rate did not differ between the 2 environments. Oxygen consumption respiratory exchange ratio and plasma concentrations of epinephrine, norepinephrine, lactate, and glucose were greater in the cold environment than the thermoneutral environment during low intensity exercise but did not differ between the environments during higher intensity exercise. There was a trend toward decreased plasma β-hydroxybutyrate and free fatty acid concentrations in the cold compared with the thermoneutral environment, whereas plasma glycerol concentrations did not differ between the 2 environments.

Conclusions.—During high-intensity exercise, heat loss is offset by heat production, so that simultaneous exposure to cold does not alter physiologic responses to exercise. During lower-intensity exercise in the cold environment, however, heat production did not offset heat loss, leading to reduced rectal temperature and increased carbohydrate metabolism and sympathoadrenal activity. These perturbations may indicate a potential detrimental effect of prolonged exercise in a cold environment.

▶ Despite the mild British climate, there have been a surprisingly large number of deaths from hypothermia among hill walkers in both England and Scotland. Factors contributing to such incidents included a lack of adequate protective or waterproof clothing and additional coverings for an emergency such as a physical injury, together with a lack of food reserves and a low level of fitness in those attempting arduous mountain journeys. Ambient temperatures on days when incidents occurred have sometimes been as high as 5°C, but the victim's heat loss has commonly been increased by rain, which soaked the clothing and largely destroyed its insulation. Often, the problem was exacerbated by high winds and the pumping of air underneath the clothing during climbing.[1] In 1 of the incidents investigated by Pugh,[1] fitter walkers were able to complete an extensive hill walk without problems. Those who were in poorer condition generated less heat and thus were not able to generate enough heat to prevent problems of hypothermia from developing. The present report offers an up-to-date laboratory simulation of this type of situation, with participants walking on a treadmill for 45 minutes out of each hour at a pace corresponding first to 60% and then to 30% of maximal oxygen intake in a wet and windy environment at an ambient temperature of 5°C. While the rapid pace was maintained, participants kept their core temperatures at 38.3°C, but values fell by about 1.5°C over 4 hours at the slower pace (which probably would have been the choice of unfit participants in the fatal hill walks). As cooling occurs, there is an increased secretion of noradrenaline. In theory, this should mobilize fat, but such a response was not observed in the present study, perhaps because cooling caused vasoconstriction in the fat deposits. The metabolic cost of shivering was met mainly from glycogen reserves; during a mountain walk, this would further impair the performance of the unfit individual, lengthening the time needed to reach the safety of the home base.

R.J. Shephard, M.D., Ph.D., D.P.E.

Reference

1. Pugh LGCE: Cold stress and muscular exercise, with special reference to accidental hypothermia. *Br Med J* 2:333–337, 1996.

Thermal and Metabolic Responses to Cold-water Immersion at Knee, Hip, and Shoulder Levels

Lee DT, Toner MM, McArdle WD, et al (Queen's College of the City Univ of New York, Flushing; United States Army Research Inst of Enviromental Medicine, Natick, Mass)

J Appl Physiol 82:1523–1530, 1997   7–8

Background.—Compensatory responses are commonly inadequate for maintaining body temperature during cold-water immersion, particularly with large portions of the body immersed and decreasing water temperatures. There is evidence that the majority of heat loss during cold-water immersion occurs from the trunk. When exercise is performed, however, peripheral muscles are more highly perfused, leading to an acceleration of heat loss. Previous studies explored the effects on heat loss of cold-water immersion at only a single level, failing to address the effects of immersion level on thermal balance. The effects of immersion level on thermoregulation were studied.

Methods.—Eight men were immersed in water at 15°C and then 25°C, to the level of the knee, hip, and then shoulder, at rest and during exercise on a cycle ergometer at 35% of peak oxygen consumption, for up to 135 minutes. Rectal, esophageal, and skin temperatures, as well as cutaneous heat flow and oxygen intake, were monitored.

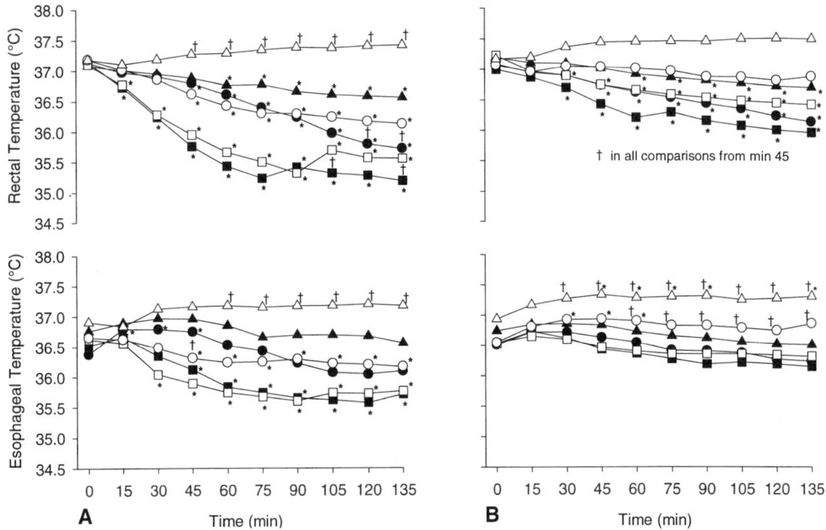

FIGURE 2.—Rectal temperature at 15°C (**A, top**) and 25°C (**B, top**) and esophageal temperature at 15°C (**A, bottom**) and 25°C (**B, bottom**) water. *Asterisk*, significantly different from control-air value (minute 0); *dagger*, significantly different between exercise and rest, $P < 0.05$; *black square*, shoulder with rest; *white square*, shoulder with exercise; *black circle*, hip with rest; *white circle*, hip with exercise; *black triangle*, knee with rest; *white triangle*, knee with exercise. (Courtesy of Lee DT, Toner MM, McArdle WD, et al: Thermal and metabolic responses to cold-water immersion at knee, hip, and shoulder levels. *J Appl Physiol* 82:1523–1530, 1997.)

Results.—Rectal and esophageal temperatures were lowest during immersion to the shoulders and highest during immersion to the knee, regardless of exercise and water temperature, with the exception that esophageal temperature was not significantly affected by immersion level at 25°C. (Fig 2). Rectal temperature did not decline below pre-treatment temperatures during immersion to the knee at 15°C or 25°C or to the hip at 25°C, during exercise. Esophageal temperature did not decrease below pre-treatment levels during immersion to the knee or hip at 15°C during exercise and during all conditions at 25°C. Metabolic heat production was greater during exercise under all conditions, and was greater during exposure to the shoulders than to the knee or hip during rest and exercise at 15°C and during rest, but not exercise, at 25°C. The increase in heat production induced by exercise was lower during immersion to the shoulders than to the knee or hip at both water temperatures.

Conclusions.—Caution is necessary when describing thermal balance using body temperature measured at a single site in humans exercising during cold-water immersion. The responses of rectal and esophageal temperatures to cold-water immersion are not identical. Immersion in 25°C water above the hip and in 15°C water above the knee depresses body temperature even during light exercise, largely secondary to heat production that is inadequate to offset heat loss.

▶ The exercise scientist is often interested to examine whether physiologic responses to a bout of activity result from the increase in core temperature or from some other aspect of exercise such as a change in hormonal milieu or an increase in blood flow. One answer to this question can be sought through thermal clamping—the increase of heat loss induced by immersing the individual in cold water is used to offset the increase in metabolic heat production.[1] However, it is relatively tricky to find an appropriate water temperature that will clamp core temperatures in both thin and fat individuals, and as the present authors demonstrate with partial immersion, there may be substantial differences in the response of rectal and esophageal temperatures. The rectal temperature is influenced more by conditions in the lower half of the body, although the trends in rectal and esophageal temperature measurements are similar. When exercise is performed in an immersion tank, it is also important to ensure that electrical equipment is well-grounded. An electrically braked cycle ergometer can be used if it is isolated from the individual by a positive pressure tank.[1] If exercise is light (35% of maximal oxygen intake in the experiments of Lee et al.), or the clamping is over-zealous, shivering increases body heat production in an attempt to sustain core temperature.

R.J. Shephard, M.D., Ph.D., D.P.E.

Reference

1. Cross MC, Radomski MW, VanHelder WP, et al: Endurance exercise with and without a thermal clamp: Effects on leukocytes and leukocyte subsets. *J Appl Physiol* 81:822–829, 1996.

Association Between Raised Body Temperature and Acute Mountain Sickness: Cross Sectional Study

Maggiorini M, Bärtsch P, Oelz O (Univ Hosp, Zurich, Switzerland; Univ Clinic of Medicine, Heidelberg, Germany; Stadtspital Triemli, Zurich, Switzerland)
BMJ 315:403–404, 1997   7–9

Introduction.—Acute mountain sickness has long been associated with fever. A study was made of the association between acute mountain sickness and body temperature and of high altitude pulmonary edema and body temperature.

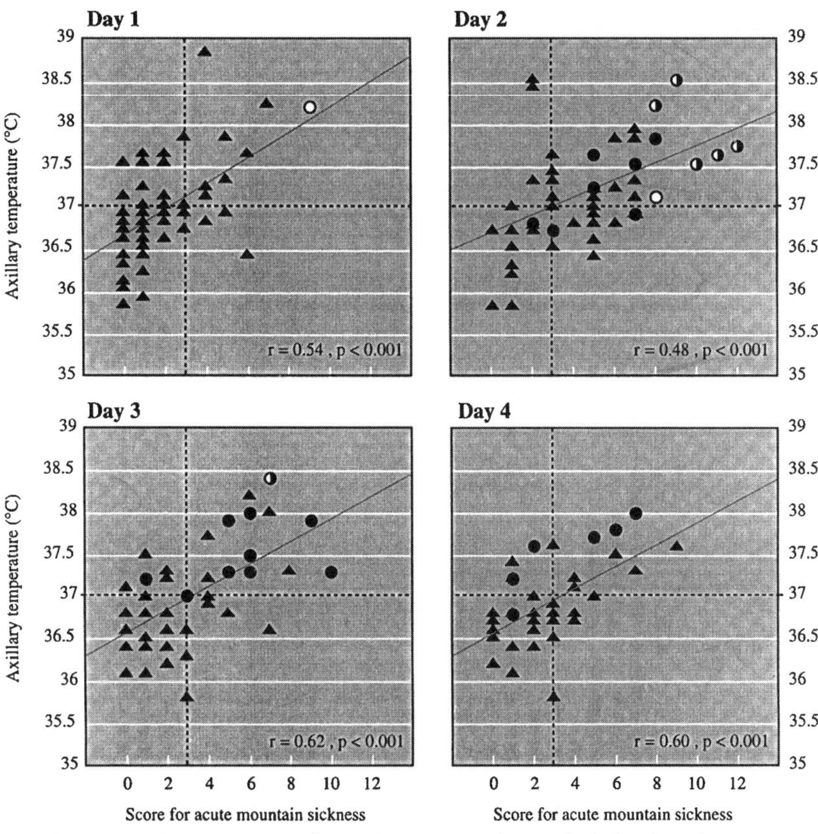

FIGURE 1.—Body temperatures and scores for mountain sickness at high altitude on day 1 (N = 60), day 2 (N = 57), day 3 (N = 50), and day 4 (N = 44). Some climbers had same body temperature and same score. *Oblique line* is regression line. (This article was first published in Maggiorini M, Bärtsch P, Oelz O: Association between raised body temperature and acute mountain sickness: Cross sectional study. *BMJ* 315:403–404, 1997, and is reproduced by permission of the BMJ.)

Methods.—Sixty climbers ascended to a mountain hut at 4,559 meters above sea level within 22 hours and stayed there for 72 hours. The climbers were examined at low altitude, 2–6 hours after arrival at the hut, and each morning during days 2–4. In a clinical interview, symptoms and signs of acute mountain sickness were assessed and scored. Climbers were classified as healthy, having mild acute mountain sickness, or, having severe acute mountain sickness. Climbers were considered to have high altitude cerebral edema if they had at least 3 of the following symptoms: headache resistant to paracetamol, dizziness, ataxia, and vomiting

Results.—Three of the 60 climbers had to be evacuated because of pulmonary or cerebral edema on the second day, 7 were evacuated on the third day, and 5 on the fourth day. Chest radiography was used to diagnose pulmonary edema in 22 climbers. Healthy climbers and those with mild mountain sickness had a mean increase in temperature of 0.5°C. Those with acute mountain sickness had a mean increase in temperature of 1.2°C, and those with cerebral edema had a mean increase of 1.7°C (Fig 1).

Conclusion.—In climbers studied at low and high altitude, there was a strong relationship between body temperature, hypoxemia, and severity of acute mountain sickness. After rapid ascent to high altitude, a rise in temperature is a sign of acute mountain sickness and is associated with the severity of hypoxemia.

▶ Reasons why pulmonary edema can complicate severe mountain sickness remain the subject of debate. Given that there can also be cerebral edema, a change in fluid balance at the tissue/capillary interface seems the most plausible explanation, with fever arising from secondary infection. However, several cytokines can also influence the function of cerebral thermoregulatory centers, and a triggering of cytokine release by either local hypoxemia or hypoxia-related muscle injury could be the initiating factor for both pulmonary edema and fever. Irrespective of mechanisms, a rising body temperature is an adverse sign in those affected by mountain sickness.

R.J. Shephard, M.D., Ph.D., D.P.E.

Magnetic Resonance Imaging of Osteonecrosis in Divers: Comparison With Plain Radiographs

Shinoda S, Hasegawa Y, Kawasaki S, et al (Atsumi Hosp, Japan; Nagoya Univ, Japan)
Skeletal Radiol 26:354–359, 1997   7–10

Objective.—Whereas radiographic evaluation has traditionally been used to diagnose dysbaric osteonecrosis in divers, type A lesions can be overlooked. Because MRI has been used in the early diagnosis of idiopathic avascular necrosis of the femoral head, its diagnostic value in detecting bone lesions in divers was compared with radiography.

Methods.—Conventional radiography and MRI were performed on the shoulder, hip, and knee joints of 23 male scuba divers, aged 25 to 60 years. Clinical symptoms, personal history, and imaging results were compared.

Results.—Magnetic resonance imaging located 27 bone lesions in 39 proximal humeri, 17 lesions in 36 proximal femurs, 13 lesions in 32 distal femurs, and 12 lesions in 32 proximal tibias. There were 22 type E humeral lesions and 10 type E femoral lesions; metaphyseal type M, diaphyseal type D, and E lesions were seen in 27 proximal humeri, 17 proximal femurs, 13 distal femurs, and 12 proximal tibias. Morphologic patterns were diffuse and of low-intensity, with unclear and irregular borders. Radiographic evaluation showed 14 humeral type A lesions, 2 femoral type A lesions, 5 proximal humeral type B lesions, 6 proximal femoral type B lesions, 5 distal femoral type B lesions, and 2 proximal tibial type B lesions. Radiographic and MRI findings corresponded for type A and E lesions of the humerus but not for the femur. Type B and type M and D lesions corresponded for the proximal humerus and femur but not for the distal femur and proximal tibia.

Conclusion.—Divers with osteonecrosis diagnosed in 1 site should have an MRI of the hip joint. Magnetic resonance imaging can be used for early detection of femoral head osteonecrosis and should also be performed on shoulder joints of divers who dive deeper than 15 m.

▶ Magnetic resonance imaging appears to be a very sensitive technique in the detection of osteonecrosis. Assuming that it is not overdiagnosing this condition, there is a great deal of work to be done in educating scuba enthusiasts to regulate their dives more carefully.

R.J. Shephard, M.D., Ph.D., D.P.E.

Extraocular Circadian Phototransduction in Humans

Campbell SS, Murphy PJ (Univ Med School, White Plains, NY)
Science 279:396–399, 1998

7–11

Background.—In humans, an endogenous circadian clock determines physiological and behavioral rhythms. The photoreceptors that entrain the mammalian biological clock may not be the same cells that mediate vision. In some totally blind persons, bright light suppresses melatonin output in the absence of conscious light perception. The response of the human circadian clock to extraocular light exposure was investigated.

Methods and Findings.—Thirty-three phase-shifting trials were performed in 15 healthy adults, aged 22 to 67 years. Body temperature and melatonin concentrations throughout the circadian cycle were measured before and after light pulses applied behind the knee, in the popliteal region. The timing of the light pulse was found to be systematically associated with magnitude and direction of phase shifts, resulting in the

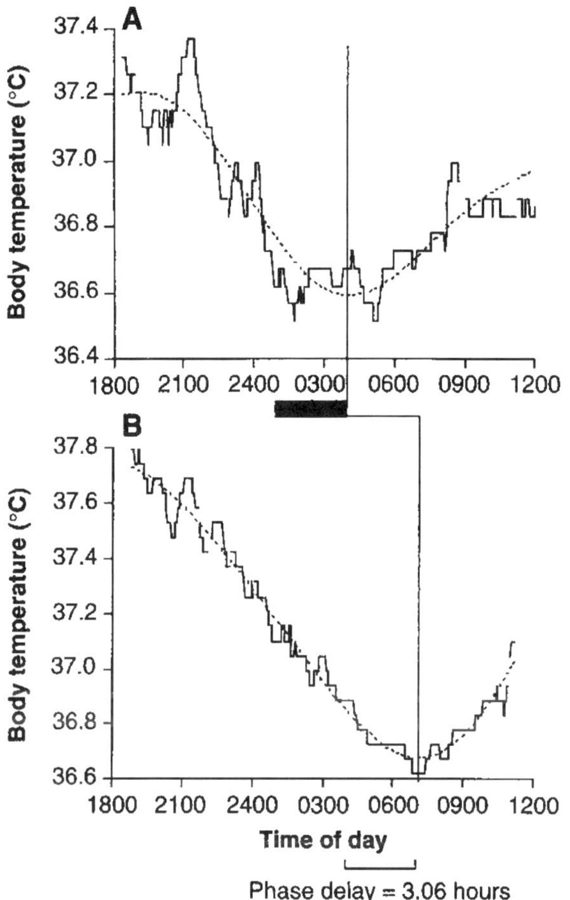

FIGURE 1.—Example of a delay in circadian phase in response to a 3-hour bright light presentation to the popliteal region. Light was presented on 1 occasion between 0100 and 0400 after night 2 in the laboratory (black bar) while the participant (a 29-year-old male) remained awake and seated in a dimly lit room (ambient illumination < 20 lux). The circadian phase was determined by fitting a complex cosine curve (dotted line) to the raw body core temperature data (solid line). Resulting phase estimates are indicated by vertical lines. The baseline (night 1) circadian phase A occurred at 0404; the circadian phase after light presentation B (last 24 hours in the laboratory) occurred at 0708. The phase angle between the midpoint of the light stimulus and the fitted body temperature minimum at baseline was 1.57 hour. The resulting phase advance was 3.06 hours. (Reprinted with permission from Campell SS, Murphy PJ: Extraocular circadian phototransduction in humans. *Science* 279:396–399, copyright 1998, American Association for the Advancement of Science.)

production of a phase response curve. Examples of phase shifts in individuals are given in Figures 1 and 2.

Conclusions.—These findings challenge the notion that mammals are not capable of extraretinal circadian phototransduction. This has impor-

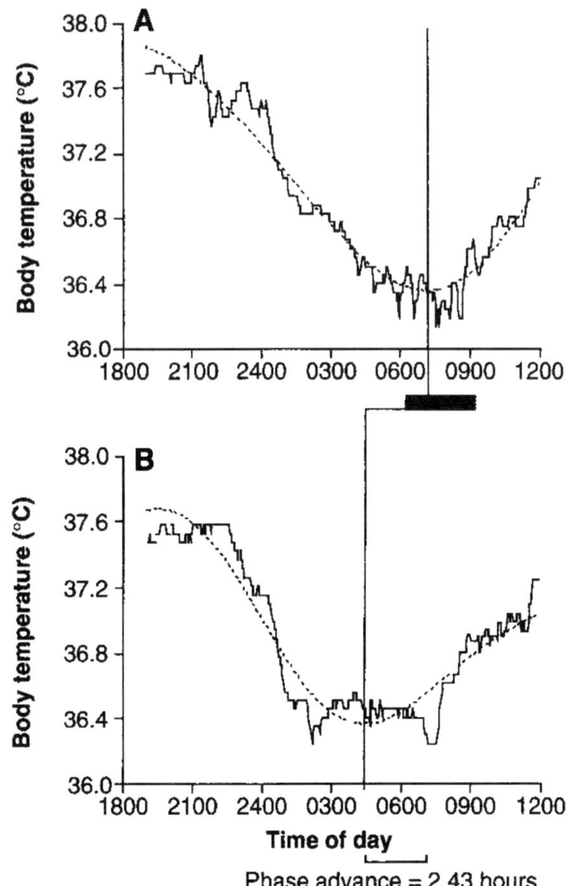

FIGURE 2.—Example of an advance in circadian phase in response to a 3-hour bright light presentation to the popliteal region. Light was presented on 1 occasion between 0600 and 0900 after night 2 in the laboratory (black bar) while the participant (a 44-year-old male) remained awake and seated in a dimly lit room (ambient illumination < 20 lux). The circadian phase was determined by fitting a complex cosine curve (dotted line) to the raw body core temperature data (solid line). Resulting phase estimates are indicated by vertical lines. The baseline (night 1) circadian phase A occurred at 0713; the circadian phase after light presentation B (last 24 hours in the laboratory) occurred at 0453. The phase angle between the midpoint of the light stimulus and the fitted body temperature minimum at baseline was 0.28 hour. The resulting phase advance was 2.334 hours.

tant implications for the development of more effective treatments for sleep and circadian rhythm disorders.

▶ The results here are bizarre but barely believable. Evidently, resetting your body clock is more than meets the eye. If crabs have clock sensors on their tails and fruit flies have time-keeping genes on their wings, humans have time sensors behind their knees. In this novel experiment, shining a bright light for 3 hours on the backs of knees (the popliteal space) shifted the nadir of body temperature by up to 3 hours. In other words, bright light behind the knees can advance or delay the circadian phase by up to 3 hours. Possibly, light behind the knees activates a blood-born photoreceptor (e.g., hemoglobin) to increase levels of nitric oxide that go to the brain and shift the clock. If this work holds up, it will be a bombshell. Night workers can shift their clocks to fit their work. Travelers can board planes to far-off locales, strap bands on their knees, sleep while light shifts their clocks, and arrive refreshed yet in sync with the locals. Just in case this study can't be duplicated, a practical review of causes and prevention of travel fatigue and jet lag in athletes has recently appeared.[1]

E.R. Eichner, M.D.

Reference

1. Reilly T, Atkinson G, Waterhouse J: Travel fatigue and jet-lag. *J Sports Sciences* 15:365–369, 1997.

A Relationship Between Heat Loss and Sleepiness: Effects of Postural Change and Melatonin Administration
Kräuchi K, Cajochen C, Wirz-Justice A (Psychiatric Univ Clinic, Basel, Switzerland)
J Appl Physiol 83:134–139, 1997   7–12

Objective.—Both exogenous and endogenous melatonin lowers core body temperature in human beings by decreasing heat production or increasing heat loss. Lying down also induces hypothermia. The phase-advancing effects and thermoregulatory effects of melatonin were separated, and their relation to sleepiness was investigated.

Methods.—In a double-blind, placebo-controlled, cross-over study, 8 healthy male students, aged 21 to 31 years, received either 1 melatonin (5 mg) or 1 placebo capsule per day in random order with a 1-week washout period in between. Heart rate, rectal temperature, skin temperatures (1 cm above the navel, middle of the instep, and sole of the left foot), and subjective sleepiness ratings were continuously monitored from 9 AM to 10 PM while the volunteers were sitting and from 10 AM to 5 PM while the volunteers were lying down. Melatonin was administered at 1 PM. Salivary melatonin concentration was determined every 45 minutes right after volunteers subjectively rate their sleepiness. The effect of postural change after lying down and the effect of melatonin were analyzed statistically.

Results.—Whereas rectal temperature decreased significantly after lying down, reaching a minimum at 60 to 90 minutes after lying down, foot and stomach temperatures increased significantly after lying down in all volunteers. Melatonin significantly increased sleepiness and significantly reduced rectal temperature compared with placebo. The heat loss and decrease in core body temperature were compared for the natural and pharmacologic increase in sleepiness. The decrease in rectal temperature after lying down lasts about 2 hours and can be attributed to heat loss resulting from reflexive skin vasodilation. Heart rate slowing and skin blood flow increases are induced by reduced sympathetic outflow and sleepiness increases. Melatonin increases foot temperature and decreases rectal temperature, possibly by acting not only on specific melatonin receptors but also on supposed melatonin receptors of arteriovenous anastomosis that regulate heat loss and induce sleepiness about 40 minutes after administration.

Conclusion.—Hypothermia appears to be related to sleepiness and is mediated through distal skin vasodilation as core body temperature decreases. Whether melatonin can induce sleepiness when peripheral heat loss is limited is being studied.

▶ If you want to get to sleep fast, take your socks off. That's the moral of this study on posture, melatonin, temperature, and sleepiness. Lying down cools down core temperature by reflexive skin vasodilation that "heats your feet" so they shed heat from your body. This "postural hypothermia" lasts about 2 hours and makes you sleepy. The same cooling and parallel sleepiness occurs after taking melatonin, perhaps because melatonin interacts with putative receptors in arteriovenous anastomoses of the skin circulation. Either way—lying down or taking melatonin—the consequent hypothermia seems functionally related to sleepiness.

E.R. Eichner, M.D.

Roles of Intensity and Duration of Nocturnal Exercise in Causing Phase Delays of Human Circadian Rhythms

Buxton OM, Frank SA, L'Hermite-Balériaux M, et al (Univ of Chicago; Northwestern Univ, Evanston, Illinois; Université Libre de Bruxelles, Belgium)
Am J Physiol 273:E536–E542, 1997   7–13

Objective.—Nighttime exercise can alter circadian rhythm the next day by 1 to 2 hours, as determined by an analysis of nocturnal elevation of plasma thyrotropin (TSH) and melatonin levels. These phase shifts were observed when individuals exercised 2 to 5 hours before minimal core body temperature was reached. Smaller phase delays were recorded when exercise was undertaken near the temperature minimum time. The phase-shifting effects of exposure to a 1-hour high intensity nocturnal exercise session were compared with the phase-shifting effects of a 3-hour nocturnal exercise session and continuous bed rest.

Methods.—Eight normal male volunteers, aged 20 to 30 years, participated in 3 2-night studies separated by at least 2 weeks where circadian rhythms were measured in the absence of exercise, with a 3-hour low-intensity exercise session, or with a 1-hour high intensity exercise session. TSH and melatonin levels in venous blood were measured at 20-minute intervals between 4 PM and 4 AM, at hourly intervals between 4 AM and 4 PM, and at 20-minute intervals between 4 PM and 4 AM. Core body temperature was measured throughout. Sleep onset and offset were recorded.

Results.—Core body temperature increases averaged 0.80 for the low-intensity exercise and 1.75 within 90 minutes after beginning high-intensity exercise. The rise in TSH was delayed by 18 minutes at baseline, 78 minutes with low-intensity exercise, and 95 minutes with high-intensity exercise. Both low-intensity and high-intensity TSH values were significantly different from baseline values but not from each other. The delays in the rise of melatonin were 23 minutes at baseline, 63 minutes with low-intensity exercise, and 55 minutes with high-intensity exercise. The low-intensity delay in melatonin rise but not the high-intensity rise was significantly different from baseline values. One hour of high-intensity exercise was as effective as 3 hours of low-intensity exercise in altering circadian rhythm.

Conclusion.—Single high-intensity exercise sessions may be beneficial as a method for acclimating night workers to a new dark-light cycle.

▶ This study extends research suggesting that nocturnal exercise can delay the circadian phase in human beings. By using noctural onsets of thyrotropin and melatonin as markers, it is shown here that high-intensity exercise (including 40 minutes at 75% of VO_2 max) for 1 hour equals low-intensity exercise for 3 hours in delaying circadian phase. The practical point is that night workers who want to stay alert on the job yet be ready to sleep when they get home in the morning can help their cause by exercising for an hour or so at their mid-shift "lunch" break. Exactly how exercise delays the circadian phase is unclear; maybe the exercise-evoked increase in body temperature plays a role. If airlines put stairclimbers or exercycles on big planes, passengers could exercise on long flights to ward off jet lag and reduce the threat of deep venous thrombosis.

E.R. Eichner, M.D.

8 Women, Children, and Aging

Comparison of Injury During Cadet Basic Training by Gender
Bijur PE, Horodyski M, Egerton W, et al (Albert Einstein College of Medicine, Bronx, NY; Univ of Florida, Gainesville; US Military Academy, USAMEDDAC, West Point, NY; et al)
Arch Pediatr Adolesc Med 151:456–461, 1997   8–1

Introduction.—The number of women in the U.S. military has increased fivefold since 1973. Investigations performed primarily by army researchers have reported an excess of injuries in women during basic training. The current state of risk injury by gender was assessed during cadet basic training at the United States Military Academy at West Point. The contribution of pretraining conditioning and height to the male-female differential in injuries was also examined.

Methods.—The mean age of 473 male and 85 female cadets taking cadet basic training the summer before freshman year was 18.4 years. Cadets were followed for rate of injuries resulting in 1 or more days of excuse from physical activities per 100 cadets and the rate of injuries resulting in hospitalization for 1 or more nights per 100 cadets. The extent to which pretraining conditioning and height account for the association between gender and injuries was assessed using the ordinary least-squares multiple regression.

Results.—The injury rate of women was 2.5 times that of men. Women had 3.9 times as many injuries that resulted in hospitalization of 1 or more nights. Women had significantly more stress fractures and stress reactions than their male counterparts. Height was not significantly correlated with the total rate of injuries, the rate of injuries resulting in hospitalization, or the incidence of multiple injury episodes for either men or women. Multiple injury episodes were significantly correlated with 2-mile run performance in women, but not in men.

Conclusion.—Findings regarding the differences in injury rates by gender are in keeping with earlier reports. Pretraining conditioning, but not height, was significantly related to rate of injury.

▶ The observation that women have a higher risk for injury during military training than men is in keeping with the existing literature dealing with the subject. The attempt on the part of the authors to explain this on the basis of pretraining conditioning, "psychological stresses," the fact that ". . . equipment used by women was designed for men," or "the difference in height between men and women" is not only absurd, it is not supported by data.

J.S. Torg, M.D.

Stress Fractures in Female Athletes: Diagnosis, Management and Rehabilitation
Brukner P, Bennell K (Olympic Park Sports Medicine Centre, Melbourne, Victoria, Australia; Univ of Melbourne, Victoria, Australia)
Sports Med 24:419–429, 1997   8–2

Background.—In women, stress fractures account for a greater proportion of injuries than in men. This article reviews the diagnosis, imaging modalities, and treatments used for stress fracture in female athletes.

Diagnosis.—When first seen, most athletes with stress fracture report pain with an activity that increases with continued activity. Thus, taking a pain history is essential, as is determining any predisposing factors such as changes in training or equipment (such as shoes), diet, medications, or menstruation. Physical examination typically reveals localized bony tenderness at the fracture site and, occasionally, redness, swelling, or periosteal thickening. If the stress fracture involves the lower limb, biomechanical testing must be part of the physical exam. The differential diagnosis includes muscle or tendon injury, compartment syndrome, traction periostitis, bone tumor (particularly osteoid osteoma), and infection. The diagnosis is usually made clinically, with diagnostic tests used mainly to confirm the diagnosis.

Imaging Modalities.—Although radiography rarely shows any abnormalities in stress fractures, confirming signs when visible include new periosteal bone formation, sclerosis, a callus, or a fracture line. A triple phase bone scan can show injury as early as 48 hours, and all 3 phases of the scan will be positive. However, a bone scan is very unspecific and the actual fracture is not visible. Thus changes in isotope bone scans must be correlated with clinical features to pinpoint the site of the fracture. Computed tomography can help differentiate stress fracture from other conditions that show increased uptake on bone scan and from a stress reaction. Also, magnetic resonance imaging can differentiate stress fracture from bone tumors or an infectious process. Specific findings on magnetic resonance imaging include new bone formation and marrow and periosteal hemorrhage and edema.

Treatment.—Stress fractures are treated by resting from the aggravating activity. Pain is treated with analgesics or nonsteroidal anti-inflammatory drugs while the athlete keeps fit with activities such as cycling, swimming, water running, and upper-body weights. Once the pain is clear, the aggravating activity can be resumed gradually, and usually athletes can return to

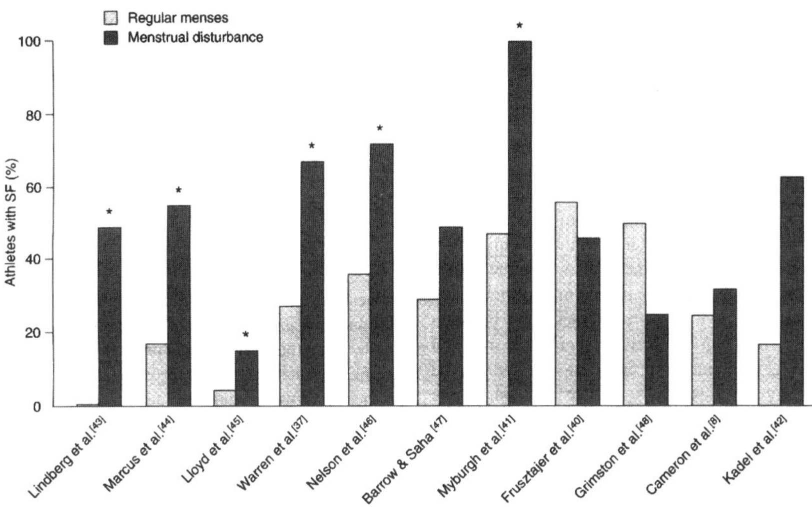

FIGURE 3.—Cross-sectional studies where the percentage of athletes with stress fractures (*SF*) could be compared in groups with and without menstrual disturbances. *p less than 0.05. (Courtesy of Brukner P, Bennell K.: Stress fractures in female athletes. Diagnosis, management and rehabilitation. *Sports Med* 24:419–429, 1997.)

performance within 6 to 8 weeks. Stress fractures of the neck of the femur, the anterior cortex of the tibia, the navicular, and the second and fifth metatarsals require further treatment because they tend to develop delayed union or nonunion. To keep the stress fracture from recurring, the causes of the injury must be identified and corrected. In particular, stress fractures seem to be more common in women with menstrual disturbances (Fig 3). Furthermore, biomechanical injuries such as excessively supinated or pronated feet can contribute to stress fractures.

▶ It's refreshing to find an article on sports injuries in female athletes that spends more time discussing the identification and treatment of the injury than in trying to explain why women are more at risk for that particular injury. The authors also seem to appreciate the fact that the female athlete is as eager to return to her sport as is the male athlete. It's too bad that this article won't be readily available to athletes and their coaches. The material would be understandable to most nonphysicians and would provide the athlete and coach with knowledge essential to understanding this all too common sports injury.

B.L. Drinkwater, Ph.D.

Knee Injuries in Women Collegiate Rugby Players

Levy AS, Wetzler MJ, Lewars M, et al (American Orthopaedic Rugby Football Association, Philadelphia)
Am J Sports Med 25:360–362, 1997

8–3

Introduction.—With 267 women's collegiate and noncollegiate rugby clubs, women's rugby is the fastest growing form of rugby in North America. The frequency and types of knee injuries in women's collegiate rugby were assessed and compared with data on injuries in other NCAA women's sports.

Methods.—Female rugby players who played in the 4 seasons between 1992 and 1994 completed questionnaires regarding position and playing experience. They were asked to provide documentation for surgical procedures and diagnostic imaging. A knee injury was defined as "any injury to the knee region that resulted in a player missing one game or two practices."

Results.—Forty-two of 50 clubs responded to questionnaires. Eighthundred ten female collegiate rugby players were assessed. Of 58,296 exposures at games and practices, there were 76 knee injuries (rate of 1.3 per 1,000 exposures). The highest incidence of injuries was anterior cruciate ligament (ACL) tears (21 tears, incidence 0.36 per 1,000 exposures). Sixty-seven percent of ACL tears occurred in rugby backs.

Conclusion.—The knee injury rate for women's collegiate rugby is similar to rates of other women's collegiate sports. The 21 ACL tears (0.36 incidence per 1,000 exposures) is a slightly higher rate than what is reported for women's soccer and basketball (0.31 and 0.29, respectively). It would be useful to compare these rates with those of male rugby players to determine whether field conditions or training programs contribute to knee injuries in rugby.

▶ Although this study did not compare the ACL injury rates between women and men, the high incidence of ACL injuries in rugby compared with women's soccer and basketball emphasizes once again the importance of determining why women appear to be at high risk and what, if anything, can be done to prevent these injuries.

B.L. Drinkwater, Ph.D.

A Rigorous Comparison Between the Sexes of Results and Complications After Anterior Cruciate Ligament Reconstruction

Barber-Westin SD, Noyes FR, Andrews M (Deaconess Hosp, Cincinnati, Ohio)
Am J Sports Med 25:514–526, 1997

8–4

Introduction.—There is a higher relative incidence of anterior cruciate ligament (ACL) injuries in women than in men, yet a review of 20 recent publications on results of central-third patellar tendon autogenous ACL

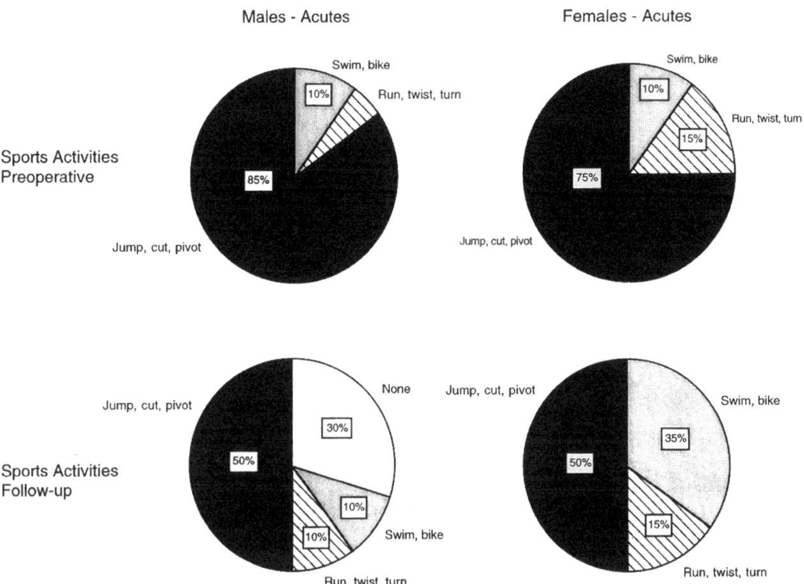

FIGURE 7.—The type of sports activities patients participated in before the reconstruction and at follow-up are shown for patients who were operated on for acute ACL ruptures. There was no statistically significant difference in the activity levels preoperatively. At follow-up, 6 (30%) men were no longer participating in sports activities because of reasons other than the knee condition. All the women had returned to some type of athletic activity. *Acutes,* Acute subgroup. (Courtesy of Barber-Westin SD, Noyes FR, Andrews M: A rigorous comparison between the sexes of results and complications after anterior cruciate ligament reconstruction. *Am J Sports Med* 25:514–526, 1997.)

reconstructions indicates that twice as many men as women had surgery and were followed-up in formal investigations. Ninety-four male and female patients (47 each sex) were evaluated to determine if differences existed between the sexes in complications and outcome of ACL reconstruction. This is the first known report in English literature in which this issue is addressed.

Methods.—Men were matched with women for age and time of interval between injury and surgery, then for preoperative activity level, months of follow-up, condition of articular cartilage, and number of operative procedures done before ACL reconstruction. There was arthroscopic evidence of complete ACL rupture in all patients. Knee displacement testing was performed and differences in measurements of the affected and ipsilateral leg were compared. Isometric testing was performed in samplings of patients from each subgroup: 19 female chronic group, 16 male chronic group, 10 female acute group, and 17 male acute group. Comprehensive knee examination included knee joint effusion, range of knee motion, patellofemoral and tibiofemoral crepitus, and alignment-related factors. Ability of surgery to restore normal knee motion was classified as functional, partially functional, or failed. Classification of the condition of the articular cartilage was done during ACL reconstruction. Rehabilitation for this cohort started with exercise the day after reconstruction and included immediate knee motion in a range of 0 to 90 degrees and immediate partial weightbearing.

Results.—There were no significant differences in mean anteroposterior displacement values between men and women with chronic ACL deficiency; the acute subgroup in mean follow-up anteroposterior displacement values; preoperative or follow-up between both sexes in pivot shift test grading; differences between men and women in either subgroup in the percentage of knees in the functional, partially functional, or failed categories; between sexes in either subgroup in the percentage of patients who had moderate patellofemoral crepitus at follow-up; sexes in the percentage of patients who had anterior knee pain at follow-up; sexes in either subgroup in strength deficits of the quadriceps and hamstring muscles; or between sexes in the number of knees with noteworthy articular cartilage deterioration. There was a significant difference in the activity levels and frequency of participation between preinjury and postoperative follow-up in the acute subgroup (Fig 7).

Conclusion.—There were no sex or subgroup (acute vs chronic) differences in patellofemoral complications, objective variables, subjective variables, knee motion, or sports activity levels in patients undergoing ACL reconstruction. Equal consideration should be given to young athletes of both sexes when contemplating operative treatment for ACL injuries. Athletes from both sexes had similar goals and athletic pursuits at an average follow-up of 2 years.

▶ About the only good news to come out of the ACL injury controversy is the report by these authors that there is no difference between the sexes in the outcome or complications resulting from ACL surgery. It is, however, disconcerting that they suggest that the sex of the athlete may have been used as a selection factor in deciding which athletes undergo ACL reconstruction. One can only hope this was a hypothetical consideration, not a practice.

B.L. Drinkwater, Ph.D.

Osteoarthrosis of the Hip in Women and Its Relationship to Physical Load From Sports Activities

Vingård E, Alfredsson L, Malchau H (Karolinksa Hosp, Stockholm; Natl Inst for Working Life, Solna, Sweden; Karolinska Inst, Solna, Sweden; et al)
Am J Sports Med 26:78–82, 1998   8–5

Background.—Previous studies have shown an association between osteoarthrosis of the hip in men who are currently active athletes. However, few studies have investigated sports activities of women and their relationship to osteoarthrosis. These authors studied women with osteoarthrosis of the hip and investigated both their previous athletic activities and the combined physical load from sports and other activities.

Methods.—Two groups of women, aged 50–70 years, were examined: 230 women who had received total hip replacement due to osteoarthrosis of the hip, and 273 age- and geographic area–matched controls without hip problems. Telephone interviews were used to gather data on sports participation before the age of 50 years. Participation was categorized as low (less than 100 hours/week), medium (100 to 800 hours/week), or high (more than 800 hours/week). Data regarding occupational histories to determine total workload were also gathered. Analyses were adjusted for age, body mass index at 40 years old, occupational workload, smoking status, and hormone therapy.

Findings.—Compared with the low-exposure group of women with osteoarthritis, women with a high sports exposure had a relative risk of 2.3 and those with a medium exposure had a relative risk of 1.5 of developing osteoarthritis of the hip. Furthermore, the risk for osteoarthrosis of the hip increased as workloads from both sports and occupational activities increased. Women having high sports exposure and high occupational workloads had a 4.3 relative risk compared with women with low sports and occupational workloads. The numbers of women participating in individual sports were too small to determine whether certain sports put the participant at greater risk.

Conclusions.—Prior medium-to-high participation in sports activities seems to be a moderate risk factor for the development of osteoarthrosis of the hip in older women. The etiologic fraction (that is, the proportion of cases that could have been prevented if the exposed women had not been exposed) for the women with high sports exposure is 57%. More research is needed to understand the negative effects of sports participation on osteoarthritis vis à vis its beneficial effects in preventing osteoporosis, ischemic heart disease, diabetes, bowel disorders, and other conditions.

▶ It is highly unlikely that any woman will give up her participation in sports because she might need a hip replacement at some time in the future. Nor should she. "Exposure," the total number of hours spent participating in sports, did not differentiate between the 15 sports plus "others" listed. Four hours of soccer or jogging was equivalent to 4 hours playing golf or swimming. Neither was there any indication of the skill level of the participant or the age when they were participating in their sport. Before one concludes that sport is a risk factor for "severe osteoarthrosis of the hip," more definitive and carefully designed studies need to be done.

B.L. Drinkwater, Ph.D.

Effect of Training on the Aerobic Power and Anaerobic Performance of Prepubertal Girls

McManus AM, Armstrong N, Williams CA (Univ of Exeter, Devon, UK)
Acta Paediatr 86:456–459, 1997   8–6

Introduction.—Few trials have tried to elucidate maturational status and reported the responses of prepubertal children to carefully controlled exercise training programs. The purpose of this study was to assess the effects of exercise training on the aerobic and anaerobic performance of 15 prepubertal girls from each of 3 urban schools.

Methods.—Schools were randomly assigned to sprint running group (SR), cycle ergometer exercise group (CEE), or control group. Mean ages of SR, CEE, and controls were 9.8, 9.3, and 9.6 years, respectively. Students underwent assessment of peak VO$_2$ with an incremental, discontinuous treadmill test to voluntary exhaustion. Anaerobic performance was calculated with the peak power in 5 seconds and the mean power over a 30-second period obtained during a Wingate Anaerobic Test. Girls in the CEE group cycled 3 times weekly for 8 weeks for 20 minutes to maintain heart rates at 80% to 85% maximal heart rate. Girls in the SR group participated in 3 sessions each week for 8 weeks. Distance covered in 10 and 30 seconds was used as a target to be beaten in subsequent runs. Girls in the control group were asked to continue their usual exercise level for 8 weeks and were retested at completion of follow-up.

Results.—All research subjects were prepubertal. There was a 23% attrition rate (favorable rate when compared with other exercise training trials with prepubertal girls). There was a disappointing loss of 8 research subjects in the control group. Girls in both exercise training groups had significant increases in peak VO$_2$ and in peak power in 5 seconds. There were no significant changes between preexercise and posttraining mean power over a 30-second period in the SR or CEE groups. Girls in the control group had no significant changes in aerobic power or anaerobic performance (Table 2).

Conclusion.—It is possible for prepubertal girls to increase their peak VO$_2$ and peak power in 5 seconds after both continuous cycling and sprint running exercise training programs. For long-term health and well-being, it is important to encourage positive attitudes about physical activity and promote exercise programs devoted to improving aerobic and anaerobic performance in children.

TABLE 2.—Aerobic and Anaerobic Data Pretraining and Posttraining

| | | Treatment group | | |
		Cycle ergometer trained ($n = 12$)	Spring running trained ($n = 11$)	Control ($n = 7$)
Peak V̇o$_2$	Pretraining	1.30 (0.19)	1.54 (0.24)	1.49 (0.15)
(1 min^{-1})	Posttraining	1.43 (0.20)*	1.67 (0.22)*	1.46 (0.15)
Peak power in 5 s	Pretraining	219.8 (56.7)	291.4 (59.9)	297.5 (75.2)
(W)	Posttraining	264.1 (62.9)*†	319.8 (57.4)*†	309.3 (49.9)
Mean power over 30 s	Pretraining	175.1 (48.8)	229.6 (35.2)	210.7 (38.1)
(W)	Posttraining	174.3 (39.5)†	236.1 (36.5)†	205.7 (26.5)

Values are mean (SD).
*Significant at $P < .05$.
†$n = 10$.
(Courtesy of McManus AM, Armstrong N, Williams CA: Effects of training on the aerobic power and anaerobic performance of prepubertal girls. *Acta Paediatr* 86:456–459, 1997.)

Responses of Young Girls to Two Modes of Aerobic Training
Welsman JR, Armstrong N, Withers S (Univ of Exeter, Devon, UK)
Br J Sports Med 31:139–142, 1997   8–7

Introduction.—The responses of young children, particularly young girls, to aerobic exercise are not well understood. The physiologic effects of 2 different modes of aerobic exercise on aerobic fitness and blood lipid levels was assessed in healthy 9– to 10-year-old girls.

Methods.—Thirty children each were randomly selected from 2 middle schools. Twenty girls in each school were assigned to a training group of either cycle ergometry or a variety of aerobic activities (aerobics) (mean ages 10.1 and 10.2 years, respectively, and 10.2 years for control). The remaining 20 girls formed a control group. All research subjects participated in a progressive treadmill running test to exhaustion to determine oxygen uptake (peak VO_2). Plasma total cholesterol and high-density lipoprotein cholesterol were measured. Each exercise group met 3 times weekly for 8 weeks. In the cycle ergometry class, participants exercised for 20 minutes at about 80% peak heart rate. The aerobics group met for 40 minutes doing aerobic exercises for 2 days and a variety of aerobics, strength, and muscular endurance components for 1 day. Controls were asked to continue their usual daily activities.

Results.—There were no significant changes in peak VO_2 or peak respiratory exchange ratio in any group; peak heart rate in the cycle group decreased significantly. There were no significant changes in plasma total

TABLE 2.—Peak Exercise Responses and Blood Lipid Pretraining and Posttraining

	Aerobics (n=17)	*Cycle ergometer (n=18)*	*Control (n=16)*
Peak $\dot{V}O_2$ (litres/min)			
Pre	1.58 (0.26)	1.76 (0.18)	1.72 (0.35)
Post	1.61 (0.23)	1.79 (0.14)	1.72 (0.37)
Peak heart rate (beats/min)			
Pre	208 (8)	210 (6)	208 (10)
Post	206 (7)	203 (4.3)*	209 (8)
Peak RER			
Pre	1.05 (0.04)	1.1 (0.04)	1.08 (0.06)
Post	1.05 (0.04)	1.05 (0.03)	1.07 (0.04)
Peak blood lactate (mmol/l)			
Pre	6.5 (1.4)	7.6 (1.9)	7.6 (2.4)
Post	6.6 (1.2)	6.1 (1.8)	7.4 (1.7)
Total cholesterol (mmol/l)			
Pre	Not sampled	5.12 (0.75)	5.50 (1.05)†
Post		4.67 (0.58)	4.96 (1.05)
HDL cholesterol (mmol/l)			
Pre	Not sampled	1.70 (0.88)	1.67 (0.42)†
Post		1.50 (0.43)	1.69 (0.27)

Values are mean (SD).
*Significantly different ($P < .01$) from pretraining values.
†$n = 8$.
Abbreviation: RER, Respiratory exchange ratio. *HDL*: high-density lipoprotein; *RER*: respiratory exchange rate; VD_2: volume of oxygen utilization.
(Courtesy of Welsman JR, Armstrong N, Withers S: Responses of young girls to two modes of aerobic training. *Br J Sports Med* 31:139–152, 1997.)

cholesterol or high-density lipoprotein cholesterol in the cycle group (Table 2).

Conclusion.—The major finding was the lack of change in peak aerobic fitness in either the cycle or aerobics exercise groups after 8 weeks of thrice weekly exercise.

▶ McManus et al. (Abstract 8–6) are undoubtedly correct in suggesting that the emphasis in this age group should be on encouraging a positive attitude toward physical activity. However, because many girls this age are engaging in youth soccer, swimming, gymnastics, etc., it is also important to understand their potential and limitations in regard to training programs established by their coaches. The McManus et al. and Welsman et al. studies used similar protocols for cycle ergometer training but reached different conclusions. McManus et al. found an increase in VO_2 peak; Welsman et al. did not. The question of how girls this age respond to aerobic training remains a question.

B.L. Drinkwater, Ph.D.

Training Effects of Short and Long Bouts of Brisk Walking in Sedentary Women

Murphy MH, Hardman AE (Univ of Ulster, Jordanstown, Co Antrium Northern Ireland; Loughborough Univ, UK)

Med Sci Sports Exerc 30:152–157, 1998   8–8

Background.—Many studies have shown the fitness benefits of brisk walking in sedentary women. The effects of short and long bouts of brisk walking in this population were compared.

Methods.—Forty-seven women, mean age 44.4, were assigned by random to 3 10-minute walks per day, 1 30-minute walk per day, or no training. Brisk walking was done at 70% to 80% of maximal heart rate, on 5 days wk^{-1}, typically at speeds ranging from 1.6 to 1.8 m/sec^{-1} (3.5 and 4.0 mph). The study lasted 10 weeks.

Findings.—Twelve women in each walking group and 10 control subjects completed the study. Compared to the control group, women in both walking groups had increased $\dot{V}O_{2max}$ and $\dot{V}O_2$ at a blood lactate concentration of 2 $mmol/L^{-1}$. These values did not differ significantly between the walking groups. Changes in heart rate during standard, submaximal exercise and resting systolic blood pressure did not differ between the walking and control groups. The sum of 4 skinfold thicknesses declined in both walking groups. However, body mass and waist circumference declined significantly only in the women in the short-bout walking group. Short- and long-bout walkers did not differ in anthropometric changes.

Conclusions.—Short bouts of brisk walking result in fitness improvements similar to those of long bouts of brisk walking in sedentary women. Short bouts of walking are at least as effective as long bouts in reducing body fat.

▶ This study examines the question of whether short bouts of walking taken at intervals throughout the day can have effects on physical fitness comparable to those produced by the longer continuous bouts traditionally prescribed. Comparison between 2 groups of walkers and a control group revealed no significant differences in fitness parameters between the 2 walking programs. This study suggests that 3 10-minute walking bouts per day are as effective as 1 30-minute bout, which may be good news for those who have difficulty in finding a 30-minute block of time in a busy day. The shorter bouts were also found to be as effective in decreasing body fatness as long bouts of similar duration in these groups of subjects. This study emphasizes that duration of individual exercise bouts is less important than the actual participation in sessions of brisk walking by sedentary women. Health care professionals need to continue to emphasize that brief walks to the store, or parking the car some distance from the mall entrance, or brisk walks through the malls will all make a contribution to fitness and body composition.

M.J.L. Alexander, Ph.D.

Gender Differences in Rowing Performance and Power With Aging

Seiler KS, Spirduso WW, Martin JC (Univ of Texas, Austin)
Med Sci Sports Exerc 30:121–127, 1998   8–9

Background.—Indoor rowing is a sport that can be used to assess the functional impact of global changes in the cardiovascular and skeletal muscle systems during aging. Gender differences in rowing performance and power with aging were explored.

Methods.—Data were obtained from a composite ranking of regional, national, and international indoor rowing competitions. The competitive indoor rowing performance times of 2,487 men aged 24–93 years and 1,615 women aged 24–84 years were analyzed.

Findings.—Age was correlated only modestly with performance in men and women. When regression analysis was limited to only the 95th percentile of each 2-year age increment (in 119 men and 79 women), age strongly predicted performance variance in both sexes. Performance declined in a curvilinear manner among the top men. Performance decline was 3% per decade between the ages of 24 and 50 years, compared to 7% between the ages of 50 and 74 years. Performance decline in women was linear throughout the 50-year age span (Fig 5).

Conclusions.—Men and women appear to lose absolute power at a similar rate across the age span analyzed in this study. However, their pattern of performance decline and maintenance of relative power differ. Differences in the effect of aging on performance across endurance sports appear to be caused more by physics than physiology.

▶ It has been widely reported that there are general declines in physical performance with increasing age; however, there are some exceptions with

a.

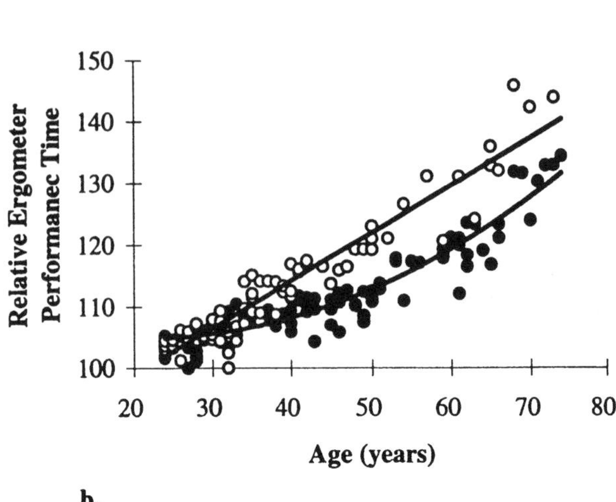

b.

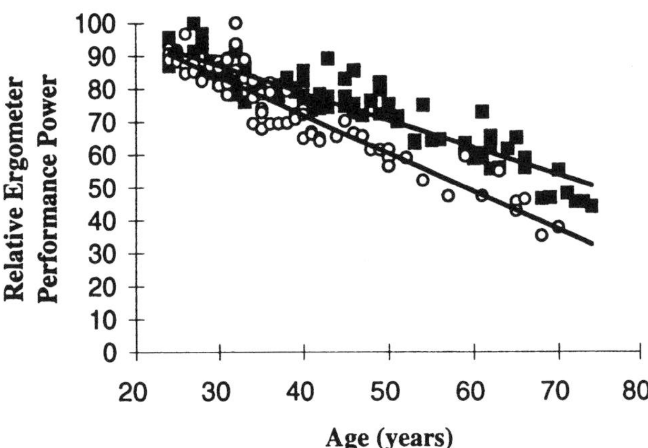

FIGURE 5.—Performance time (**A**) and power (**B**) of best male (*filled symbols*) and female (*open symbols*) age groups relative to the best overall young individal rowers. Each age group mean is divided by the fastest young male or female result, respectively, to determine performance across age relative to the best absolute performance. Values are expressed in percent. (Courtesy of Seiler KS, Spirduso WW, Martin JC: Gender differences in rowing performance and power with aging. *Med Sci Sports Exerc* 30:121–127, 1998.)

physically active subjects in older decades. Competitive indoor rowing is a popular fitness activity that has a large range of age groups participating. Examination of rowing performance data from a large number of male and female subjects revealed that age was only a modest predictor of rowing performance. Differences in stature, training volume, and technique created large variability independent of age, so analysis was performed on only those subjects above the 95th percentile in each age category. When only the top performers were analyzed, age predicted 90% of the differences in performance time and average power. For the top men, performance was a curvilinear function of age, whereas, for women, the pattern of performance decline was linear. This difference was explained on the basis of the different shape of the power-velocity curve for older men and women, than for younger men. The best men and the best women at any age perform at different positions on the power-velocity curve, suggesting that gender-related strength and power differences produce differences in rowing performance.

M.J.L. Alexander, Ph.D.

The Effects of Oral Contraceptives on Delayed Onset Muscle Soreness Following Exercise
Thompson HS, Hyatt J-P, De Souza MJ, et al (Univ of Massachusetts, Amherst; New Britain Gen Hosp, Conn)
Contraception 56:59–65, 1997   8–10

Background.—Exercise can damage muscles and cause an efflux of the intramuscular protein creatine kinase into the serum. Estrogen treatment may attenuate this efflux and thus protect skeletal muscle from damage. If so, then perhaps oral contraceptives (OCs) containing estrogen would protect women from muscle damage after exercise. This premise was tested in OC users and in non-OC users with normal menstrual cycles.

Methods.—The recreationally active premenopausal subjects (mean age 23.5) fell into 2 groups: 7 OC users and 6 eumennorheic women. Each performed a 50-minute bench stepping exercise at a cadence of 70 beats/min and a height equal to 110% of the distance from the subject's knee to foot arch. Heart rates were kept within 10% of the subject's age-predicted maximum heart rate. Both groups were tested when their estrogen levels were highest (day 18 for the OC users and during the midluteal portion for the non-OC users). Subjects rated their muscle soreness before exercise; immediately thereafter; and at 48, 76, and 92 hours after exercise on a 10-point scale with 1 being normal and 10 being very, very sore. Soreness, range of motion, dynamic and isometric strength, circumference, and serum creatine kinase activity were tracked as measures of muscle damage.

Findings.—Estrogen levels during testing did differ significantly between the groups, as expected. At 48 hours, the hamstrings, quadriceps, gluteal, and calf muscles were significantly more sore than at baseline in both groups, and hamstring range of motion was significantly less at 48, 72, and 96 hours in both groups. However, the only measure of muscle damage that differed significantly between the groups was quadriceps muscle soreness. At 48 hours after exercise, both perceived peak soreness of the quadriceps with palpation and global quadriceps soreness with movement were significantly greater in the non-OC users than in the OC users (Fig 2).

Conclusions.—Fifty minutes of bench stepping induced significant quadriceps soreness at 48 hours in both groups, but the OC users felt

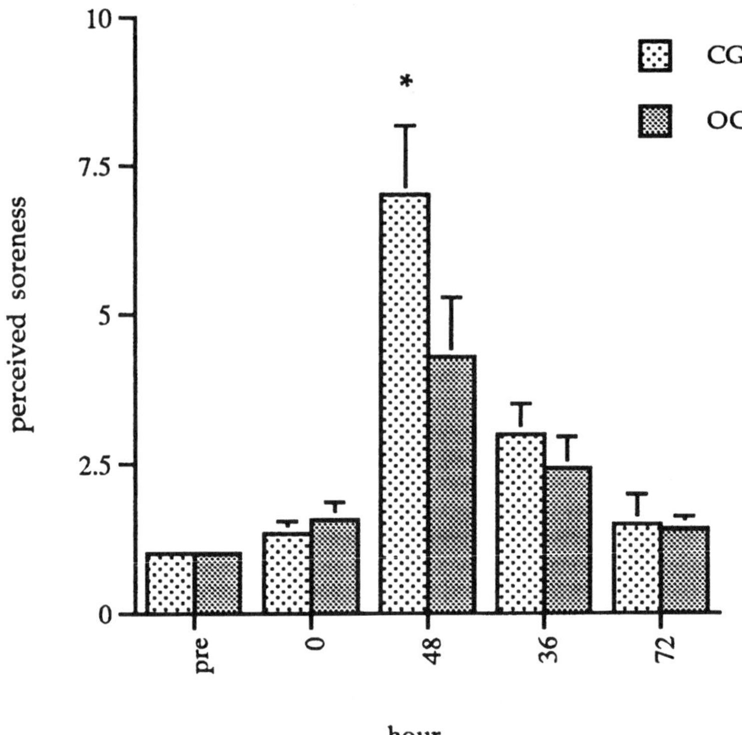

FIGURE 2.—Mean global quadricep soreness with movement at baseline, immediately post-exercise, and 48, 72, and 96 hours after exercise. Soreness scale: 1 = normal and 10 = very, very sore. *Abbreviations:* CG, eumenorrheic controls; OC, oral contraceptive users. * *P* less than 0.01 between groups. (Courtesy of Thompson HS, Hyatt J-P, De Souza MJ, et al. The effects of oral contraceptives on delayed onset muscle soreness following exercise. *Contraception* 56:59–65, copyright 1997 by Elsevier Science, Inc.)

significantly less sore than the non-OC users. This muscle soreness was not associated with an increase in serum creatine kinase activity, which means quadriceps damage after bench stepping is not associated with enzyme release. One possible explanation for the differences in soreness is that OC users may have a higher pain threshold due to chronically elevated opioid peptide levels.

▶ With the rapid increase of women's participation in masters competition, the response of users and non-users of hormone replacement therapy among postmenopausal masters athletes would be interesting to observe.

B.L. Drinkwater, Ph.D.

Relationship Between Physical Activity Related Energy Expenditure and Body Composition: A Gender Difference
Westerterp KR, Goran MI (Maastricht Univ, The Netherlands; Univ of Alabama, Birmingham)
Int J Obes 21:184–188, 1997   8–11

Introduction.—Exercise is thought to be an important factor in the prevention of obesity. A negative correlation has been found between physical activity and the degree of obesity. The measurement of average daily metabolic rate and basal metabolic rate is often used in the calculation of energy expenditure for physical activity and body composition or percentage of fat. To examine the relationship between physical activity and percentage of body fat more thoroughly, after correcting for age, average daily metabolic rate, basal metabolic rate, age, and percentage of body fat of individuals were analyzed.

Methods.—There were 290 participants, 18–49 years old, with 146 women and 144 men. The participants' body mass ranged widely, including morbidly obese individuals and anorectics with a minimal fat mass. Observations on average daily metabolic rate, basal metabolic rate, and percentage of body fat were made and analyzed.

Results.—In women, age explained 3% to 7% of the variation in percentage of body fat. In men, age explained 5% to 20% of the variation in percentage of body fat. In men, the explained variation in percentage of body fat was raised by adding physical activity, with a lower percentage of body fat being related to a higher level of physical activity. In women, however, body composition had no relationship to physical activity. Percentage of body fat increased significantly with increasing age in a subset of individuals who had body mass range between 20 and 35 kg/m^2.

Conclusion.—Men have a significant inverse cross-sectional relationship between percentage of body fat and activity energy expenditure, whereas women do not seem to have such a relationship. Unless accompanied by a restriction of energy intake, exercise is not effective in reducing body fat in females.

▶ There have been periodic suggestions that body fat is more stable in women than in men.[1] Anthropological justification for such a difference might be found in the energy needs of pregnancy and lactation. The present report seems to support this view, finding a significant inverse relationship between energy expenditure and percentage of body fat in men but not in women. Problems in measuring activity patterns cannot explain the gender difference in the present study, because energy expenditures were monitored using the doubly labeled water technique. Men compensate less for changes in energy expenditure than do women,[2] and much of a man's fat is stored in the abdominal region, where it is more readily mobilized.[3] Regression techniques found that physical activity, as measured by doubly labeled water, explained only 12% of the variation of fatness in the men. However, a weakness in this conclusion is that age was also included in the regression analysis; age may serve as a surrogate of both decreasing physical activity and increasing fatness, and if so, activity could be accounting for a much larger fraction of the observed obesity in men.

R.J. Shephard, M.D., Ph.D., D.P.E.

References

1. Murray SJ, Shephard RJ, Greaves S, et al: Effects of cold stress and exercise on fat loss in females. *Eur J Appl Physiol* 55:610–618, 1986.
2. Tremblay A, Déspres JP, Leblanc C, et al: Sex dimorphism in fat loss in response to exercise training. *J Obes Weight Regul* 3:193–203, 1984.
3. Egger G, O'Neill M, Bolton A, et al: Results of an abdominal obesity reduction program for men only: The gutbuster 'waist' loss program. *Int J Clin Obes* 19(S2):37, 1995.

Energy Expenditure of Swimmers During High Volume Training
Trappe TA, Gastaldelli A, Jozsi AC, et al (United States Olympic Training Ctr, Colorado Springs, Colo; Univ of Texas, Galveston)
Med Sci Sports Exerc 29:950–954, 1997   8–12

Purpose.—Competitive swimmers now train at a volume of 20 km/d, or 5 to 6 h/d. Such high-duration training can deplete muscle carbohydrate stores, which may affect the response to training. Optimal adaptation to training must include proper nutrition in terms of amount and composition. The doubly labeled water (DLW) method is a useful tool for assessing energy costs. This method was used to determine total energy requirements of female swimmers performing high-volume training.

Methods.—The study including 5 elite female swimmers from the U.S. Swimming National Team. After giving a saliva sample for background enrichment, the swimmers were given a dose of DLW. An initial saliva sample was taken after at least 4 hours of equilibration and on the morning of the fifth day after DLW dosing. The subjects completed dietary records to obtain an estimate of energy intake and food quotient during the 5-day study period. Assessments of resting energy expenditure were made on a nontraining day. During the study, the athletes trained for 5 to 6 hours, swimming a mean of 17.7 km/d.

Results.—The swimmers' mean total energy expenditure during the study was 23.4 MJ/d, while estimated energy intake was 13.1 MJ/d. The mean 10.3 MJ/d difference between these values translated into an energy balance of −43% (Table 2).

Conclusions.—These findings suggest that elite female swimmers training at a high volume have a significant negative energy balance. This result could be related to either underreporting of food intake by the athletes or true undereating. Though underreporting is possible, it might be difficult for athletes training at such a high volume to meet the energy requirements of their training program.

TABLE 2.—Total Energy Expenditure, Resting Energy Expenditure, and Energy Intake

Subject	TEE (MJ·d^{-1})	REE (MJ·d^{-1})	TEE/REE	EI (MJ·d^{-1})	Energy Balance (%)
1	26.5	8.3	3.2	14.0	−47
2	26.8	9.5	2.8	15.9	−41
3	20.3	6.7	3.0	11.4	−44
4	16.7	6.5	2.6	10.6	−37
5	26.7	7.6	3.5	13.8	−48
Mean	23.4	7.7	3.0	13.1	−43
±SE	2.1	0.5	0.2	1.0	2

Abbreviations: TEE, total energy expenditure; *REE*, resting energy expenditure; *EI*, energy intake.
(Courtesy of Trappe TA, Gastaldelli A, Jozsi AC, et al: Energy expenditure of swimmers during high volume training. *Med Sci Sports Exerc* 29:950–954, 1997.)

▶ Although the authors believe that part of the energy deficit may be due to underreporting of food consumed, they do note that it might be difficult for the swimmers to meet their energy needs during high-volume intensive training. These results are an excellent example of the point made by Loucks et al. in a previous article that athletes may be eating what would be a normal diet for the average women (in this case 3,136 kcal·d) and still have an energy deficit because of the energy requirements of their training (5,593 kcal·d). Whether this deficit has affected the menstrual cycle of these women was not reported.

B.L. Drinkwater, Ph.D.

A Cross-sectional Study on Body Composition and Energy Expenditure in Women Athletes During Aging

Ryan AS, Nicklas BJ, Elahi D (Univ of Maryland, Baltimore; Baltimore Veterans Affairs Med Ctr, Maryland)
Am J Physiol 271:E916–E921, 1996   8–13

Introduction.—An increase in obesity and central body fat is associated with aging, which predisposes individuals to cardiovascular disease, hypertension, dyslipidemia, and diabetes mellitus. This may be altered by increased physical activity. However, no studies have been conducted to examine women athletes and regional fat distribution. With aging males, resting metabolic rate declines 1% to 2% per decade. A study sought to determine whether an increase in intra-abdominal adipose tissue and a decrease in fat-free mass that occur during aging can be prevented in women athletes. Substrate oxidation and resting metabolic rate were determined in highly trained women over a wide age span.

Methods.—In 43 highly trained women and in 14 sedentary women aged 18–69, the relationships between total and regional body composition, intra-abdominal adipose tissue, resting metabolic rate, and substrate oxidation were examined. The controls were divided into 2 age groups: 18–29 and 40–50, whereas the athletes were divided into 4 age groups: 18–29, 30–39, 40–49, and 50–69.

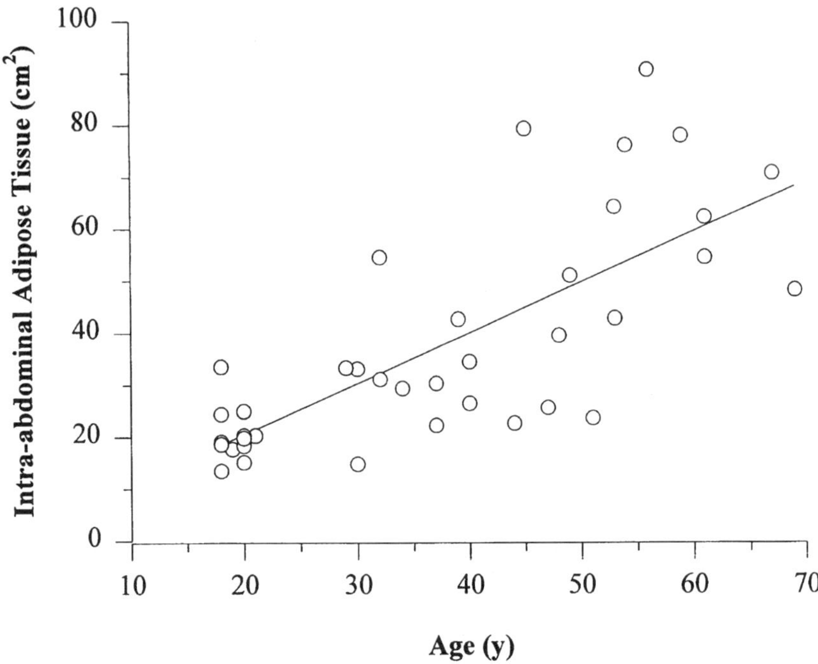

FIGURE 1.—Relationship between age and intra-abdominal adipose tissue area in women athletes (r = 0.75, P < 0.0001). (Courtesy of Ryan AS, Nicklas, BJ, Elahi D: A cross-sectional study on body composition and energy expenditure in women athletes during aging. *Am J Physiol* 271:E916–E921, 1996. Copyright the American Physiological Society.)

Results.—In the athletes, maximal oxygen consumption declined with age. In all groups of athletes, maximal oxygen consumption was higher than in controls. Between the youngest and the oldest athletes, no differences in percent fat and fat-free mass were found. In controls, percent body fat and total fat mass were higher than in athletes for older and younger women; however, body mass index was less than 25 kg/m² in all women. In young athletes, fat-free mass was higher than in young control subjects. Intra-abdominal adipose tissue increased with age (Fig 1), but sagittal diameter and subcutaneous abdominal fat did not, despite no increase in percent fat among athletes. In younger and older controls, intra-abdominal adipose tissue and subcutaneous abdominal fat were higher than in younger and older athletes. The decline in resting metabolic rate in the athletes was independently predicted by age and fat-free mass. Fat oxidation was highest in the youngest athletes and declined with age.

Conclusion.—Intense long-term exercise in women athletes prevented the decline in fat-free mass with age. Low intra-abdominal adipose tissue stores were found in endurance-trained women, and this may potentially reduce subsequent risk associated with the metabolic syndrome.

▶ Perhaps the most interesting outcome of this study is the finding that the waist-to-hip ratio (WHR) did not differ across age or between athletes and controls. Yet intra-abdominal fat increased with age in both athletes and controls and was markedly higher in controls than in athletes. Obviously, WHR is not a good indicator of visceral adiposity for women. The good news is that older athletes were able to maintain the same low percent body fat and fat-free mass as the younger athletes.

B.L. Drinkwater, Ph.D.

Prescribing Exercise Intensity for Older Women
Kohrt WM, Spina RJ, Holloszy JO, et al (Washington Univ, St Louis)
J Am Geriatr Soc 46:129–133, 1998   8–14

Introduction.—Exercise intensity is usually assessed by measuring heart rate. Under current American College of Sports Medicine (ACSM) guidelines, relative exercise intensities calculated by the heart rate reserve method are regarded as equivalent to values calculated by maximal aerobic power. Maximal heart rate and maximal aerobic power both decline with age. This study assessed the relationships between common methods of prescribing exercise intensity in older women.

Methods.—The study included 112 women, aged 60–72 years, who did not exercise regularly. All were healthy nonsmokers. A treadmill walking test was performed to determine maximal aerobic power and heart rate. On a separate day, the women performed a treadmill exercise protocol consisting of 4 6-minute stages of level walking at speeds of 67, 80, 94, and 107 m/min. The stages were separated by 10-minute rest periods. Measurements of maximal aerobic power were made during the last 2 minutes of each exercise stage. An ACSM equation was used to calculate the predicted rate of oxygen uptake for each subject at each stage. The measured and predicted aerobic power values at each stage were then compared.

Results.—At all stages, the relationships between percent of maximal heart rate—assessed by measured or predicted HR max—and percent maximal aerobic power were similar to those used in the ACSM guidelines. However, the values for percentage of maximal aerobic power and percentage of heart rate reserve were not equivalent. Values for rating of perceived exercise appeared to be lower than described in the ACSM guidelines. At all stages, measured oxygen uptake significantly exceeded the values calculated by the ACSM equation for prediction of energy expenditure during walking.

Conclusions.—Heart rate expressed as a percentage of maximal heart rate appears to be an appropriate method of prescribing exercise intensity in healthy but sedentary older women. Methods based on percentage of heart rate reserve are not appropriate, as this value is not equivalent for percentage of maximal aerobic power for such women. The result would be exercise at a higher than expected percentage of maximal aerobic power, based on ACSM guidelines. Ratings of perceived exercise could be a useful adjunct for monitoring of exercise intensity. These and previous findings suggest that adults aged 60–80 years can exercise at relatively higher intensities than younger people.

▶ The women in this study were not only older women but older *sedentary* women. An average $\dot{V}O_2$ max of 19.9 mL·kg^{-1}·min^{-1} certainly confirms the fact that these women did not exercise regularly, if at all. Although it is important to identify differences in physiologic responses that are a result of the aging process, it is equally important to differentiate between the effect of age vs. age plus inactivity. There are many older women today who are training and competing in a wide variety of sports. Results based on studies of sedentary women may or may not apply to them.

B.L. Drinkwater, Ph.D.

Physical Activity and Mortality in Postmenopausal Women
Kushi LH, Fee RM, Folsom AR, et al (Univ of Minnesota, Minneapolis)
JAMA 277:1287–1292, 1997   8–15

Introduction.—Numerous studies show that physical activity has beneficial health effects. Most studies on the association of physical activity with mortality have been conducted among men, and results indicate that exercise reduces coronary artery and overall mortality. The association between physical activity and mortality was evaluated prospectively in postmenopausal women.

Methods.—Study participants were members of the Iowa Women's Health Study, were recruited in January 1986, were aged 55–69 years, and held a valid Iowa driver's license in 1985. Approximately half of these women (99,826) were selected randomly and sent a 16-page questionnaire. The final sample included 40,417 of the 41,826 women who returned the questionnaire and were postmenopausal at baseline. The survey included questions related to health habits, medical history, anthropometry, and leisure physical activity. Level of physical activity was characterized as low in 18,940 women, medium in 10,987, and high in 9,919. The status of the women was followed up for 7 years.

Results.—Relative risks (RRs) of death from all causes were calculated according to levels of physical activity, adjusting for age and multiple covariates. Higher levels of physical activity were associated with a decreased risk for death. Compared with women who reported no regular physical activity, those who did engage in such activity had a multivariate-adjusted RR of death of 0.78. Among women reporting a moderate level of physcal activity, increasing frequency (low to high) was associated with decreasing RR (1.0, 0.71, 0.63, and 0.59). A similar pattern was seen for increasing regularity of vigorous physical activity. Among women with no baseline diseases and excluding those who died in the first 3 years of follow-up, the RR of death was 0.77 for those engaging in any physical activity, compared with those performing no physical activity. These beneficial effects of physical activity were apparent in all 5-year age categories and in all quartiles of waist-to-hip ratios.

Conclusions.—Regular physical activity, even performed once a week at a moderate level, reduced mortality from any cause in postmenopausal women. Associations were strongest for 2 categories of mortality: cardiovascular diseases and respiratory illnesses. These findings confirm the benefits of regular physical activity in postmenopausal women.

▶ While the study by Stevenson et al. (Abstract 8–17) concludes that lower waist-to-hip ratios in active women were related to a more favorable SBP-related risk for cardiovascular disease (CVD), Kushi et al. report that waist-to-hip ratio had little effect on mortality risk in their cohort of postmenopausal women followed over a period of 7 years. It was physical activity per se that seemed to confer protection. While it is premature to establish abdominal obesity as a marker for CVD risk in women, it is reassuring that both studies found physically active women had a lower risk for CVD or death.

B.L. Drinkwater, Ph.D.

Greater Rate of Decline in Maximal Aerobic Capacity With Age in Physically Active vs Sedentary Healthy Women

Tanaka H, DeSouza CA, Jones PP, et al (Univ of Colorado, Denver)
J Appl Physiol 83:1947–1953, 1997   8–16

Introduction.—Maximal aerobic capacity, as determined by maximal oxygen uptake (VO_{2max}), decreases with advancing age in both sexes. The rate of decline in VO_{2max} with age has been shown in cross-sectional studies to be greater in physically active women compared with sedentary women. The rate of decline in VO_{2max} with age was evaluated prospectively in a well-controlled, laboratory-based trial of physically active and sedentary women.

Methods.—Of 156 healthy women aged 20 to 75 years, 84 were endurance-trained athletes (ET) and 72 were non-obese and sedentary. About 10 women were included in each 10-year age period for both groups. Women in the ET group had been training at least 2 years and were actively competing in road-running races. Women in the sedentary group were not involved in regular exercise. A continuous incremental treadmill protocol was used to assess VO_{2max}. Five-site skinfold measurements were used to determine percent body fat.

Results.—With advancing age, body mass and percent body fat rose in the sedentary group. For the ET group, body mass and fat-free mass did not decline with age, but percent body fat was positively correlated with age. At all ages, VO_{2max} was higher in the ET group. The rate of decline in VO_{2max} was significantly greater in the ET group (-5.7 mL·kg^{-1}·min^{-1}·decade^{-1}) than S (-3.2 mL·kg^{-1}·min^{-1}·decade^{-1}) (Fig 1). The relative percent rate of decline in VO_{2max} from mean levels at about age 25 years was

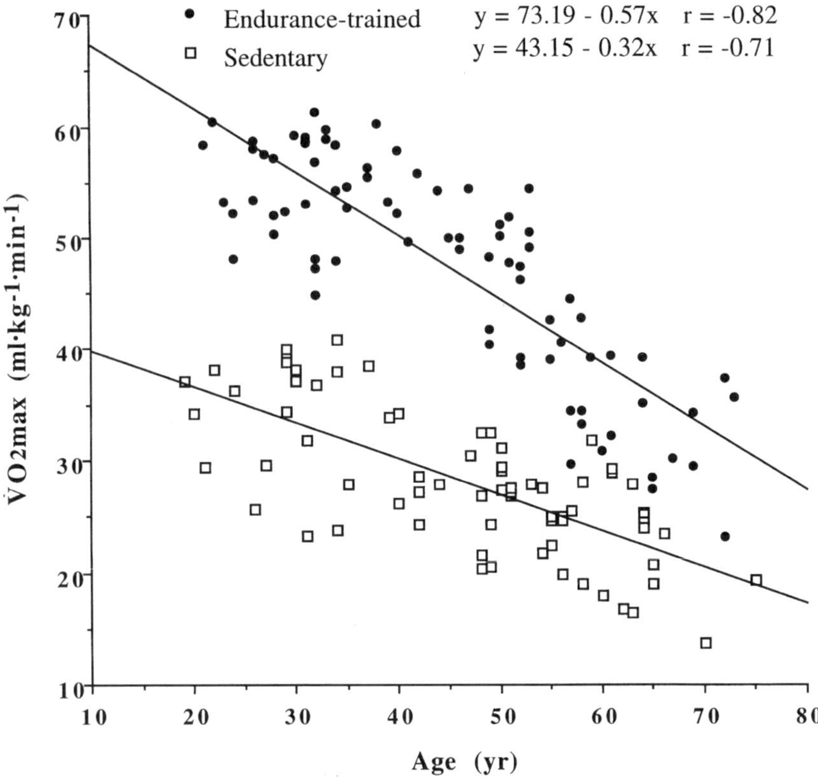

FIGURE 1.—Relations between maximal oxygen uptake (VO_{2max}) and age in endurance-trained and sedentary women. Rate of decline in VO_{2max} with age was greater in ET women than in sedentary women ($P < .01$). (Courtesy of Tanaka H, DeSouza CA, Jones PP: Greater rate of decline in maximal aerobic capacity with age in physically active vs sedentary health women. *J Appl Physiol* 83:1947–1953, 1997.)

similar for ET ($9.7\%\cdot$decade^{-1}) and S ($9.1\%\cdot$decade^{-1}). Maximum heart rate was inversely related to age for the ET and sedentary groups. Age-related reductions in maximal heart rate were similar for both groups. Age was the primary predictor and percent body fat was the secondary predictor of VO_{2max} for both groups.

Conclusion.—These results support earlier findings that absolute, but not relative, rates of decline in VO_{2max} with increasing age were greater in the ET group. This higher rate of decline in VO_{2max} in the ET group was not correlated with greater changes in body mass or composition, maximal heart rate, or training factors. It might be attributed to their higher baseline levels as young adults.

▶ Although the authors mention that some subjects were using hormone replacement therapy, it is not clear whether there was an effect of therapy on VO_{2max} in either group. A closer look at the data suggests that the endurance athletes maintained their VO_{2max} from age 20 to 49 years (-3.6

mL·kg^{-1}·min^{-1}) while the decrement for the sedentary women was twice that (-7.9 mL·kg^{-1}·min^{-1}). After age 50, the VO$_{2max}$ of the endurance-trained women dropped by 8.7 mL·kg^{-1}·min^{-1} while that of the sedentary women decreased only slightly (-1.5 mL·kg^{-1}·min^{-1}). An obvious question would seem to be, do menopausal changes affect the aerobic power of endurance athletes more than sedentary women, and what role might HRT play in these changes?

B.L. Drinkwater, Ph.D.

Blood Pressure Risk Factors in Healthy Postmenopausal Women: Physical Activity and Hormone Replacement

Stevenson ET, Davy KP, Jones PP, et al (Univ of Colorado, Boulder)
J Appl Physiol 82:652–660, 1997

8–17

Introduction.—Cardiovascular diseases (CVDs) are the primary cause of death in middle-aged and older female Americans. Postmenopausal women who participate in regular physical activity have a decreased risk of CVD. Sedentary and physically active females were evaluated to determine if those who were physically active had more favorable blood pressure–related risk factors for CVD than their healthy non-obese, less active counterparts.

Methods.—Of 52 healthy, non-obese women, 18 were highly physically active (mean age 55 years) and 34 were sedentary to minimally active (mean age 59 years). Eight of the physically active (44%) and 17 of the sedentary women (50%) were currently taking hormone replacement therapy for at least 1 year. Blood pressure recordings were taken with the subject supine, sitting, and standing with conventional sphygmomanometry and over a 24-hour period of normal daily activity. Systolic blood pressure (SBP) was taken during submaximal and maximal exercise. Increases from preexercise to submaximal and maximal exercises were determined.

Results.—Women in both groups were similar in age, height, and estimated fat-free mass. Active women had significantly lower measures of body mass index, waist-to-hip ratio, body weight, sum of skinfolds, estimated percent body fat, and waist circumference than controls (Table 1). Groups were similar in casual levels of supine, sitting, and standing blood pressure. Active women had lower SBP variability than controls during daytime and nighttime hours, but there were no group differences in SBP variability over the full 24-hour period. Diastolic BP (DBP) variability was lower in active women; the difference was significant during daytime hours. The SBP response to submaximal treadmill exercise was lower in physically active vs sedentary women. In univariate analysis, the blood pressure–related CVD risk factors that correlated with physical activity and VO$_{2max}$ levels were daytime SBP and DBP variability, absolute level of SBP at the submaximal workload of 6.4 metabolic equivalent, and increase in SBP from preexercise levels to the submaximal exercise workload. The

TABLE 1.—Subject Characteristics in Physically Active Women vs. Controls

	Active Women	Controls
n	18	34
Age, yr	55 ± 1	59 ± 1
Height, cm	167 ± 1	164 ± 1
Weight, kg	57.7 ± 1.2*	68.8 ± 1.6
BMI, kg/m^2	20.7 ± 0.3*	25.6 ± 0.5
Sum of skinfolds, cm	66.9 ± 5.8*	153.2 ± 6.3
Estimated %body fat	18.2 ± 1.3*	34.2 ± 1.1
Estimated fat-free mass, kg	47.0 ± 0.9	44.9 ± 0.9
Waist circumference, cm	70 ± 1*	84 ± 2
Waist-to-hip ratio	0.74 ± 0.01*	0.80 ± 0.01
Estimated energy expenditure, kcal · kg^{-1} · day^{-1}	45 ± 1*	35 ± 1
$\dot{V}O_{2max}$, ml · kg^{-1} · min^{-1}	43.7 ± 2.1*	24.2 ± 0.8

Values are mean ±SE.
*P < .01.
Abbreviations: BMI, Body mass index; VO_{2max}, maximal oxygen consumption.
(Courtesy of Stevenson ET, Davy KP, Jones PP: Blood pressure risk factors in healthy postmenopausal women: Physical activity and hormone replacement. *J Appl Physiol* 82:652–660, 1997.)

VO_{2max} was a significant predictor of 24-hour SBP variability and SBP before treadmill exercise and at maximal exercise. Waist circumference was the primary predictor of all SBP-related CVD risk factors. Daytime and 24-hour DBP loads were substantially lower in those receiving hormone replacement therapy.

Conclusion.—Highly physically active women seemed to have more favorable SBP-related CVD risk factors relative to healthy non-obese but less-active women of the same age. This finding could be partly mediated by a lower level of abdominal fat estimated by waist circumference. Hormone replacement recipients had lower DBP loads and a strong tendency for lower levels of 24-hour and nighttime DBP.

▶ Not only did the physically active women differ from the controls in activity level and aerobic power, but they also differed in many variables related to body mass and body fat (Table 1). Generalizing from results obtained from a group of women who had been training an average of 16 years and running 31 miles/week to what is generally accepted as a definition of "physically active" postmenopausal women would be a mistake. The interaction of physical activity and hormone replacement therapy would have been of interest. However, the authors elected to combine the athletes and controls into either an HRT or non-HRT group—perhaps because of the small sample size in each category.

B.L. Drinkwater, Ph.D.

Effects of Diet and Exercise on Energy Expenditure in Postmenopausal Women
Thompson JL, Gylfadottir UK, Moynihan S, et al (Stanford Univ, Palo Alto; Univ of North Carolina, Charlotte)
Am J Clin Nutr 66:867–873, 1997   8–18

Introduction.—It has been suggested that exercise training can prevent the decline in resting metabolic rate (BMR) during dietary restriction. Exercise increases metabolically active fat-free mass and has a long-term carryover effect on BMR. The effects of 24 weeks of a moderate diet plus exercise program or diet-only program on BMR, bone mineral density, energy expenditure during daily activities, muscle strength, and maximal oxygen consumption (VO_2max) were assessed in 40 menopausal women.

Methods.—Research subjects of 120% to 140% of ideal body weight and a mean age of 65 years were assigned to either the diet plus exercise program or 1 of 2 groups in the diet only program: 1 group was asked to consume 2,092 kJ/d (group D-2,092) (500 kcal/d) less than needed for weight maintenance and the other group was asked to consume 2,929 kJ/d (group D-2,929) (700 kcal/d) less than needed for weight maintenance. Women in the diet plus exercise group were asked to consume 2,092 kJ/d less than required for weight maintenance. The diet program met the American Heart Association's guidelines of 30% fat, 50% to 55% carbo-hydrates, and 10% to 15% protein. Women in the diet and exercise group walked 3 times weekly and participated in strength-training twice weekly. Indirect calorimetry was used to measure BMR for 3 consecutive morn-ings. Expired gases were analyzed to determine energy expenditure (EE): resting while sitting, standing, and at 1.4 and 2.4 mph on the treadmill. Dual-energy X-ray absorptiometry was used to measure body composition and total bone mineral density.

Results.—All groups had significant decreases in body weight, body fat mass, and percentage body fat. There was a small but significant reduction in fat-free mass. Bone mineral density did not change in any group. Values for BMR were significantly lower for all 3 groups at 12 and 24 weeks compared with baseline. There were no significant changes in EE during resting or standing, but it was lower over time for sitting and walking at 1.4 and 2.4 mph. There were no significant changes in VO_2max for any groups. There were significant increases in strength from baseline to final evaluation ranging from 19% for military press to 164% for leg curl. Seven of 12 females in the diet and exercise group reported continuing exercising on their own.

Conclusion.—Postmenopausal women can lose significant body weight and body fat without a big drop in BMR. Women in the D-2,929 group had a bigger decrease in EE than women in the diet plus exercise and D-2,092 groups at rest and during walking. The addition of exercise to a moderate energy deficit diet may help conserve EE. Addition of exercise helped research subjects achieve continued weight loss after program cessation. Those who did not exercise or continue to exercise tended to gain weight. This cohort did not have a plateau in strength that has been observed in elderly women after 8 weeks of strength training. These are important findings because it is crucial that women who are overweight and postmenopausal maintain BMR and bone mass while losing body fat.

▶ Most women who attempt to lose weight through severe caloric restriction find it very difficult to maintain the weight loss. The results of this study suggest that less severe caloric restriction might prevent large decreases in BMR. That, together with an exercise program, may lead to more success in maintaining weight loss.

B.L. Drinkwater, Ph.D.

Low Energy Availability, Not Stress of Exercise, Alters LH Pulsatility in Exercising Women

Loucks AB, Heath EM (Ohio Univ, Athens)
J Appl Physiol 84:37–46, 1998

8–19

Background.—The occurrence of amenorrhea in female athletes has been explained by the "exercise stress hypothesis," under which the stress of exercise activates the hypothalamic-pituitary-adrenal (HPA) axis, leading to disruption of pulsatile gonadotropin-releasing hormone (GnRH) secretion, leading to disruption of pulsatile luteinizing hormone (LH) secretion. A competing hypothesis is the "energy availability hypothesis," under which disruption of the GnRH pulse generator is caused by an unknown signal reflecting insufficient energy for both reproduction and locomotion. These hypotheses were evaluated by testing the independent effects of energy availability and exercise stress on LH pulsatility in exercising women.

Methods.—Nine healthy, sedentary, regularly menstruating women, aged 18–29 years, participated in the study. Customary 24-hour energy expenditure was estimated by having the subjects wear a physical activity monitor for 2 days. The women then performed intense exercise of 30 kcal/kg lean body mass/day at 70% of aerobic capacity for 4 days, starting on day 5, 6, or 7 of the menstrual cycle. Exercise energy expenditure was calculated by subtracting estimated habitual energy expenditure from the controlled energy expenditure during exercise. On days 8, 9, or 10 of the menstrual cycle, LH was assayed in blood drawn every 10 minutes for measurement. Frequent measurements of serum cortisol, follicle-stimulating hormone, estradiol, growth hormone, and glucose were performed on the same day. On the 4 exercise days and the sampling day, the subjects were randomized to receive a liquid diet designed to provide a balanced or deprived energy availability: 45 or 10 kcal/kg LBM/day, respectively. This permitted testing of the effects of low energy availability on LH pulsatility. The effects of exercise stress on LH pulsatility were assessed by comparing values to those reported for nonexercising women with similar controlled energy availability.

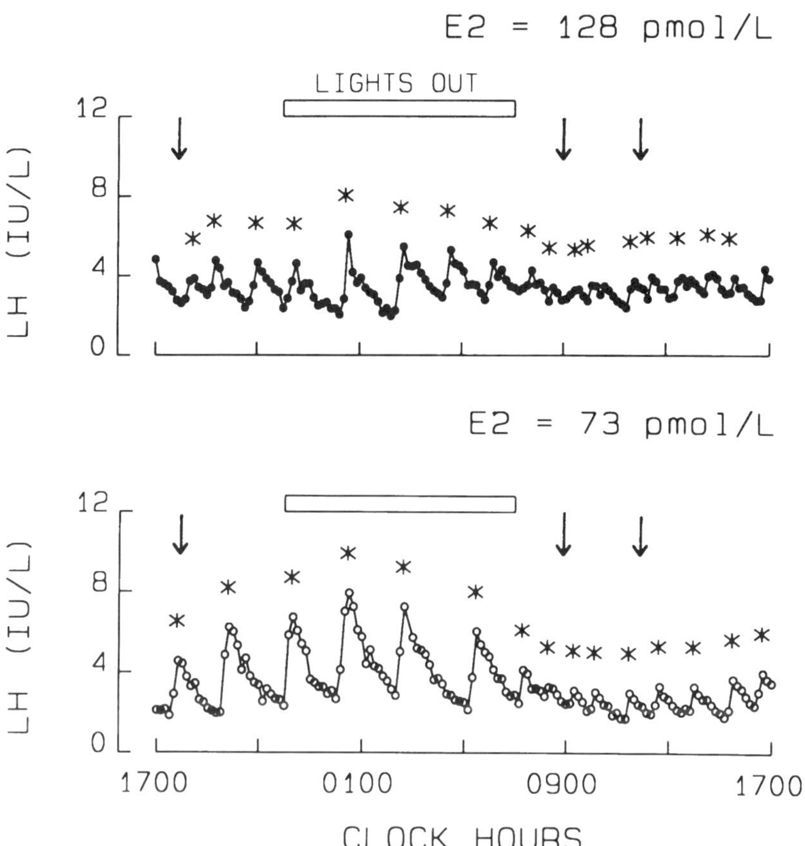

FIGURE 4.—Representative 24-hour luteinizing hormone (LH) pulsatile patterns after the 2 energy availability treatments. Blood samples were drawn at 10-minute intervals for 24 hours, *A*, LH pulsatile pattern after balanced energy availability treatment. *B*, LH pulsatile pattern after low energy availability treatment. Estradiol (E_2) concentrations are 24-hour transverse mean of measurements at 6-hour intervals. *Open bar*, sleep. *Arrows*, meal administrations. *LH pulses. (Courtesy of Loucks AB, Heath EM: Low energy availability, not stress of exercise, alters LH pulsatility in exercising women. *J Appl Physiol* 84:37–46, 1998.)

Results.—Assessment of metabolic responses suggested that low energy availability caused by exercise energy expenditure reduced T_3 by 18%, IGF-I by 26%, and insulin by 34%, compared with baseline. At the same time, 24-hour pooled growth hormone concentration rose by 26% and 24 hour mean serum cortisol concentration by 11%. Low energy availability caused by exercise energy expenditure caused a 10% reduction in LH pulse frequency over 24 hours (Fig 4). This effect was 60% smaller than that of low energy availability caused by dietary energy restriction. The effect of low energy availability on LH pulse frequency was apparent only during the waking hours. Twenty-four–hour LH pulse amplitude was increased by 36%.

The stress of exercise had no effect on T_3, insulin, insulin-like growth factor, growth hormone, or cortisol levels in either the balanced- or low-energy availability groups. In neither group did exercise stress lead to suppression of 24-hour pulse frequency, awake or during sleep. Exercise stress had no effect on LH pulse amplitude, on 24-hour LH transverse mean, on E_2, or on 24-hour follicle-stimulating hormone transverse mean.

Conclusions.—Intense exercise in sedentary women does not affect LH pulsatility independently of its effect on energy availability. The effect of exercise energy expenditure on LH pulsatility is not as great as that of an equivalent degree of dietary energy restriction. Low energy availability caused by exercise energy expenditure is also associated with reductions in T_3, insulin, and IGF-I and with increases in cortisol and growth hormone. Female athletes may experience disruptions of reproductive function even in the absence of dietary restriction. To avoid such problems, women athletes may have to learn to eat when they are not hungry, just as they have learned to drink when they are not thirsty.

▶ It is difficult to overemphasize the importance of the studies coming from this laboratory. The pervasive—and difficult to eradicate—belief that it is "strenuous" exercise that results in disruption of the female reproductive cycle is a consistent theme in most lay articles addressing this issue. The series of carefully designed studies from Loucks et al. should be required reading before anyone speaks to the topic of "athletic amenorrhea."

B.L. Drinkwater, Ph.D.

Effects of Estrogen Replacement Therapy on Dehydroepiandrosterone, Dehydroepiandrosterone Sulfate, and Cortisol Responses to Exercise in Postmenopausal Women
Johnson LG, Kraemer GR, Kraemer RR, et al (Southeastern Louisiana Univ, Hammond; Texas Tech Univ, Amarillo)
Fertil Steril 68:836–843, 1997   8–20

Introduction.—Normal serum levels of cortisol are maintained with aging, unlike the progressive decline of adrenal androgens dehydroepiandrosterone (DHEA) and DHEA sulfate (DHEAS). The effects of hormone replacement therapy (HRT) on DHEA, DHEAS, and cortisol responses to treadmill exercise were assessed in 16 healthy postmenopausal women.

Methods.—Seven research subjects had been receiving HRT (conjugated estrogen tablets or estropipate tablets) for a mean of 7.64 years, and 9 received no HRT. Mean age of women who were receiving HRT or were untreated was 50.43 and 53 years, respectively. Research subjects underwent determination of body composition and VO_{2max}. Before treadmill testing, they were asked to refrain from exercise and alcohol intake for 48 hours and to fast overnight. Blood samples were obtained from an intravenous catheter before, during, and 30 minutes after treadmill testing. The

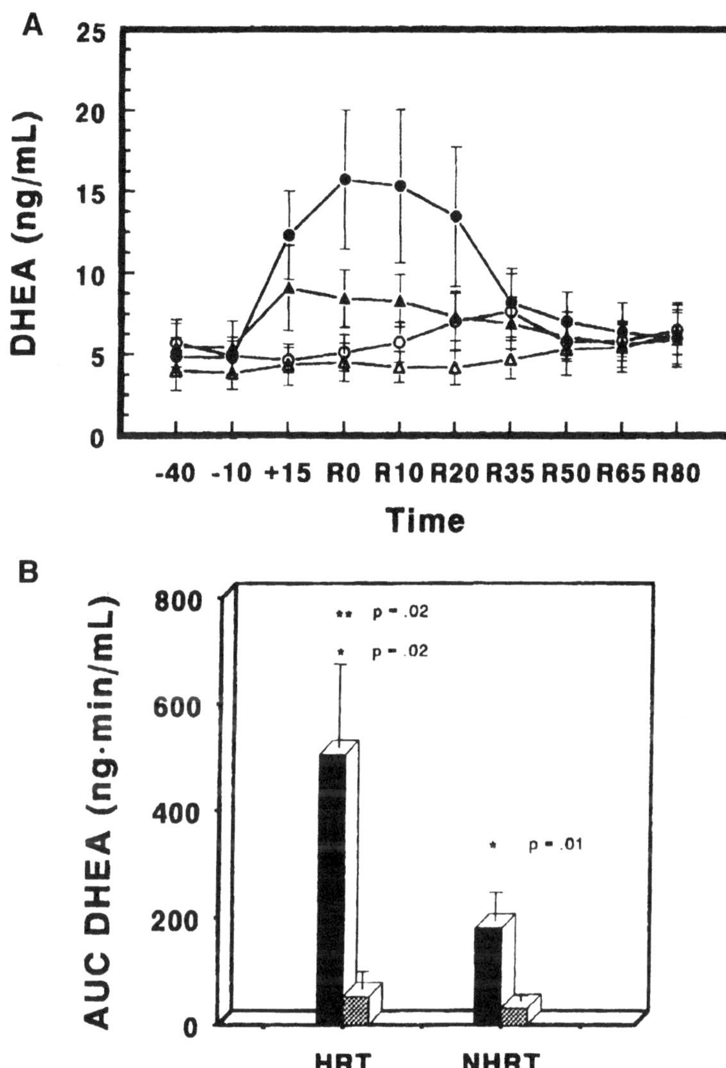

FIGURE 2.—(A), Mean DHEAS concentration (± SE) for the HRT group (*circles; n* = 7) and the untreated (NHRT) group (*triangles; n* = 9) during the exercise (*open squares*) and control (*open circles and triangles*) trials; (B), HRT and untreated DHEA area under the curve concentrations for the exercise (*solid squares*) and control (*solid circles and triangles*) trials; statistical significance noted between (**) and within (*) groups. (Courtesy of Johnson LG, Kraemer GR, Kraemer RR: Effects of estrogen replacement therapy on dehydroepiandrosterone, dehydroepiandrosterone sulfate, and cortisol responses to exercise in postmenopausal women. *Fertil Steril* 68:836–843, 1997. Reprinted with permission of the publisher, the American Society for Reproductive Medicine [formerly the American Fertility Society].)

same blood sampling protocol without exercise was used in a control session with the same research subjects 1 month later. Plasma volume changes were calculated from the hematocrit and hemoglobin values to control for hemoconcentration/hemodilution. The area under the curve was determined for DHEA, DHEAS, and cortisol for the experimental and control trials.

Results.—Baseline concentrations of FSH (mIU/mL), LH (mIU/mL), and estradiol (pg/mL) were within normal limits of expected values for post-menopausal women. Serum DHEA concentration peaked at 15.74 and 9.08 ng/mL, respectively, immediately after exercise for women receiving HRT and those not treated (a significant difference); DHEA and cortisol area under the curve were significantly greater for women treated with HRT compared with the untreated group (Figure 2). The DHEAS AUC was not significantly greater for the HRT than the untreated group during the exercise trial.

Conclusion.—Estrogen replacement therapy enhances DHEA and cortisol but not DHEAS responses to exercise. Further investigation is needed to determine if higher DHEA levels ameliorate the aging process.

▶ The role of hormone replacement therapy (HRT) in decreasing the risk of degenerative changes and disease in postmenopausal women is a challenging area for research. Although the results of this study may seem to be quite straightforward, it should be noted that only 2 of the 7 women in the HRT group were HRT subjects. Five of the women were using estrogen only and would best be described as ERT subjects. Although the authors do not believe the lack of ovaries affected the results, they do not address the possible effect of a progestin on their dependent variables.

B.L. Drinkwater, Ph.D.

Effects on Bone Mineral Density of Low-dosed Oral Contraceptives Compared to and Combined With Physical Activity

Hartard M, Botterman P, Bartenstein P, et al (Technical Univ of Munich)
Contraception 55:87–90, 1997   8–21

Background.—The development of postmenopausal osteoporosis is in large part determined by the maximum bone mineral density (BMD) measured when a person is 20 to 30 years old. Studies have shown that physical activity correlates significantly with BMD. Another significant determinant of BMD is the estrogen level, and oral contraceptives (OCs) with high levels of ethinylestradiol have been shown to protect bone mass in the premenopausal woman. However, the effects of current low-dose OCs on BMD in younger women are not known. This study assessed BMD in women based on their activity level and their use of low-dose OCs.

Methods.—One hundred twenty-eight women, 20–35 years old, were divided into 4 groups based on the duration of physical activity and OC use. Long-term exercise was defined as $\geq$ 3 years of regular exercise for $\geq$ 2 hours/week. Long-term OC use was defined as $\geq$ 3 years of OC use. Group A consisted of 30 women with long-term exercise (mean 9.45 $\pm$ 4.32 years) and short-term use of OCs (1.6 $\pm$ 1.69 years). Group B consisted of 37 women with long-term exercise (10.4 $\pm$ 4.14 years) and long-term OC use (8.2 ± 4.14 years). Group C consisted of 31 women with short-term exercise (3.26 ± 3.69 years) and long-term OC use (7.9 ± 2.88 years). Group D consisted of 30 women with short-term exercise (3.5 ± 3.5 years) and short-term OC use (1.5 ± 1.73 years). All participants had normal medical and gynecologic status. DXA was used to assess BMD in both the right and left femoral necks and the anteroposterior and lateral spine (L2–L4).

Findings.—Physical activity had more of an effect on BMD than OC use (Table 2). In all the regions examined, BMD was highest in group A. BMD at the right and left femoral neck was significantly higher in Group A (long-term exercise, short-term OC use) than in the other 3 groups. Except for 1 significant difference in the anteroposterior lumbar spine between Groups B and C (both with long-term OC use), BMD between Groups B and C did not differ significantly. Similarly, BMD between Groups B and D and between Groups C and D did not differ significantly.

Conclusions.—The less active women (Groups C and D) showed no benefit from either short-term or long-term OC use. This finding supports other data showing that long-term, low-dose OCs do not affect the BMD of young women, and thus do not protect younger women from developing osteoporosis in later life. In fact, despite the long-term exercise in Group B, the long-term use of OCs seems to have attenuated the beneficial effect of exercise on BMD. This finding has clinical implications in decid-

---

TABLE 2.—Number of Subjects, History of Exercise and Oral Contraceptive (OC) Intake, and Bone Mineral Density of the Right and Left Femoral Neck and Lumbar Spine in Group A (Long-term Exercise and Short-term OC Intake), Group B (Long-term Exercise and OC Intake), Group C (Short-term Exercise and Long-term OC Intake), and Group D (Short Term Exercise and OC Intake)

Group	A	B	C	D
n	X (30) ±SD	X (37) ±SD	X (31) ±SD	X (30) ±SD
Exercise (years)	9.45* 4.32	10.40* 4.14	3.26 3.69	3.50 3.53
OC (years)	1.60 1.69	8.20† 2.43	7.90† 2.88	1.50 1.73
Right neck (g/cm²)	0.971‡ 0.131	0.903 0.124	0.907 0.103	0.903 0.095
Left neck (g/cm²)	0.984‡ 0.129	0.915 0.127	0.898 0.099	0.904 0.097
L2–L4 ap (g/cm²)	1.177§ 0.150	1.144‖ 0.130	1.072 0.124	1.085 0.120
L2–L4 lat (g/cm²)	0.858¶ 0.124	0.788 0.100	0.796 0.120	0.780 0.075

*$p < 0.05$ (A to C and D, B to C and D).
†$p < 0.05$ (B to A and D, C to A and D).
‡$p < 0.05$ (A to B, C, and D).
§$p < 0.05$ (A to C and D).
‖$p < 0.05$ (B to C).
¶$p < 0.05$ (A to B and D).
(Courtesy of Hartard M, Bottermann P, Bartenstein P, et al. Effects on bone mineral density of low-dosed oral contraceptives compared to and combined with physical activity. *Contraception* 55:87–90, copyright 1997 by Elsevier Science Inc.)

ing how much estrogen to administer to amenorrheic female athletes who are participating in extensive endurance training.

▶ There has been some concern expressed about the wisdom of using oral contraceptives (OC) or other exogenous estrogens to prevent bone loss in amenorrheic adolescent athletes. Might the OCs actually inhibit the development of peak bone mass in these young women? This study suggests that it is indeed possible that they do. More effort needs to be directed toward encouraging resumption of normal menses in adolescents and younger women rather than relying on hormonal supplementation to prevent bone loss—an avenue which may also prevent normal bone acquisition.

B.L. Drinkwater, Ph.D.

Effect of Two Training Regimens on Bone Mineral Density in Health Perimenopausal Women: A Randomized Controlled Trial
Heinonen A, Oja P, Sievänen H, et al (UKK Inst for Health Promotion Research, Tampere, Finland)
J Bone Miner Res 13:483–490, 1998
8–22

Objective.—Bone mineral density (BMD) has a major effect on the risk of fractures among the elderly. Though the BMD response to exercise has been studied in postmenopausal women, there are few data on the effects in perimenopausal women. Two types of exercise—calisthenics and endurance training—were compared for their effects on BMD in perimenopausal women.

Methods.—The randomized, controlled trial included 105 healthy, sedentary women aged 52–53. They were assigned to an endurance training group, a calisthenics training group, and a control group. Within each group, some women were postmenopausal or perimenopausal and were not taking estrogen replacement therapy (nonestrogen category), while others were still menstruating regularly or were taking estrogen replacement (estrogen category). The 2 exercise groups were to exercise 4 times weekly for 18 months. The endurance training group performed various types of exercise at 55% to 75% of VO_{2max}, according to individual assessments. The calisthenics group performed strength-endurance exercises designed to load the muscles of the trunk, pelvis, hip, and lower limbs with ordinary pace. The control group performed once-weekly stretching exercises. Dual-energy x-ray absorptiometry was performed to evaluate BMD of the lumbar spine, right femoral neck, calcaneus, and dominant distal radius at intervals before, during, and at the end of the exercise program.

Results.—The final analysis included 27 subjects in the control group, 26 in the calisthenics group, and 23 in the endurance group. Bone mineral density of the femoral neck followed a linear trend in the endurance group, suggesting maintenance of the baseline value. No significant training effect was apparent for the calisthenics group. Neither exercise group showed

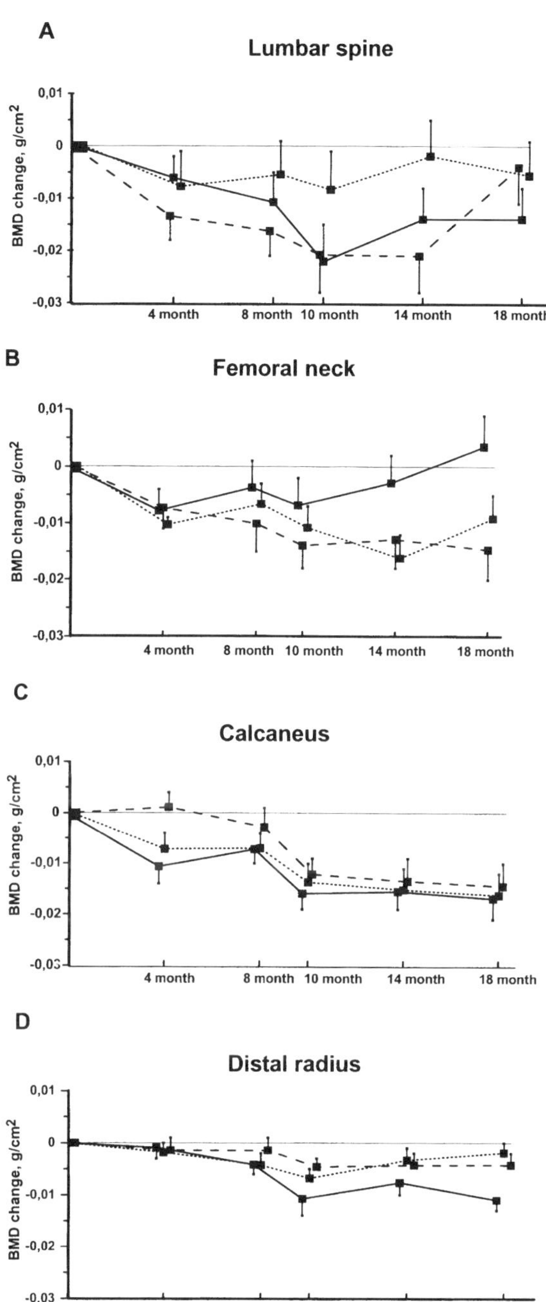

FIGURE 2.—The estimated changes in the BMD (GLM analysis) at A, the lumbar spine, B, the femoral neck, C, the calcaneus, and D, the distal radius during the study period. The solid line represents the endurance group, the dashed line the calisthenics group, and the dotted line the control group. Bars indicate standard error of estimates. (Courtesy of Heinonen A, Oja P, Sievänen H, et al: Effect of two training regimens on bone mineral density in healthy perimenopausal women: A randomized controlled trial. *J Bone Miner Res* 13:483–490, 1998. Reprinted by permission of Blackwell Science, Inc.)

any significant training effect on BMD of the lumbar spine or calcaneus. The endurance group showed a significant negative trend in BMD at the distal radius (Fig 2). Fifteen percent of the endurance group, 11% of the calisthenics group, and 9% of the control group showed a significant increase in VO_{2max}.

Conclusions.—An 18-month program of relatively intense exercise training can preserve BMD of the femoral neck in perimenopausal women. The multiexercise endurance training regimen used in the current study appears to be safe and feasible in this group of women. Follow-up studies are needed to see if endurance training can prevent fractures of the femoral neck in older women.

▶ There are many reasons for women of all ages to engage in physical activity on a regular basis. However, it is hard to see how a 0.4% increase in femoral neck BMD after 18 months of endurance training at the same time that BMD is decreasing at other skeletal sites will encourage sedentary women to become and remain active. I don't think anyone doubts that physically active women have a higher bone density than sedentary women. The vital question is whether they can sustain this advantage during the postmenopausal years without the benefit of estrogen.

B.L. Drinkwater, Ph.D.

High-Impact Exercise Promotes Bone Gain in Well-trained Female Athletes
Taaffe DR, Robinson TL, Snow CM, et al (Stanford Univ, Calif; Univ of South Alabama, Mobile; Oregon State Univ, Calif)
J Bone Miner Res 12:255–260, 1997   8–23

Background.—Any factor that maximizes peak bone mass and reduces loss of bone mass before and after menopause will help to prevent osteoporosis. Gymnastics is associated with high-impact loading strains on bone, which may have powerful bone-promoting effects. Previous studies have shown that collegiate gymnasts have greater regional and total body bone density than runners, swimmers, or nonathletic women, independent of menstrual cycle status. This study analyzed the effects of gymnastics and other athletic activities on buildup of bone mineral density (BMD) over time.

Methods.—The study included 106 young women of varying athletic activity; those in cohort I were observed for 8 months and those in cohort II for 12 months. Cohort I included 26 gymnasts, 36 runners, and 14 nonathletic women; cohort II included 8 gymnasts, 11 swimmers, and 11 nonathletic women. Some of the athletes, but none of the controls, were taking oral contraceptives. All women completed a detailed questionnaire regarding health; exercise, including sport-specific and supplementary training; and menstrual history, particularly amenorrhea and oligomenorrhea. Dual-energy x-ray absorptiometry was performed at the beginning

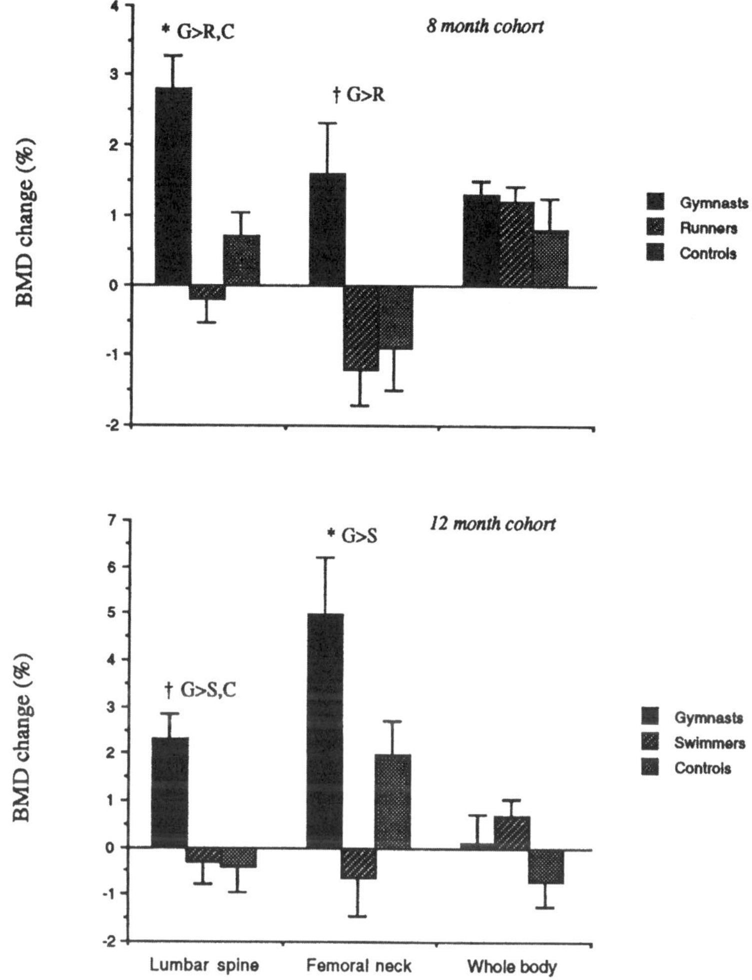

FIGURE 1.—Percent change in lumbar spine, femoral neck, and whole body BMD for 8-month (top panel) and 12-month (bottom panel) cohorts. $^*p < 0.001$, $†p < 0.01$. Values are mean ± SEM. (Courtesy of Taaffe DR, Robinson TL, Snow CM, et al: High-impact exercise promotes bone gain in well-trained female athletes. *J Bone Miner Res* 12:255–260, 1997. Reprinted by permission of Blackwell Science, Inc.)

and end of follow-up to assess BMD of the lumbar spine, femoral neck, and whole body. Data from the whole-body scan were used to calculate bone-free lean tissue mass, fat mass, and percent body fat.

Results.—The gymnasts were of similar age and body composition to the athletic and control groups but had a later age at menarche. Absolute and relative fat mass were lower in the athletes than controls. The gymnasts and swimmers began sport-specific training before menarche; these groups trained approximately 20 hr/week during the study, including 3 hr/week of weight training and 2.5 hr/week of aerobic activity. The runners ran about 43 miles/week, with a similar amount of weight training. At baseline, menstrual cycle irregularities were reported by 28% of runners, 35% of gymnasts, and 27% of swimmers.

In cohort I at baseline, gymnasts had the higher BMD values and runners the lowest. In cohort II, femoral neck BMD was higher in gymnasts than in swimmers and nonathletes. Over time, changes in bone density were unaffected by menstrual status or oral contraceptive use. Gymnasts had significantly greater bone gain at follow-up than the other athletes or nonathletic controls (Fig 1). The runners, swimmers, and controls showed no significant change in BMD. Change in whole-body BMD was no different among groups in either cohort. However, at 8 months, both the gymnasts and runners showed gains in BMD that were significantly greater than zero.

Conclusions.—The mechanical loading associated with gymnastics appears to increase BMD at clinically relevant sites—i.e., the lumbar spine and femoral neck—in young women. Gymnasts continue to show bone gain over time, despite their initially high BMD values and regardless of their menstrual status. Thus high-impact loading, and not selection bias, appears to account for the high BMD values observed in women gymnasts. High skeletal impacts appear to have a particularly osteotropic effect; muscle-strengthening activities do not appear to contribute significantly.

▶ Several previous studies also have reported that the bone density (BMD) of swimmers does not differ from that of sedentary controls. This lack of an osteogenic effect from an aquatic activity is usually ascribed to the buoyancy provided by the water. Apparently, 3 hours per week of weight training did not completely offset the negative effect of the weightless environment of the pool.

Considering the importance of understanding the role menstrual status plays in the acquisition and maintenance of BMD, the more information we can obtain the better. For example, it would be interesting to know if the athletes with the menstrual cycle irregularity were the women using oral contraceptives. It would seem preferable when possible not to combine amenorrheic, oligomenorrheic, and eumenorrheic women in a single group. With the small number of women in each menstrual category, it is not surprising that the BMD differences between groups were not significant.

B.L. Drinkwater, Ph.D.

Exercise and Bone Mineral Density in Mature Female Athletes
Dook JE, Henderson JNK, Price RI (Edith Cowan Univ, Joondalup, Western Australia; Sir Charles Gairdner Hosp, Nedlands, Western Australia)
Med Sci Sports Exerc 29:291–296, 1997   8–24

Introduction.—Aging-related reductions in bone tissue and muscle strength can lead to loss of independence and low quality of life in old age. Weight-bearing exercise has important effects on bone mineral density. Understanding of this relationship is essential to strategies to maintain skeletal strength among women, particularly those entering menopause. The BMD effects of high-impact, medium-impact, and nonimpact athletic training over many years—compared with no training—were studied in mature women.

Methods.—The athletic participants were drawn from participants in the Australian Masters Games. All were older than 40 and had their last menstrual period within the previous year. All had trained for at least 20 years in their chosen sport, either netball or basketball (considered high-impact sports), running or field hockey (considered medium-impact sports), or swimming (considered a nonimpact sport). All participants met competition standards and had started their sport before 13 years of age. Twenty women in each impact category were identified, along with a control group of sedentary women. All subjects underwent dual-energy x-ray absorptiometry to measure BMD, total body fat, and total lean mass. Muscle strength assessment included isometric muscle strength of the dominant arm flexors and leg extensors, measured at 90 degrees of flexion. Daily calcium intake was estimated as well. The effects of training in the various impact categories on BMD were analyzed.

Results.—The 4 groups were similar in age, height, weight, calcium intake, and alcohol intake; the athletes had a higher activity level than the controls. In all 3 groups of athletes, corrected lean body mass was significantly higher than in controls. Fat mass was higher in the controls than in the exercise groups. Leg extensor strength was greater in the high-impact group than in the control group. There were no other significant differences between groups in leg extensor strength, and no differences in arm

TABLE 2.—Whole Body, Regional Arm, and Regional Leg BMD, Fat Mass, Height-corrected Lean Mass, Leg Extensor Strength, and Arm Flexor Strength for the Four Study Groups

	HIGH (netball, basketball)	MED (running, hockey)	NON (swimming)	CON (sedentary)
Whole body BMD	1.15*†	1.12*	1.06	1.02
$(g{\cdot}cm^{-2})$	(0.08)	(0.10)	(0.08)	(0.07)
Regional leg BMD	1.20*†	1.18*†	1.11	1.05
$(g{\cdot}cm^{-2})$	(0.09)	(0.09)	(0.09)	(0.08)
Regional arm	0.73*	0.71*	0.71*	0.67
BMD $(g{\cdot}cm^{-2})$	(0.05)	(0.05)	(0.05)	(0.05)
Fat mass (kg)	20.3*	19.5*	19.5*	26.4
	(6.2)	(5.3)	(8.1)	(4.8)
Corrected lean	41.3*	41.0*	42.7*	37.5
mass (kg)	(2.3)	(2.2)	(2.7)	(2.3)
Leg extensor	352*	323	305	264
strength (N)	(104)	(81)	(58)	(57)
Arm flexor	207	209	200	190
strength (N)	(75)	(42)	(39)	(41)

*P < 0.05 compared with CON.
†P < 0.05 compared with NON.
Data are expressed as mean (SD).
(Courtesy of Dook JE, Henderson JNK, Price RI: Exercise and bone mineral density in mature female athletes. *Med Sci Sports Exerc* 29:291–296, 1997.)

flexor strength. Whole-body and regional leg BMD were higher in the high-impact group than in the nonimpact and control groups. These values were also significantly higher in the medium-impact group than in the control group (Table 2). These differences were significant after correction for other predictors of BMD, including height, corrected lean mass, and leg extensor strength. Corrected regional arm BMD did not differ significantly among groups.

Conclusions.—Mature women with a long history of participation in high-impact or medium-impact sports show greater whole-body and regional BMD than control women who have not participated in any regular sporting activity. For women participating in nonimpact activities, such as swimming, BMD is no greater than in controls. Non-weight-bearing activities may not provide sufficient strain to affect bone remodeling, the findings suggest. The BMD effect of high-impact activity is independent of variations in muscle strength. Women who regularly participate in high-impact exercise during their premenopausal years have greater BMD than nonathletes.

▶ To participate in this study, an athlete must have started in her sport before age 13 years. Several recent studies have suggested that physical activity during childhood and adolescence has a more positive and longer-lasting effect on bone than exercise commenced during the adult years. This raises the question of how much of the difference in bone mineral density between athletes in the high and medium impact groups and the nonimpact and control groups was due to a lifetime of activity and how much was due to their activity during childhood and adolescence.

B.L. Drinkwater, Ph.D.

Bone Mineral Density and Risk of Breast Cancer in Older Women
Cauley JA, for the Study of Osteoporotic Fractures Research Group (Univ of Pittsburgh, Pa; et al)
JAMA 276:1404–1408, 1996   8–25

Objective.—Bone mineral density (BMD) may be a useful indicator of exposure to estrogen in older women. If so, then women with higher levels of BMD should be at increased risk of breast cancer. This prospective study evaluated the effects of baseline BMD in older women on the incidence of breast cancer at 3 years' follow-up.

Methods.—The study included 9,704 women aged 65 or older. Women who died before follow-up, who developed breast cancer within 1 year of baseline, or who were taking estrogen replacement therapy at baseline were excluded. This left 97 women who developed breast cancer within 3 years' follow-up and 6,757 controls. OsteoAnalyzers were used to determine baseline bone mass at the distal radius, mid radius, and calcaneus. In addition, BMD of the proximal femur and lumbar spine was measured using dual-energy x-ray absorptiometry. Other variables analyzed included weight, height, reproductive and menopausal history, family history of breast disease, history of osteoporosis or spine fracture, smoking, alcohol, and exercise. The link between BMD and breast cancer was analyzed by proportional hazards regression models. The final multivariate model included adjustment for age, body mass index, exercise, smoking, age at menarche, age at menopause, and other factors.

Results.—The study cohort's average incidence of breast cancer was 4.3/1,000 person-years. At all sites, mean BMD was significantly greater in women who developed breast cancer than in those who did not. Each 1-standard deviation increase in BMD was associated with a 30% to 50% increase in relative risk of breast cancer. The risk estimates were little affected by further adjustment for obesity or family history of breast cancer.

Conclusions.—Older women with high BMD of the radius, hip, or spine are at increased risk of breast cancer, these findings indicate. The study is the first to demonstrate a link between BMD and breast cancer. Efforts to identify common factors should provide useful insights into causation and prevention. The findings suggest the need to reevaluate the risks and benefits of hormone replacement therapy in terms of BMD, osteoporosis, breast cancer, and coronary heart disease.

▶ A number of studies have suggested a link between a woman's lifetime exposure to estrogen and her risk for breast cancer. In this study, the authors use bone density (BMD) as a surrogate marker for exposure to estrogen. Interestingly, the variables usually used to indicate lifetime exposure to estrogen, age at menarche and menopause and nulliparity, did not differ between cancer cases and controls. Nor is a low BMD an insurance against breast cancer as cancer cases can be observed in each quartile of BMD. In fact, in 3 of the 5 sites there is no apparent difference in incidence rates between the fourth and fifth quartile. Considering the fact that current estrogen users were excluded from the study and there was no difference between groups in past or never use of estrogen, it seems premature to conclude that these data shed any new light on, "... the balance of risks and benefits of hormone replacement therapy."

B.L. Drinkwater, Ph.D.

Bone Health Is Not Affected by Luteal Phase Abnormalities and Decreased Ovarian Progesterone Production in Female Runners

De Souza MJ, Miller BE, Sequenzia LC, et al (Univ of Connecticut, Farmington; Univ of California, Davis)
J Clin Endocrinol Metab 82:2867–2876, 1997   8–26

Background.—Female athletes are at increased risk of decreased bone mineral density (BMD) due to the chronic hypoestrogenemia that occurs with amenorrhea. Other menstrual alterations, such as short and inadequate luteal phases, may not be clinically apparent, yet they, too, may

TABLE 1.—Subject Characteristics

	SedOvul	ExOvul	ExLPD	Probability
	(n = 9)	(n = 14)	(n = 10)	
Demographics				
Age (yr)	26.4 ± 1.3	30.4 ± 1.4	25.2 ± 2.1	0.065
Height (cm)	164.0 ± 1.6	167.0 ± 2.2	161.8 ± 1.9	0.195
Weight (kg)	63.6 ± 5.5	60.4 ± 2.2	58.3 ± 2.4	0.577
Body fat (%)	26.5 ± 2.7	21.1 ± 1.5*	19.0 ± 1.3†	0.022
Reproductive characteristics				
Age of menarche (yr)	13.8 ± 0.5	13.0 ± 0.4	12.9 ± 0.3	0.340
Reproductive age (yr)	12.7 ± 1.2	16.9 ± 1.4	12.9 ± 2.2	0.179
Cycle parameters				
Menstrual cycle length (days)	28.6 ± 0.7	27.6 ± 0.7	26.9 ± 0.8	0.394
Day of LH surge	15.8 ± 0.7	14.7 ± 0.7	17.9 ± 0.7‡	0.018
Number of bleeding days	5.3 ± 0.2	5.0 ± 0.3	5.5 ± 0.4	0.383
Follicular phase length (days)	15.8 ± 0.7	14.7 ± 0.8	20.5 ± 1.7§	0.001
Luteal phase length (day)	12.8 ± 0.5	12.8 ± 0.4	6.4 ± 1.5§	0.0002
Training characteristics				
VO$_2$ peak (mL/kg/min)	30.2 ± 1.6	40.9 ± 1.5*	42.9 ± 1.5†	
Running/week (km)	2.1 ± 1.8	32.3 ± 3.7*	25.6 ± 5.6†	0.00006
Training/week (h)	0.5 ± 0.3	4.7 ± 0.7*	4.5 ± 0.6†	0.00007
Resting heart rate (bpm)	74.3 ± 2.3	60.7 ± 2.4*	61.8 ± 1.2†	0.0003
Resting systolic blood pressure (mmHg)	109.8 ± 3.1	115.9 ± 2.9	111.4 ± 2.3	0.502
Resting diastolic blood pressure (mmHg)	65.5 ± 2.5	77.5 ± 2.2	67.2 ± 2.8	0.018

Values are mean ± SEM.
*SedOvul vs. ExOvul.
†SedOvul vs. ExLPD.
‡ExOvul vs. ExLPD.
§SedOvul and ExOvul vs. ExLPD.
(Courtesy of De Souza MJ, Miller BE, Sequenzia LC, et al. Bone health is not affected by luteal phase abnormalities and decreased ovarian progesterone production in female runners. *J Clin Endocrinol Metab* 82:2867–2876, 1997, copyright The Endocrine Society.)

affect bone density. This study examined whether decreased progesterone production is associated with BMD.

Methods.—The subjects were 33 women 18 to 35 years old who were in good health and free of chronic disease, whose menstrual status had not changed in the past year, who had not used hormone therapy for the past year, who had no eating or depressive disorders for 3 years, and who had not taken any drugs that affect calcium metabolism for 3 years. The women were categorized into 3 groups matched for age, height, weight, and reproductive maturity: 9 sedentary eumenorrheic women who performed ≤1 hour/week of aerobic activity for the past year (SedOv group), 14 runners who ran ≥ 2 hr/week for the past 12 months who had normal menstrual cycles (ExOv group), and 10 runners who had luteal phase defects (ExLPD). Luteal phase defects included a short luteal phase (< 10 days) or inadequate progesterone production (< 3 μg/mg creatinine for at least 3 days in the midluteal phase). Over 3 menstrual cycles, subjects provided daily urine samples that were analyzed for free luteinizing hormone, estrone conjugates (E1C), and pregnanediol 3-glucuronide (PdG; adjusted for creatinine). They also provided weekly blood and urine samples that were evaluated for biochemical markers of bone metabolism, estradiol, progesterone, follicle stimulating hormone, and luteinizing hor-

TABLE 3.—Bone Parameters

	SedOvul	ExOvul	ExLPD	Probability
	(n = 9)	(n = 14)	(n = 10)	
Bone mineral density				
Whole body (g/cm^2)	1.144 ± 0.323	1.194 ± 0.039	1.146 ± 0.022	0.472
Lumbar spine L2–4 (g/cm^2)	1.026 ± 0.041	1.093 ± 0.037	1.034 ± 0.029	0.345
Femoral neck (g/cm^2)	0.875 ± 0.053	0.910 ± 0.059	0.883 ± 0.019	0.673
Biochemical bone markers				
BSAP (U/L)	15.1 ± 1.9	15.9 ± 1.3	17..6 ± 1.2	0.521
Osteocalcin (ng/mL)	7.0 ± 0.5	6.6 ± 0.3	7.2 ± 0.5	0.567
CICP (ng/mL)	107.5 ± 11.5	124.8 ± 12.1	114.7 ± 6.6	0.598
DPD (nM/mM Cr)	7.4 ± 0.3	6.0 ± 0.4	6.2 ± 0.5	0.070
NTx (nM BCE/mmol Cr)	55.7 ± 9.3	49.6 ± 7.1	54.6 ± 5.5	0.814

Values are mean ± SEM.

(Courtesy of De Souza MJ, Miller BE, Sequenzia LC, et al. Bone health is not affected by luteal phase abnormalities and decreased ovarian progresterone production in female runners. *J Clin Endocrinol Metab* 82:2867–2876, 1997.)

mone. BMD was measured using total body, lumbar spine, and right proximal femur scans.

Findings.—Mean PdG production during the luteal phase had a significant inverse correlation with the kilometers run per week and the hours per week spent in physical activity (Table 1). PdG production was significantly lower in the ExLPD and ExOvul groups compared with the SedOvul group (2.4 ± 0.4, 3.5 ± 0.3, vs 5.1 ± 0.6 ng/ml creatinine). Luteal phases were significantly shorter and follicular phases were significantly longer in the ExLPD group. Despite their longer follicular phases, the ExLPD group had significantly lower E1C production during the early follicular phase than the SedOvul group (22.2 ± 2.1 vs 27.1 ± 2.0 µg/ml creatinine). However, BMD and bone metabolism between the 3 groups did not differ (Table 3).

Conclusions.—Indicators of bone metabolism did not differ despite significant differences in progesterone production between the groups. Disturbances in the luteal phase occurred even when the volume of training was not severe (4.5 hours/week over 25.6 km/week). Progesterone does not seem to have an independent effect on bone health; estradiol is probably the primary ovarian steroid that affects bone health, and the 3 groups had similar estradiol environments overall.

▶ Although De Souza and colleagues were unable to find any evidence that decreases in ovarian progesterone production had an effect on bone mineral density (BMD), it is unlikely that this study will put an end to the controversy on the effect of luteal phase abnormalities on bone. In spite of a rigorous selection of subjects, the careful delineation of the hormonal status of these women, and the lack of any evidence linking progesterone to bone turnover, some will point to the relatively small number of subjects and single BMD measurement as reasons to question the result. Fortunately, this is the third study to cast serious doubt on the theory that luteal phase disturbances—

and, in particular, a decrease in progesterone—are associated with a loss of bone mass.

B.L. Drinkwater, Ph.D.

National Survey on Gender Differences in Cardiac Rehabilitation Programs: Patient Characteristics and Enrollment Patterns
Thomas RJ, Miller NH, Lamendola C, et al (Northwestern Univ, Chicago; Stanford Univ, Palo Alto, Calif; Cardiovascular Medicine and Coronary Interventions, Redwood City, Calif; et al)
J Cardiopulmon Rehabil 16:402–412, 1996   8–27

Objective.—Cardiac rehabilitation (CR) programs have been shown to improve functional capacity, psychosocial well-being, and some manifestations of coronary heart disease (CHD). Few studies have evaluated the benefits to women of CR. A U.S. national survey of CR programs studied the number of men and women in such CR programs in 1990; any sociodemographic and clinical characteristics that differed between men and women; the predicted vs. actual male-to-female ratio of CR enrollees; the percentage of eligible individuals enrolled in CR; and the CR breakdown by gender, race, age, and region of the country.

Methods.—Five hundred of the 1,864 registered CR programs were surveyed by means of 2 questionnaires; and the number of patients with myocardial infarction (MI), percutaneous transluminal coronary angioplasty (PTCA), and coronary artery bypass surgery (CABS) among the enrollees was estimated.

Results.—There were 163 responses (32.6%). The response rate was significantly lower in the South. All programs offered outpatient CR. There were 1,322 women and 1,418 men in the programs. Compared with men, women were significantly older (63.7 vs. 60.6 years); significantly more likely to represent a minority (9.3% vs. 4.9%); significantly less likely to be married (59.2% vs. 87.4%); and significantly more likely to have CHD risk factors including hypertension (60.3% vs. 48.5%) and hyperlipidemia (59.7% vs. 51.6%). Women were significantly less likely to be current smokers (9.2% vs. 11.6%) or former smokers (46.5% vs. 65.4%). Women were significantly less likely to have had an MI (30.2% vs. 34.7%) or CABS (35.9% vs. 44.3%) but more likely to have had a diagnosis of angina pectoris (16.7% vs. 8.3%) or recent PTCA (15.9% vs. 12.6%). Significantly fewer women than men were enrolled in phase II CR programs (64.2 vs. 24.1). The post-MI and post-CABS female-to-male enrollment ratios were 0.33 and 0.30, respectively. Enrollment was less likely for patients over 65 years of age who were nonwhites, or Southerners.

Conclusion.—Women, nonwhites, the elderly, and Southerners are less likely to be enrolled in CR programs. Methods need to be developed to increase enrollment in these programs for these underserved populations.

▶ Given the well-established benefits of postcoronary rehabilitation, it is disturbing that in the United States, CR programs are attended by only 13.3% of male and 6.9% of female patients after MI. Probably the main factor limiting participation is the reluctance of many health insurance agencies to reimburse for rehabilitation services. Other considerations include the extent of physician encouragement and the ability to find time and transportation to what may be a relatively distant rehabilitation center. Patients may decide that it does not make a great deal of sense to spend 2 or 3 hours in traveling to attend a half-hour exercise class, particularly if they are expected to make this journey 3 to 5 times a week; the opportunity cost is much lower for a home program which receives occasional reinforcement through center visits and telephone contacts.

Time conflicts (for example, the preparation of meals for spouse and children or rigidly-timed hourly employment) probably restrict female program participation more than that of men. Programs may also be seen as male oriented, with little opportunity to pursue the types of activity that appeal to women, such as dancing and aerobics classes with a musical accompaniment. All of these issues need to be addressed if participation is to be increased to a level that will have a sizable impact upon community health.

R. Shephard, M.D., Ph.D., D.P.E.

Benefits of Cardiac Rehabilitation and Exercise Training in Elderly Women
Lavie CJ, Milani RV (Ochsner Clinic and Alton Ochsner Medical Found, New Orleans, La)
Am J Cardiol 79:664–666, 1997   8–28

Objective.—Cardiac rehabilitation and exercise training programs improve exercise capacity, obesity indices, plasma lipids, behavioral characteristics, and quality of life, reducing subsequent hospitalization costs and the morbidity and mortality of coronary artery disease (CAD). Because there is little information on the benefits of therapy in women, the benefits of cardiac rehabilitation programs in elderly women were compared with those of other patients with CAD.

Methods.—Results of a phase II cardiac rehabilitation and exercise training program were compared for 70 women, over 65 years of age, and 574 other patients with CAD (91% men) referred 4 to 8 weeks after a CAD event. Patients receiving lipid medication were excluded from the study. The program consisted of 12 weeks, totalling 36 education and exercise sessions. Baseline and final data were compared. Behavioral and quality-of-life parameters were evaluated in 52 elderly women and 296 other patients with CAD.

Results.—At baseline, elderly women had significantly lower exercise capacity and body mass indices and a significantly higher percent body fat, total cholesterol, low-density lipoprotein (LDL) cholesterol, and high-

TABLE 2.—Improvements in Exercise Capacity, Obesity Indices, and Lipids After Cardiac Rehabilitation and Exercise Training Programs in Elderly Women (n=70)

Parameter	Before Rehabilitation	After Rehabilitation	% Change	p Value
Exercise capacity, estimated METs	4.7 ± 1.7	6.1 ± 2.4	+30	<0.0001
Body mass index (kg/m^2)	25.5 ± 4.4	24.9 ± 4.7	−2*	<0.05
Percent body fat	31.7 ± 7.5	28.5 ± 7.3	−10*	<0.0001
Total cholesterol (mg/dl)	223 ± 43	220 ± 45	−1.5	0.50
Triglycerides (mg/dl)	171 ± 84	158 ± 79	−13	0.08
HDL cholesterol (mg/dl)	47 ± 14	49 ± 14	+3	0.24
LDL cholesterol (mg/dl)	147 ± 54	139 ± 35	−2	0.22
LDL/HDL	3.35 ± 1.47	3.06 ± 1.08	−12	<0.01

*Improvements were statistically greater ($P < 0.03$) than noted for other patients (0% and −5%, respectively, for body mass index and percent body fat). Improvements in exercise capacity and lipids were statistically similar in the 2 groups.

Abbreviations: HDL, high-density lipoprotein; *LDL*, low-density lipoprotein; *MET*, metabolic equivalent.

(Reprinted by permission of the publisher from Lavie CJ, Milani RV: Benefits of cardiac rehabilitation and exercise training in elderly women. *AMERICAN JOURNAL OF CARDIOLOGY* 79:664–666, copyright 1997 by Excerpta Medica, Inc.)

density lipoprotein (HDL) cholesterol than other patients with CAD. After training, women had significant improvements in exercise capacity, body mass index, and LDL/HDL cholesterol (Table 2). Total cholesterol, HDL cholesterol, and LDL cholesterol improved nonsignificantly. Whereas improvements in body mass index and percent body fat were significantly greater for elderly women than for other patients with CAD after rehabilitation, other improvements were similar between groups. In the subgroup of elderly women, anxiety, somatization, and total quality of life improved significantly and were similar to improvements for other CAD patients.

Conclusion.—After cardiac rehabilitation, exercise capacity and obesity measures in elderly women improve significantly, and lipid levels improve modestly. Anxiety, somatization, and total quality-of-life measures also improve significantly. These findings suggest that elderly women should be referred for cardiac rehabilitation routinely after CAD.

▶ Although there may be difficulty in persuading elderly women to attend rehabilitation programs, this report shows that faithful participants attain a substantial response, including a 30% increase in peak oxygen intake over 12 weeks and attendant improvements in quality of life. Indeed, because elderly female patients with CAD begin rehabilitation from a low level of function, the gains achieved may have a greater impact on their ability to undertake the activities of daily living than would be the case in a typical male class member.

R. Shephard, M.D., Ph.D., D.P.E.

Prevalence and Features of Joint Hypermobility Among Adolescent Athletes

Decoster LC, Vailas JC, Lindsay RH, et al (New Hampshire Musculoskeletal Inst, Manchester; Lahey-Hitchcock Clinic, Manchester, New Hampshire; Univ of Vermont, Burlington; et al)

Arch Pediatr Adolesc Med 151:989–992, 1997   8–29

Introduction.—Individuals with joint hypermobility are advised to avoid strenuous physical activity to avoid an increased risk of athletic injury. The assumption of increased risk is based on findings of joint hypermobility in the rheumatologic and pediatric literature. Comparable trials of athletes with joint hypermobility are limited. This study describes the prevalence and features of joint hypermobility in adolescent athletes.

Methods.—The widely accepted Carter-Wilkinson-Beighton method was used to measure range of motion at the knees, trunk, fingers, thumbs, and elbows bilaterally in 264 athletes. The age range of 150 males and 114 females was 12 to 19 years. On a 0 to 9 scale, 5 was considered hypermobile. Athletes were given an "injury allowance" point if they screened positive on a side with a significant prior injury.

Results.—Thirty-two of 264 athletes scored 5 or higher. Two scored positive for hypermobility by the insurance allowance, so the total was 34 athletes with hypermobility (12.9%). Significantly more females than males had hypermobility (25 [22%] *vs.* 9 [6%]).

Conclusion.—The incidence of joint hypermobility in this series of young athletes was 12.9%. Significantly more females than males had hypermobility.

Clinical Significance.—The influence of hypermobility on athletic injury rates has not been determined. This question should be answered before advising youths with joint hypermobility to avoid athletic endeavors. If the injury risk is higher, it may be better to determine a means of protecting them from undue risk and allowing them to participate in regular physical activity *vs.* the current recommendation of activity avoidance.

▶ This practical study needed doing. The follow-up study on frequency of sports injury in these athletes should clarify whether adolescent athletes with joint hypermobility really are at higher risk for athletic injury. In this preparticipation screening of 264 junior high and high school athletes, 22% of the females were hypermobile as opposed to 6% of the males. Because the sample was preponderantly white, possible racial differences in hypermobility were not addressed. No difference by sport played was seen, except as related to sex. A prior study found about 10% of ballet dancers studied were hypermobile.[1]

E.R. Eichner, M.D.

Reference

1. Klemp P, Chalton D: Articular mobility in ballet dancers: A follow-up study after four years. *Am J Sports Med* 17:72–75, 1989.

Twenty-Year Follow-up of Aerobic and Body Composition of Older Track Athletes

Pollock ML, Mengelkoch LJ, Graves JE, et al (Univ of Florida, Gainesville; Veterans Affairs Med Ctr, Gainesville, Fla)
J Appl Physiol 82:1508–1516, 1997   8–30

Background.—In aging, maximum oxygen intake ($\dot{V}O_{2max}$), pulmonary ventilation, heart rate, fat-free weight (FFW), and muscular strength decline; body fat increases. Previous suggestions of similar $\dot{V}O_{2max}$ drops for active and sedentary persons were made from cross-sectional, not longitudinal studies, and most longitudinal studies have younger subjects.

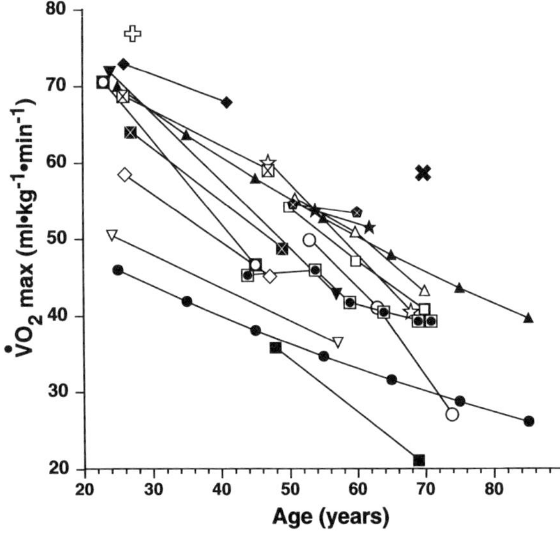

◇ Astrand et al., 1973, Athletes-Untrained (n=31)
□ Trappe et al., 1996,Highly Trained-Untrained (n=15)
⊠ Trappe et al., 1996, Fitness Trained (n=18)
⊠ Trappe et al., 1996, Highly Trained (n=10)
☆ Trappe et al., 1996, Older Fitness Trained (n=10)
◉ Kasch et al. 1995, Fitness Trained (n=12)
■ Kasch et al. 1995, Untrained (n=12)
◆ Marti et al., 1991, Athletes-Trained (n=27)
▲ Heath et al., 1981, Athlete, Norms
● Heath et al., 1981, Untrained, Norms

✖ Maud et al., 1981, Elite Older Athlete (n=1)
✚ Pollock et al., 1977, Elite Young Athletes (n=20)
⊗ Pollock et al., 1987, Highly Trained (n=11)
▼ Robinson et al., 1976, Athletes-Untrained (n=13)
▽ Robinson et al., 1976, Untrained (n=9)
★ Rogers et al., 1990, Highly Trained (n=15)
○ Pollock et al., present, Low intensity (n=2)
□ Pollock et al., present, Moderate Intensity (n=10)
△ Pollock et al., present, High Intensity ((n=9)
✚ Cooper, 1990, Norms

FIGURE 2.—Maximum oxygen uptake $\dot{V}O_{2max}$ of endurance athletes and nonathletes of various ages. Data are from studies listed (*bottom*). (Courtesy of Pollock ML, Mengelkoch LJ, Graves JE, et al. Twenty-year follow-up of aerobic power and body composition of older track athletes. *J Appl Physiol* 82:1508–1516, 1997.)

Methods.—Initial evaluation (T1) included 27 competitive male track athletes in regular training. Twenty-five were retested at 10 years (T2). A third evaluation (T3) was done on subjects between 60 and 92 years of age. At T3, subjects' activity and training levels were high, moderate, or low. The FFW was determined. Cardiorespiratory function tests included $\dot{V}O_{2max}$. Heart rate and ECG were recorded during exercise and recovery. Blood pressure was determined. Perceived exertion was evaluated each minute and at peak exercise. Strength measurements were made.

Results.—Although $\dot{V}O_{2max}$ decreased significantly throughout, change was most notable between T2 and T3, more in the low than the high and medium training groups. Pulmonary functions held steady from T1 to T2 and then dropped significantly in all groups. Maximum heart rate decreased during both intervals except in the low group. In all groups, resting heart rate increased but remained low. The high and medium groups remained lean but had significantly decreased FFW and increased body fat. Leg strength was significantly reduced after age 90, peak lumbar extension torque after age 79, and chest press strength after age 90. Figure 2 breaks down $\dot{V}O_{2max}$ data from longitudinal studies, a cross-sectional study of young distance runners, and a marathon world record holder (70 years). Declines in $\dot{V}O_{2max}$ varied between studies at rates related to initial value and physical activity reduction.

Conclusions.—Older endurance athletes had decreased physiologic capacity after 20 years (T3) despite high or moderate training. Great reduction in training was associated with much larger declines. Changes in FFW and body fat were related to aging and type of training; weight training may help maintain FFW and upper body strength, but data are not conclusive.

▶ Comparisons of the rate of aging of sedentary and athletic individuals have until recently relied largely on cross-sectional data,[1] because most longitudinal studies have studied subjects for only short periods, giving unstable values for the rate of aging. Some studies using cross-sectional data were able to control quite well for levels of habitual physical activity in their various cohorts. Such studies suggested that the rate of aging of aerobic power in athletes was only marginally less than that of the general population; lean mass was well preserved until around 70 years of age, but then there was a substantial loss despite continued physical activity. Now, longitudinal studies of greater duration are appearing, although the number of subjects discussed is still small relative to those used in the cross-sectional surveys. Pollock and associates identified 9 track competitors who had maintained an elite level of training over the age span 50–70 years. The loss of aerobic power in this group was 15% over the 20 years, a rate of about 7.5 mL/kg.min per decade, even greater than the typical value for sedentary subjects (about 5 mL/kg.min per decade). Certainly, these data do not support the idea that a continuation of training does much to inhibit the intrinsic process of aging.

R. Shephard, M.D., Ph.D., D.P.E.

Reference

1. Shephard RJ: Fitness and aging, in Blais C (ed): *Aging into the 21st Century* Downsview, ON; Captus Publications, 1991, pp 22–35.

Effects of Age, Physical Training, and Physical Fitness on Coronary Heart Disease Risk Factors in Older Track Athletes at Twenty-Year Follow-up

Mengelkoch LJ, Pollock ML, Limacher MC, et al (Univ of Florida, Gainesville)
J Am Geriatr Soc 45:1446–1453, 1997   8–31

Background.—Previous research suggests that the prevalence of coronary heart disease (CHD) risk factors may remain low if long-term physical activity is maintained. However, few longitudinal studies have been done on habitually active persons older than 65 years, and limited CHD risk factor data have been reported. Current CHD risk factor values in older male athletes were compared with those in mid-life and relationships between changes in CHD risk factors and aging, physical training, and physical fitness were examined.

Methods.—The participants were 21 men, aged 60 to 92 years, who had been assessed on 3 occasions 10 years apart. At the third assessment, the men were divided into 3 groups based on physical activity levels. The high-intensity group consisted of 9 subjects, who remained elite in national and international competition. The moderate-intensity group included 10 men, who continued frequent, rigorous endurance training but rarely competed. The low-intensity group included 2 subjects, who had greatly decreased their training volume and intensity.

Findings.—The risk factors of smoking, diabetes, and obesity had never been present in these men. The prevalence of family history of cardiovascular disease and abnormal resting ECG remained at $\leq 14\%$ through the third assessment. Average systolic and diastolic blood pressure continued to be low without medication. However, diastolic blood pressure measures showed the greatest redistribution between evaluation periods of any risk factor. Mean total cholesterol was lower at the second and third assessment than at the first assessment. Changes in VO_{2max} was associated with body weight changes and percent body fat between the first and second assessments. Age was correlated with changes in systolic blood pressure and total cholesterol between the second and third assessments.

Conclusions.—The prevalence of CHD risk factors and mean risk factor values remained low and generally stable in older athletes who had maintained habitual exercise training. Further studies on a large sample of men and women are needed to better delineate the effects of habitual exercise training on CHD risk factors.

▶ This 20-year follow-up of elite male track athletes shows "if you use it you don't lose it." No controls are available, the study group is small, and all subjects are men, so the study has its limits. But it is useful because it profiles coronary heart disease risk factors in midlife[1] and again in later life. At follow-up, 21 of the original 27 men, now ages 60–92, were profiled. Training mileage had fallen 44% and training pace had fallen 32%, but coronary heart disease risk factors remained absent or low. These athletic men even failed to show the "normal" age-related rise in resting blood pressure, probably because of exercise habits and weight-control.

E.R. Eichner, M.D.

Reference

1. Pollock ML, Miller HS, Wilmore JH: Physiological characteristics of champion American track athletes 40 to 75 years of age. *J Gerontology* 29:645–646, 1974.

Evidence for the Incompatibility of Age-neutral Overweight and Age-neutral Physical Activity Standards From Runners
Williams PT (Lawrence Berkeley Natl Lab, Calif)
Am J Clin Nutr 65:1391–1396, 1997   8–32

Introduction.—The 1995 *Dietary Guidelines for Americans* recommends physical activity together with balancing food intake to prevent weight gain. This edition uses the same definition of overweight for both younger and older adults, because age-related weight gain is not desirable. In a national cross-sectional survey of male runners, investigators tested the hypotheses that vigorous exercise prevents weight gain with age and that weight maintenance and an age-neutral adult overweight standard are consistent with a constant activity level over time.

Methods.—Study subjects were participants in the National Runners' Health Study. They completed a 2-page questionnaire. Excluded were men who were vegetarians or smokers, those who had a history of heart disease, and those taking medication to control blood pressure, cholesterol, or thyroid or insulin concentrations. Because few minorities were represented, only white men were included. The final study group consisted of 4,769 men ages 18–49 years and 2,150 men older than 49 years.

Results.—In all age categories, body mass index (BMI) and waist circumference decreased with weekly running distance (Fig 1). Both measures increased in association with age at all distance categories, and the percentage of overweight runners was greater in the 45–49-year-old age-group (30.1%) than in the younger than 30-year-old age-group (21.5%). When adjusted for age, each kilometer run per week was associated with a mean decrease of 0.033 in BMI and a mean decrease of 0.083 in waist circumference. Each additional year of age was associated with increases in BMI, waist circumference, and hip circumference. Running greater distances did not protect men from the effects of greater weight and upper body adiposity on cholesterol and blood pressure. The runners who were 50 years of age or older exhibited a decrease in BMI, a finding also reported in older sedentary men.

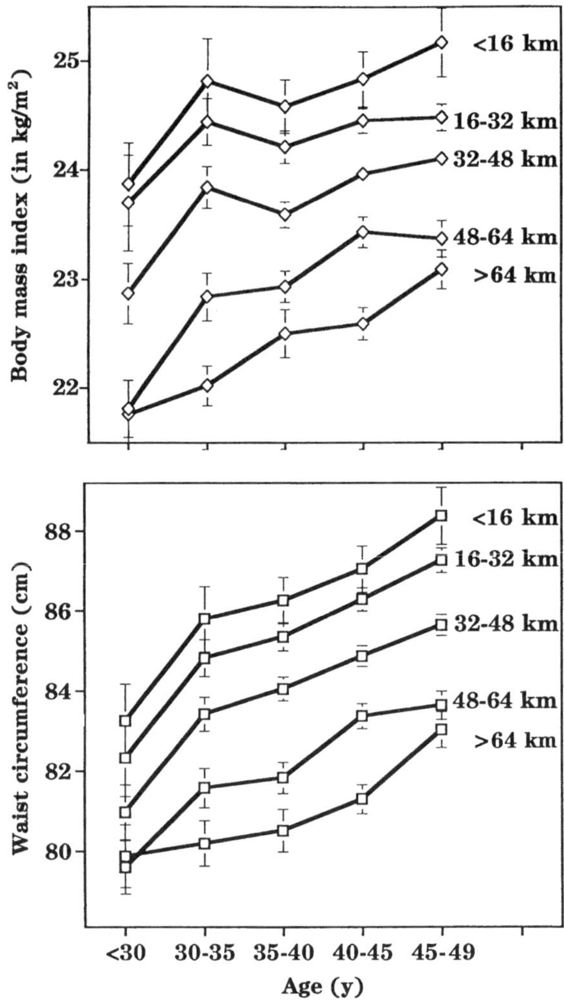

FIGURE 1.—Cross-sectional relations of mean BMI and waist circumference versus age, stratified by weekly running distance. The 64–80 and >80 km/wk categories were combined because of the small sample sizes that result when they are stratified by age. In men 50 years of age and older, each additional year of age was associated with a calculated decrease of 0.057 ± 0.008 in BMI ($P < 0.0001$). (Courtesy of Williams PT: Evidence for incompatibility of age-neutral overweight and age-neutral physical activity standards from runners. *Am J Clin Nutr* 65:1391–1396, 1997. Copyright *Am J Clin Nutr*, American Society for Clinical Nutrition.)

Conclusion.—Men who run consistent weekly distances (whether shorter or longer distances) through middle age can be expected to have an increase in total weight and waist circumference. An annual increase in distance by 2.24 km/week can compensate for the anticipated weight gain. Thus, when promoting an age-neutral adult overweight standard, substantial increases in activity over time should be recommended.

▶ It is a matter of common experience that most of the population accumulates body fat as they grow older, but it is less clear whether public health workers should adjust acceptable body mass indices to take account of this trend. Williams makes the interesting observation that even runners who are covering a distance of 80 km or more per week show increases of waist circumference and BMI with aging. However, because they start from very low values for each of these variables, they remain much thinner than the general population, even in old age. The mechanisms of fat accumulation are still debated, but likely candidates seem to be decreases in testosterone and growth hormone secretion. Given its association with cardiac risk factors, the accumulation of fat is unlikely to be benign, even in runners, and dietary recommendations should thus note the need to reduce food intake and/or increase energy expenditure to avoid an accumulation of fat with aging.

R. Shephard, M.D., Ph.D., D.P.E.

Physical Activity, Functional Limitations, and the Risk of Fall-related Fractures in Community-dwelling Elderly
Stevens JA, Powell KE, Smith SM, et al (Natl Ctr for Injury Prevention and Control, Atlanta, Ga; American Cancer Society, Atlanta, Ga)
Ann Epidemiol 7:54–61, 1997   8–33

Introduction.—Among elderly individuals, the risk of fracture after a fall is related to lack of bone strength, the risk of falling, and ineffective protective neuromuscular reactions when a fall occurs. Regular physical activity, which modifies all 3 factors, may reduce the risk of fractures. A case–control study was designed to examine the association of vigorous and mild physical activity with fall-related fractures.

Methods.—The source of data for analysis was the Study to Assess Falls among the Elderly (SAFE), a population-based study conducted among community-dwelling people 65 years and older in an area of Miami Beach, Florida. Cases were those treated for a newly diagnosed fracture that resulted from an unintentional fall in or around their home during the period from November 20, 1986, to August 31, 1988. Randomly selected controls resided in the study area during this period. Interviewers met with study participants to obtain information about their level of physical activity, level of dependence, and mental competence.

Results.—After exclusions for previous disability or inadequate data, the response rate was 65.7% (471/717) for cases and 67.0% (712/1,060) for controls. Interviews took place at an average of 2.6 months after the injury for cases and 1.9 months for controls. Cases had a total of 523 fractures, nearly one third of which were hip fractures. Cases and controls were similar in age and ethnicity, but cases tended to have a lower body mass index and a lower mental status score. A lower proportion of cases participated in physical activity, and a greater proportion had a functional limitation. Activity data were reported by a surrogate for 12% of cases versus 5% of controls. Vigorous activity was associated with an overall

TABLE 4.—Adjusted Odds Ratios (aOR)* for the Association Between Vigorous Physical Activity and Risk of Fracture Stratified by ADL Score

	ADL = 0		ADL ≥0	
	aOR	95% CI	aOR	95% CI
Vigorous activity	0.6	(0.4–0.8)	3.2	(1.1–9.8)
Female	1.3	(0.9–1.8)	0.6	(0.2–1.5)
Age				
75–84	1.2	(0.9–1.6)	0.5	(0.2–1.2)
≥85	1.3	(0.8–2.1)	0.3	(0.1–1.0)
Low mental				
status score	2.0	(1.3–3.3)	1.5	(0.7–3.3)
Quetelet index,				
Lowest 25%	1.4	(1.0–1.9)	1.5	(0.7–3.5)
Highest 25%	0.9	(0.6–1.3)	0.3	(0.1–0.8)

*Odds ratio adjusted for sex (M/F), age (65–74, 75–84, ≥85 years), mental status score (≤12, >12), and Quetelet index (lowest 25%, middle 50%, highest 25%).

(Courtesy of Stevens JA, Powell KE, Smith SM, et al: Physical activity, functional limitations, and the risk of fall-related fractures in community-dwelling elderly. *Ann Epidemiol* 7:54–61, 1997. Reprinted by permission of the publisher. Copyright 1997 by Elsevier Science Inc.)

30% decreased risk of fracture (Table 4), but the presence of any limitation of activities of daily living (ADL) significantly increased the risk of serious fracture among those reporting vigorous activity. Mild exercise did not reduce fracture risk.

Conclusion.—Among elderly individuals with no limitations in ADL, vigorous exercise was associated with a lower risk of fall-related fracture. Those with limitations may increase their risk of fracture with vigorous exercise.

▶ Sports physicians with an interest in gerontology have long maintained that an active lifestyle is helpful in preventing falls among the elderly. This article challenges this traditional viewpoint. Although a 30% reduction in the risk of falls is shown by those who engage in vigorous physical activity, those who report only moderate physical activity have no significant advantage over sedentary controls. Even more disquieting is the finding that those who are currently experiencing limitations in 1 or more ADL, yet choose to engage in vigorous activity, have a substantially increased risk of falls (an odds ratio of 2.6). These data were obtained by retrospective questionnaire, and 1 limitation of the present research is sample size. Relatively few individuals had difficulty with either 1 (39 cases) or more (40 cases) ADL. It is also difficult to make retrospective surveys of the elderly because memory may be impaired, and in some of the present subject pool, it was necessary to translate questions into Spanish or to use proxy information obtained from a relative. Despite these problems, it seems desirable to look more critically at the question of which members of the elderly population can reduce their incidence of falls by undertaking vigorous exercise.

R. Shephard, M.D., Ph.D.

Skeletal Muscle Mass and the Reduction of VO$_{2max}$ in Trained Older Subjects

Proctor DN, Joyner MJ (Mayo Clinic, Rochester, Minn)
J Appl Physiol 82:1411–1415, 1997   8–34

Introduction.—Maximal O$_2$ intake declines with aging. Reduced cardiac output, increased body fat, and reduced peripheral O$_2$ extraction are all associated with this decline, but little is known about the relationship between VO$_{2max}$ and muscle mass as a function of age. There has also been confusion about how to express and compare VO$_{2max}$ change with aging. The role of skeletal muscle in the decline of VO$_{2max}$ was examined.

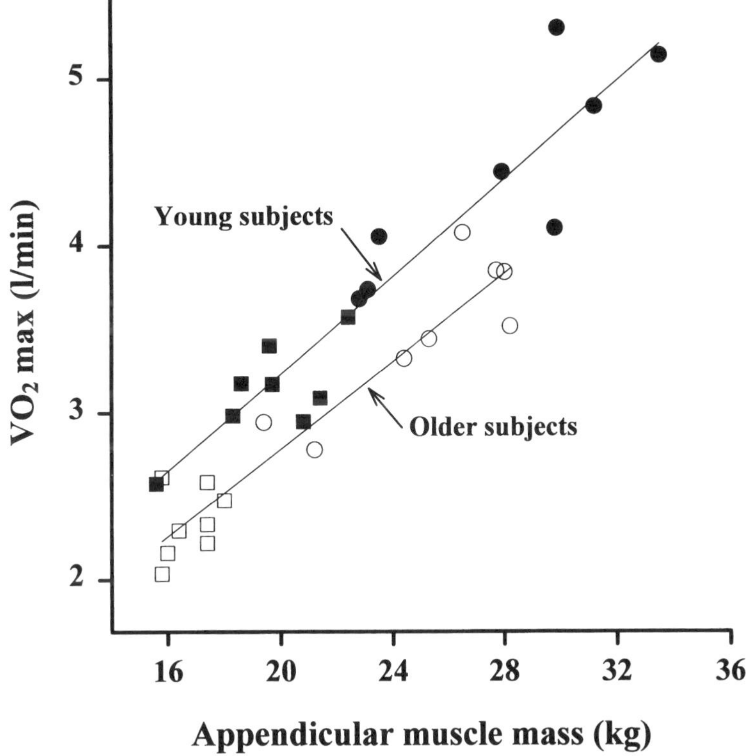

FIGURE 1.—Individual maximal O$_2$ uptake (VO$_{2max}$) values plotted against appendicular muscle mass. *Black square*, young women; *black circle*, young men; *white square*, older women; *white circle*, older men. Analysis of covariance indicated that regression line of older participants (VO$_{2max}$ = −0.08 + 0.14 · muscle mass) was 0.5 ± 0.09 L/min less for a given muscle mass than it was for young participants (VO$_{2max}$ = 0.42 + 0.14 · muscle mass). Age difference = 0.05 ± 0.09 L/min. This demonstrates that aerobic capacity per kilogram of appendicular muscle is reduced in highly trained older men and women. (Courtesy of Proctor DN, Joyner MJ: Skeletal muscle mass and the reduction of VO$_{2max}$ in trained older subjects. *J Appl Physiol* 82:1411–1415, 1997.)

Methods.—In 32 chronically endurance-trained participants, the relationships between several indices of muscle mass were examined using dual-energy x-ray absorptiometry and treadmill VO_{2max} measurement. The participants were divided into 4 groups of 8: young men (20–30 years), older men (56–72 years), young women (19–31 years), and older women (51–72 years).

Results.—In the older men, VO_{2max} per kilogram body mass was 26% lower than in the young men (45.9 vs. 62.0 mL·kg^{-1}·min^{-1}) and 22% lower in older women than younger women (40.0 vs. 51.5 mL·kg·$^{-1}$·min^{-1}). (Fig 1). When VO_{2max} was expressed per kilogram of appendicular muscle mass, the age difference was reduced to 14% for men and 13% for women. In the older participants, whole body VO_{2max} was 0.50 ± 0.09 L/min less than in the younger participants when appropriately adjusted for age and gender differences in appendicular muscle mass by analysis of covariance. In both genders, the effect was similar.

Conclusion.—A reduced aerobic power per kilogram of active muscle independent of age-associated changes in body composition, such as replacement of muscle tissue by fat, may be the cause of the reduced VO_{2max} seen in highly trained older men and women in comparison with their younger counterparts. The reduced aerobic power per kilogram of muscle likely results from age-associated reduction in maximal O_2 delivery because skeletal muscle adaptations to endurance training can be well maintained in older individuals.

▶ Causes of the age-related decline in maximal oxygen intake remain a matter of debate. One study suggested that when aerobic power was expressed in relative units (mL/[kg·min]), at least half of the apparent effect of aging was attributable to an increase in body fat content and a reduction in habitual physical activity.[1] The present report is based on cross-sectional comparison. It suggests that after adjustment for differences in lean body mass, old people have substantially lower maximal oxygen intakes (measured in absolute units, L/min). This confirms the view that aging is associated with a deterioration in the pumping ability of the heart and/or local muscle blood flow, although it leaves unanswered the possibility that part or all of the deterioration results from a lessening of habitual physical activity rather than from some intrinsic feature of the aging process.

R. Shephard, M.D., Ph.D., D.P.E.

Reference

1. Jackson AS, Beard EF, Wier LT, et al: Changes in aerobic power of men ages 25–70 yr. *Med Sci Sports Exerc* 27:113–120, 1995.

Low Levels of Physical Activity in 5-Year-Old Children
Salbe AD, Fontvieille AM, Harper IT, et al (NIH, Phoenix, Ariz)
J Pediatr 131:423–429, 1997   8–35

Objective.—The total energy expenditure (TEE) of 5-year-old children is significantly lower than that recommended by the World Health Organization, primarily because of reduced physical activity. The Pima Indians of Arizona have the highest prevalence of obesity and non-insulin-dependent diabetes mellitus in the world despite the fact that their resting metabolic rate (RMR) is similar to that of white children. Whether 5-year-old children have a lower physical activity energy expenditure (AEE) than that recommended by WHO and whether Pima Indian children have a lower AEE than white children was investigated.

Methods.—TEE using the double-labeled water method, RMR using indirect calorimetry, and physical activity were measured during the summers of 1991 through 1995 in 43 white and 84 Pima Indian 5-year-old children. Energy expended during physical activity was calculated [AEE = TEE − (RMR + 0.1TEE), where 0.1TEE represents the thermic effect of food]. Parents filled out a physical activity questionnaire estimating the number of hours per week each child spent in physical and sedentary activities.

Results.—TEE and RMR values were similar for both groups. Boys in both groups had significantly larger AEE levels than girls, with weight or fat-free mass accounting for a significant 54% of the variance. After adding fat mass to the equation, boys and girls had similar TEE values. For RMR, weight and fat-free mass accounted for 63% and 66% of the variance. When fat mass and sex were added to the equation, there was no difference between the races. Both races and sexes had similar AEE values and had engaged in similar amounts of recreational activities with boys participating in significantly more physical activities than girls.

Conclusion.—Both Pima Indian and white children had similar TEE, RMR, AEE, and physical activity levels that were significantly lower than World Health Organization recommendations for their age group. It appears that the increased incidence of obesity in Pima Indian children is the result of increased dietary intake, particularly of high-fat foods. Encouraging more physical activity in these children may help prevent obesity.

▶ The Pima Indians of Arizona have among the world's highest rates of obesity and non-insulin-dependent diabetes mellitus. Their prevalence of diabetes nears 50% by the age of 35; in some Pima children, diabetes develops by age 10. As shown in this and prior studies Pima children are heavier and fatter than white counterparts. In a prior questionnaire study, this group found that Pima children are less active than white counterparts. But in this study, with sophisticated gauging of energy expenditure, although the Pima are heavier and fatter than white counterparts by age 5, physical activity is the same in both groups. Alas, the likely reason Pima children are obese is they eat too much. Yet both white and Pima children had surprisingly low levels of physical activity, about 25% lower than recommended. This inactivity augurs poorly for both groups over the decades. A related study from Finland finds that physical activity and especially sports play before and during puberty predict the probability of an active life in young adulthood.[1]

E.R. Eichner, M.D.

Reference

1. Telama R, Laakso L, Yang X, Viikari J: Physical activity in childhood and adolescence as predictor of physical activity in young adulthood. *Am J Prev Med* 13:317–323, 1997.

Aerobic Capacity and Cognitive Performance in a Cross-sectional Aging Study
Van Boxtel MPJ, Paas FGWC, Houx PJ, et al (Maastricht Univ, The Netherlands)
Med Sci Sports Exerc 29:1357–1365, 1997   8–36

Background.—Aging has been associated with deterioration in cognitive functions such as memory, attention, reaction time, and speed of information processing. However, age-extrinsic variables, such as physical fitness, may partly explain the increase in variability of cognitive performance within birth cohorts. The basic mechanisms proposed to explain the effect of aerobic fitness on cognitive processes include the cerebral circulation hypothesis, the neurotrophic stimulation hypothesis, and a combination. The hypothesis that cognitively demanding tasks would be sensitive to aerobic capacity was tested.

Methods and Findings.—One hundred thirty-two healthy persons, aged 24–76 years, took part in a submaximal bicycle ergometer protocol and an extensive neurocognitive assessment. Tests of intelligence, verbal memory, and simple and complex cognitive speed were administered. Findings were compared with those of age-matched subjects who did not participate in aerobic sports. In a hierarchical regression analysis, 2 of the 4 subtasks reflecting cognitive speed showed main and interaction effects, with age of aerobic capacity accounting for as much as 5% of variance in parameter scores after adjustment for age, sex, and intelligence main effects.

Conclusions.—These data are consistent with a moderator model of aerobic fitness in cognitive aging. Aerobic fitness may selectively, age-dependently act on cognitive processes, especially those requiring relatively large attentional resources.

▶ This study suggests that moving fast keeps you thinking fast. The aim was to learn whether maximal aerobic capacity (estimated from a submaximal endurance test) related to cognitive performance in a healthy, normal aging population. After adjusting for age, sex, and IQ in a regression analysis, aerobic capacity had little effect on memory or simple psychomotor speed, but accounted for some of the variance in 2 of 4 tests of information processing speed. In other words, being physically fit increased the speed of thinking by up to 5%. Another recent study claims that even a single bout of exercise can boost creativity.[1] Sixty-three college students and teachers were studied. Group scores on "creative thinking" were higher after finishing an aerobics session than after viewing an "emotionally neutral" video about rock formations. Creative thinking scores hinged on listing novel uses for cans or boxes. Don't get me wrong: I believe in staying fit. But they stacked the deck in favor of exercise by choosing a dull video. How creative would you feel after viewing a video on rocks? They should try other videos, or compare creativity after playing the piano, reading a book, or drinking coffee.

E.R. Eichner, M.D.

Reference

1. Steinberg H, Sykes EA, Moss T, et al: Exercise enhances creativity independently of mood. *Br J Sports Med* 31:240–245, 1997.

Subject Index

I

Author Index

Evans RON, 55

F

Fagoaga OR, 324
Fallon KE, 70
Farfel Z, 186
Farkas R, 113
Farrell KP, 194
Farrett WD Jr, 196
Faunø P, 25
Federico DJ, 118
Fee RM, 370
Ferrauti A, 254
Field LD, 84
Fielding RA, 226
Finlay DB, 35
Flatow EL, 86
Fleming BC, 199
Fletcher JP, 79
Folsom AR, 370
Fontvieille AM, 405
Foster K, 70
Fowler PJ, 137
Frank CB, 131
Frank SA, 348
Fricker PA, 8
Frogameni AD, 93
Frontera WR, 226
Fu FH, 295
Fujimori Y, 263
Fulcher KY, 296

G

Gammon MD, 298
Ganion LR, 249
Gardner TR, 229
Garner EB, 320
Gastaldelli A, 366
Gebhard F, 85
Gehlsen GM, 249
George KP, 109
Gfell LE, 318
Ghaderi B, 134
Gilbart MK, 157
Gill TJ, 85
Gilleard W, 121
Giovannucci E, 303
Gleim GW, 200
Glitsch U, 113
González-Alonso J, 330
Goodman RA, 61
Goran MI, 365
Gordon NF, 239
Gordon WT, 43
Graves JE, 396

Greenway M, 268
Greenway P, 268
Gregory RL, 318
Groh GI, 97
Gross JH, 36
Growney ES, 217
Gu J-W, 279
Guanche CA, 29
Guinnepain M-T, 293
Gulledge TP, 312
Gylfadottir UK, 375

H

Haahtela T, 294
Habata T, 142, 143
Hackney AC, 312
Hamill J, 192
Hamilton K, 33
Handelsman DJ, 273
Hanel B, 180
Hanselmann K-F, 114
Hansen JE, 183
Hardman AE, 360
Harms CA, 182
Harper IT, 405
Harper WM, 35
Hartard M, 380
Hartkopp A, 316
Hasegawa Y, 343
Hawkins HH, 33
Heath EM, 376
Heier KA, 130
Heine O, 255
Heinonen A, 382
Heldal M, 283
Helenius IJ, 294
Helgeson JM, 257
Heller H, 177
Helms CA, 74
Henderson JNK, 386
Henderson WR, 178
Henehan M, 19
Henriksen E, 278
Hensley MJ, 164
Henson DA, 320
Herzog RJ, 40
Hezier W, 312
Hickey GJ, 8
Hicks AL, 222
Hoag RH, 35
Hochleitner BW, 73
Holloszy JO, 369
Holmes CF, 79
Hooper SL, 314
Hopkins SR, 178
Horodyski M, 351
Houx PJ, 406

Howe CJ, 273
Hsu Y-D, 336
Hu Y-H, 260
Hughes VA, 226
Huizenga JR, 236
Hyatt J-P, 363
Hyppänen E, 170

I

Ibarra C, 146
Ienna TM, 289
Insall JN, 151
Irshad F, 77
Ishimura M, 142, 143

J

Jackson DW, 131
Jaffe MS, 11
Jannetta C, 146
Janosko K, 286
Javierre C, 235
Jen CJ, 310
Jimenez CC, 262
Jobe FW, 202
Johnson LG, 378
Johnson RJ, 7
Jones PP, 371, 373
Jones R, 19
Jones S, 314
Jordan J, 311
Joyner MJ, 403
Jozsi AC, 366
Jürgensen K, 51

K

Kaeding CC, 119
Kaikkonen A, 170
Kannus P, 170
Kanter L, 210
Kaplan PA, 45
Kaufman T, 98
Kawasaki S, 343
Keim ME, 16, 17
Kerr CG, 332
Kerr KM, 191
Kienbacher T, 217
Kiernan W, 311
Kirkland AO, 233
Kirkley A, 137
Kleiner DM, 54
Knox KE, 54
Kogan MG, 152
Kohrt WM, 369